"An essential read for anyone interested in eating disorders, this book delivers exactly what its title promises. Persano challenges the current trend toward fragmented or polarized thinking, masterfully integrating the depth of psychoanalytic understanding, clinical precision, and a keen analysis of the sociocultural dynamics that shape body image today. Using psychoanalysis as a transformative tool, it offers a treatment framework that bridges biological, psychological, and social disciplines, as well as individual and collective healing, providing a comprehensive and enlightening perspective. Truly indispensable."

Ricardo Bernardi, *MD, Senior Psychiatrist; PhD, Psychology, University of Buenos Aires; Emeritus Professor, School of Medicine, University of Uruguay; Full Member, Academy of Medicine of Uruguay; Full Member, IPA; Honorary Member, Uruguayan Society of Psychoanalysis; Associate Editor for Latin America, IJPA*

"It is the rare clinician who grasps the multiple essences of eating disorders. In this work, Humberto Persano shares with us his many decades of immersion in these patients' hidden turmoil that derives from multiple developmental levels and genetic factors. He helps us see how patients' struggles with food-related symptoms are a proxy for their affective instability, inchoate desires, familial misattunement and only knowing themselves through the imagined eyes of others. We learn how their character rigidity, while deemed a virtue, hides their feared vulnerabilities and imaginings. He outlines specific treatment techniques that are built upon the therapist's ability to maintain the patient's hope for their future. He offers us both guidelines and inspiration to remain dedicated to this challenging journey."

Harvey Schwartz, *MD; IPA in Health, Chair; Training Analyst, Psychoanalytic Association of New York and Psychoanalytic Center of Philadelphia; host, IPA Podcast* Psychoanalysis On and Off the Couch

"The present volume is the best text on eating disorders from a psychoanalytic perspective that I have encountered. While paying adequate attention to neurobiological and hormonal influences, the major emphasis is on etiological features derived from psychogenic causes. The clarity and depth of the description of clinical reality facilitates the direct application of these understandings to concrete individual cases."

Otto F. Kernberg, *M.D. Professor Emeritus, Weill Cornell Medical College; Training and Supervising Analyst, Columbia University Psychoanalytic Center for Training and Research; Honorary Vice-President of the International Psychoanalytical Association (IPA)*

Exploring Eating Disorders Through Psychoanalysis

Exploring Eating Disorders Through Psychoanalysis explores eating disorders as complex clinical conditions and uses psychoanalysis to explore the psychological factors behind them.

Humberto Lorenzo Persano considers several key factors including psychosexual aspects of the psyche, object relations, ego functioning and defence mechanisms, as well as family dynamics, attachments, and the role of early childhood trauma. The book identifies the relationship between addictions, self-harm, and impulsive behaviours for complex patients as essential in the continuation of treatment and assesses specific treatments like transference-focused therapy and mentalization-based approaches. Persano also outlines future challenges and lines of research for eating disorders and their treatment.

Exploring Eating Disorders Through Psychoanalysis will be of great interest to psychoanalysts, psychologists, and psychiatrists working with eating disorders.

Humberto Lorenzo Persano is a psychiatrist at the School of Medicine in the University of Buenos Aires, Argentina. He is a professor of Mental Health and Psychiatry, and Psychology of Nutrition as well as holding the position of Director of the Institute of Clinical Psychiatry and Mental Health. He is a member of the Argentine Psychoanalytic Association, and a training analyst, supervisor, and child and adolescent psychoanalyst at the IPA.

IPA in the Community

Series Editor: Harvey Schwartz

For more information about this series, please visit: www.routledge.com/
IPA-in-the-Community/book-series/IPAC

Exploring Eating Disorders Through Psychoanalysis

Unravelling the Psyche

Humberto Lorenzo Persano with Adrian Daniel Ventura and Carlos Daniel Kremer

Routledge
Taylor & Francis Group
LONDON AND NEW YORK

Designed cover image: Getty | Kamila Baimukasheva

First published 2026
by Routledge
4 Park Square, Milton Park, Abingdon, Oxon OX14 4RN

and by Routledge
605 Third Avenue, New York, NY 10158

Routledge is an imprint of the Taylor & Francis Group, an informa business

© 2026 Humberto Lorenzo Persano

British Library Cataloguing-in-Publication Data
A catalogue record for this book is available from the British Library

ISBN: 978-1-032-72498-0 (hbk)
ISBN: 978-1-032-72489-8 (pbk)
ISBN: 978-1-032-72499-7 (ebk)

DOI: 10.4324/9781032724997

Typeset in Palatino
by Taylor & Francis Books

With love to Lara, Franco, and Bruno.

Three extraordinary gifts that life has blessed me with, reminding me every day of the joy, love, and purpose we share together.

Contents

Preface

To introduce a moment of reflection from literature for the purpose of this book, I turn once again to a fragment of Antonio Machado's poem written in 1912: "*Traveler, there is no path, the path is made by walking. Traveler, there is no path, only wakes in the sea*"[1]. This passage encapsulates the fleeting nature of existence. The notion that the path is forged by walking suggests the transitory quality of our journey, and just as wakes in the sea disappear with time, so too do the traces of our actions, leaving us unable to retrace our steps.

However, this transience does not tell the whole story. While Machado's traveler might perceive only fading wakes, there is another layer to explore. Some footprints, laid with intention, purpose, and care, can leave a lasting, tangible impact. Acts grounded in love, creativity, and wisdom have the power to transform what appears ephemeral into something enduring.

For instance, creating institutions, nurturing ideas, or producing works of art can extend the life of our contributions far beyond their original moment. These endeavors build not just impressions, but solid foundations that continue to influence and guide future generations. In this way, what might have seemed like a brief journey becomes something substantial, a lasting imprint on the world that others can build upon.

Thus, while the traveler's steps may initially create only fleeting wakes in the sea, they can also carve out a "solid ground" for those who follow. When viewed through this lens, Machado's meditation on the impermanence of life becomes a call to live with purpose: to make the transient moments count, and to shape the future with intention. This perspective offers a sense of optimism: though our journeys may be fleeting, our actions can echo far beyond our time, leaving an enduring legacy in their wake.

The journey of this book

Writing this book has been both a deeply challenging and immensely rewarding journey, reflecting on over 25 years of institutional work

---

1   In "*Proverbios y cantares*" (1912), Machado, Antonio (1983). *Poesías completas.* Madrid: Ed. Espasa-Calpe.

dedicated to eating disorders (EDs). While my career spans more than four decades in academia and the public health system, my focus over the last quarter century has been firmly rooted in the realm of EDs.

This endeavor was particularly demanding as it required revisiting the transformative process of creating a specialized unit for eating disorders within a public psychiatric hospital. The hospital, with its longstanding history of treating psychoses—primarily in male patients—posed unique challenges. I was fortunate to receive an extraordinary opportunity from Roberto Lovalvo, then General Director of Mental Health Services in Buenos Aires City, who entrusted me with the task of transforming a unit for male acute psychiatric inpatients into a dedicated space for mental health care for EDs, incorporating both day hospital and outpatient services.

Equally crucial was the unwavering support of Miguel Ángel Materazzi, the hospital's director, and Ricardo Soriano, who assisted in establishing networks for EDs within the Buenos Aires City General Direction of Mental Health Services. Introducing adolescents and young adults, predominantly female, into such a traditionally male-oriented institution was a significant challenge. Yet, this experience provided invaluable lessons on navigating institutional resistance and implementing meaningful change within hospital dynamics.

Looking back, it is remarkable to see how much can be achieved. This journey began in 1999, when we created a new and much-needed space within the public health system. At that time, no specific facilities existed to address these conditions or serve this population. Over 25 years, our unit has treated more than 3,000 patients, ranging in age from 14 to 25 years, although initially, we worked with individuals up to 30 years old.

In 2004, we participated in the design of a new building for our unit, a project that came to fruition in 2014. The process of collaborating with the Ministry of Health authorities and architects underscored the importance of intersectoral dialogue in making informed, well-grounded decisions. Architect Erik Guth enriched this experience by encouraging me to articulate how we worked, which he translated into architectural plans. His approach—"Explain to me how you work, and I'll transform it into a visual design"—was an incredible opportunity to think ahead about creating a space that was both functional and warm, promoting recovery while meeting the needs of patients and staff. I discuss this journey in the book, particularly the role of "milieu therapy" in supporting embodiment experiences and mentalization processes for individuals with EDs. Additionally, I reflect on how bringing together diverse perspectives and disciplines within the same physical space fosters dialogue and collaboration, enhancing patient care.

My work at the university has also been instrumental in shaping this book. As a full professor at the University of Buenos Aires in the Schools of Medicine and Nutrition, I've had the privilege of introducing the topic of EDs into the academic curriculum and conducting research in the field. I have led numerous training programs for residents in psychiatry, psychology, nutrition, occupational therapy, and mental health nursing, extending these efforts across Argentina and beyond. Our team's knowledge has been disseminated through papers, book chapters, and presentations at conferences, contributing to the education of future generations of healthcare professionals. All these experiences have been synthesized into this book.

International exchanges and supervision have significantly enriched my perspective and deepened my understanding of eating disorders and psychoanalysis. I owe profound gratitude to Otto Kernberg, who has been a mentor for nearly 35 years, and to Paulina Kernberg, who guided and mentored me for almost 20 years until her passing. Their unwavering dedication, encouragement, and collaboration, both in New York and Buenos Aires, have been invaluable to my professional growth. I am also deeply thankful to Philippe Jeammet, whose guidance inspired me to take the initial steps in creating the intensive day hospital and outpatient unit for eating disorders in Buenos Aires.

My heartfelt thanks extend to Peter Fonagy, whose supervision during my training at the psychoanalytic research program at University College London profoundly shaped my clinical and theoretical approach. I am equally indebted to John Clarkin and Frank Yeomans for their generous support and guidance. I would also like to honor the memory of Sidney Blatt, Robert Emde, and Horst Kächele, whose invaluable insights and contributions profoundly shaped my work. Their legacy continues to inspire my efforts in the field.

Collaborations with Cláudio Eizirik, Giovanni Battista Foresti, Harvey Schwartz, Vittorio Lingiardi, and Nancy McWilliams have greatly enriched my experience as an author, offering me the privilege of contributing to their books and engaging in meaningful academic exchanges. I am equally grateful to Ricardo Bernardi, Adela Leibowicz Duarte, Virginia Ungar, and Mónica Eidlin for creating spaces to discuss, refine, and present ideas in various academic and institutional settings. These opportunities have been instrumental in shaping my thinking and advancing my contributions to the field.

Finally, I deeply appreciate the trust placed in me by the International Psychoanalytical Association (IPA), which has given me opportunities to serve on various committees, allowing me to share and refine my ideas while contributing to the advancement of the field. These collective experiences have profoundly shaped the work presented in this book.

I want to acknowledge my professional partner, Adrian Ventura, with whom I have shared over 35 years of collaboration. His expertise in psychotherapy and supervision has been invaluable in shaping clinical practice and mentoring young professionals. I am also deeply grateful to Carlos Kremer and David Gutnisky for their profound theoretical and clinical insights, which have significantly enriched my work.

Finally, this book would not have been possible without the invaluable contributions of an exceptional team of professionals. I am deeply grateful to psychologists Angela Cardella, Ana Carnese, and Violeta Salusky; nutritionists Natalia Valicenti, Sofía Soto, and Paula Rodríguez; occupational therapist Rosana Álvarez; nurses Nora Bardi, Julieta García, and Paola García; sociologists Delia Franco and Alberto Bialakowski; and the many others who have been part of this passionate and rewarding journey. Their dedication, expertise, and collaboration have been instrumental in shaping the work presented here.

This book is a tribute to the collective efforts and knowledge gained over decades of dedication to the treatment of eating disorders. It reflects the invaluable lessons learned from collaboration, innovation, and the commitment to making a difference in the lives of patients and their families.

About the structure of the book

This book is structured to progressively build an understanding of eating disorders (EDs), primarily focusing on anorexia nervosa (AN) and bulimia nervosa (BN). These disorders are emphasized because, while the broader realm of EDs includes conditions such as binge eating disorder, atypical eating disorders, orthorexia, night eating syndrome, emotional eating disorder, avoidant/restrictive food intake disorder, and body dysmorphophobia, AN and BN are the most prevalent in clinical settings and have distinct psychological characteristics. The chapters aim to weave together psychoanalytic insights with clinical expertise, interdisciplinary collaboration, and societal perspectives.

Chapter 1: Introduction and general aspects of eating disorders

The book begins with an overview of eating disorders as complex psychological conditions, focusing on their prevalence, defining features, and the challenges they present in clinical settings. While the primary focus is on AN and BN, other EDs are mentioned to provide a comprehensive context. The chapter emphasizes the role of psychoanalysis in understanding and treating these disorders, offering unique perspectives on the mental dynamics and psyche formation involved in disordered eating.

Chapter 2: Historical context of eating disorders

This chapter delves into the historical roots of eating disorders, tracing the conceptual evolution of AN, which has been documented extensively in medical history, and the relatively later recognition of BN. It explores societal attitudes toward body image and food across different eras and cultures, shedding light on the ways these influences shape the development of EDs. By connecting historical trends with modern cultural pressures, this chapter lays the groundwork for understanding EDs within their sociocultural contexts.

Chapter 3: Clinical manifestations of eating disorders

Focusing on the clinical presentation of AN and BN, this chapter covers the course of the disorders, their differential diagnoses, and associated comorbidities. It addresses the medical, nutritional, and psychiatric complications of EDs and explores the role of addictive behaviors, impulsivity, and self-harm in complex cases. Drawing on the expertise of psychiatrists and psychoanalysts Adrian Ventura and Carlos Kremer, it offers a nuanced approach to managing challenging patients and conceptualizing their behaviors.

Chapter 4: Psychoanalytic theory and eating disorders

This chapter introduces key psychoanalytic concepts and their relevance to EDs, tracing the evolution of these ideas from Freud's early descriptions of hysteria and psychosexual development to more contemporary theories. Topics include object relations theory, ego functioning, and the construction of identity in ED patients. The chapter also explores affect regulation and the role of emotions in the etiology and maintenance of EDs.

Chapter 5: Unconscious dynamics of eating disorders

Here, the focus shifts to the unconscious conflicts related to body image and self-esteem. It examines the hidden motivations driving disordered eating behaviors, emphasizing the symbolic meanings and metaphors embedded in ED symptoms. The chapter also discusses the mentalization process and its role in helping patients achieve greater self-awareness and insight into their internal struggles.

Chapter 6: Early development and family dynamics

This chapter explores the profound impact of early attachment experiences and family environments on the development of EDs. Topics include trauma, neglect, and dysfunctional family dynamics, as well as the interactions between parents and children that contribute to disordered eating patterns. Psychiatrist and psychoanalyst and master in family therapy Carlos Kremer lends his expertise to this exploration of family influences and their implications for treatment.

Chapter 7: Transference and countertransference

Focusing on the therapeutic relationship, this chapter delves into the dynamics of transference and countertransference in the treatment of AN and BN. It offers a historical perspective on these concepts and demonstrates their practical utility in understanding and managing the complexities of ED therapy. Insights from clinical practice are woven throughout to provide real-world relevance.

Chapter 8: Dream analysis and imagery in eating disorder treatment

This chapter examines the use of dreams and imagery as tools for understanding EDs. It explores the symbolic representations of the self, the body, and food in the dreams of ED patients, offering a psychoanalytic lens through which to interpret these often-rich sources of unconscious material.

Chapter 9: Treatment approaches in psychoanalytic therapy

This chapter delves into psychodynamic approaches for treating eating disorders (EDs), emphasizing the role of resistance and defense mechanisms in sustaining maladaptive eating behaviors. It explores evidence-based interventions, including transference-focused psychotherapy and mentalization-based therapy, within a psychoanalytic framework. With contributions from senior psychiatrist and psychoanalyst Adrian Ventura, the chapter offers practical strategies for effectively navigating both the early and advanced stages of treatment.

Chapter 10: Beyond the individual: Sociocultural factors in eating disorders

Broadening the lens, this chapter examines the role of societal pressures, media, and cultural expectations in shaping body image and disordered eating. Drawing on insights from collaboration with sociologists, it integrates psychoanalytic perspectives on these influences and discusses their implications for both understanding EDs and designing effective treatment strategies.

Chapter 11: Integration and future directions

This chapter focuses on the integration of psychoanalytic approaches within intensive day hospital programs for eating disorders (EDs) in third-level psychiatric hospital environments. Drawing on the author's experience as the former General Director of Mental Health Services in Buenos Aires, it examines the critical role of public health systems, levels of care, and the development of multidisciplinary and interdisciplinary strategies. It emphasizes the importance of establishing networks and implementing specific programs for EDs within a framework of progressive care. Additionally, the chapter addresses the significance of prevention and early intervention in community settings, highlighting their potential to mitigate the long-term impact of EDs.

Conclusion: The journey towards healing

The book concludes with a reflection on the challenging but rewarding journey of healing in EDs. It explores emerging directions in psychoanalytic treatment, the integration of interdisciplinary approaches, and the enduring importance of empathy, understanding, and innovation in helping patients rebuild their lives.

Humberto Lorenzo Persano, MD, PhD
Buenos Aires, November 2024

1 Introduction

Overview of eating disorders as complex conditions

In the mental health field, eating disorders (EDs) stand out as some of the most intricate psychological conditions, requiring nuanced analysis and deep empathetic understanding. These disorders extend far beyond issues related to food and body image; they reveal the complex landscapes of psychology, emotion, and identity. Psychoanalytic perspectives, among others, provide essential insights into these layers, illuminating the unconscious conflicts, unmet emotional needs, and relational dynamics underlying eating disorders. This overview examines the multi-dimensional nature of these conditions, emphasizing the role of psychoanalysis in understanding the inner conflicts and relational patterns involved.

EDs present a vast and complex terrain that transcends simplistic assessments and requires a nuanced, interdisciplinary approach. To fully grasp their depth, it is essential to consider a network of influences—ranging from individual psychology to social, familial, and cultural factors. Eating disorders are not merely the result of dietary choices or a preoccupation with appearance; rather, they reflect deeper psychological struggles that intersect with various dimensions of life. They reveal profound relationships with the self and with others, encompassing both the internal psyche and the external world, making it necessary to approach them holistically.

At their core, eating disorders are a manifestation of inner emotional and psychological turmoil. Unhealthy eating patterns are often the outward expression of deep-seated issues related to identity, self-esteem, and emotional regulation. Understanding these disorders thus involves exploring the emotional landscapes individuals traverse and recognizing the powerful impact of these inner experiences on their behaviors. This approach necessitates delving deeper than surface-level symptoms to engage with the personal narrative individuals construct—stories intricately woven from unconscious thoughts, past experiences, and internalized cultural influences.

DOI: 10.4324/9781032724997-1

Complex interplay of genetic, environmental, and neurological factors

EDs arise from an intricate blend of genetic, environmental, and neurological factors. Recognizing these layers is crucial to moving beyond simplistic views and fostering a comprehensive understanding of these conditions. A key aspect of this understanding involves appreciating how distorted self-image, perfectionism, and unattainable ideals are internalized, shaping individuals' mental and emotional states. Therefore, understanding eating disorders means not only identifying visible symptoms but also uncovering the hidden narratives individuals hold within themselves, often rooted in their unconscious minds.

EDs are frequently misunderstood, contributing to stigma and reductive narratives that overlook their complexity. Building a solid knowledge base is essential for effective intervention and reducing this stigma. Comprehending these disorders demands that we move beyond mere clinical descriptions to engage more deeply with the psychological and emotional dimensions they represent.

Expressions of psychological distress in anorexia, bulimia, and binge eating disorder

Each eating disorder (ED)—from anorexia nervosa (AN) and bulimia nervosa (BN) to binge eating disorder (BED)—represents a unique expression of psychological distress. The term "eating disorder" itself can be misleading, as it implies a singular focus on eating habits. However, food is often a medium through which individuals express or manage internal conflicts. Disordered eating patterns reflect external manifestations of inner struggles, intertwined with issues of control, perfectionism, and self-worth. Understanding these conditions requires recognizing how they connect to broader human experiences, encompassing pain, fear, and often-unfulfilled desires for acceptance and belonging.

AN, for example, often reflects a need for extreme control, while BN may mask feelings of shame and helplessness. BED, meanwhile, can symbolize the emptiness of unmet emotional needs. Each condition serves as a map of emotional highs and lows, underscoring the importance of understanding the psychological language embedded in these experiences. Recognizing these patterns requires a commitment to interpreting each person's unique relationship with their disorder and understanding the underlying emotional language.

Influence of societal pressures and cultural expectations

Societal pressures and cultural expectations play significant roles in the development and perpetuation of EDs. The pervasive idealization of thinness, societal norms regarding beauty, and media portrayals of "perfection" contribute to an environment that exacerbates these conditions. Beyond individual psychology, cultural standards and social expectations add layers of complexity, intensifying the pursuit of unrealistic ideals. The drive for control, the anxiety associated with these unattainable standards, and the struggle for self-acceptance are all central components in the progression of eating disorders.

At the heart of these disorders are the intertwined effects of anxiety, depression, and low self-esteem. Anxiety often manifests as rigid dietary rules or compulsive behaviors, becoming a constant companion for those struggling with these disorders. Depression adds another layer, sometimes driving individuals to seek control through eating behaviors to cope with overwhelming feelings of sadness or emptiness. Self-esteem, often shaped by social influences and personal relationships, profoundly impacts how individuals perceive themselves, contributing to the vulnerability experienced by those with eating disorders.

Body image dissatisfaction and the biological dimensions of eating disorders

Body image dissatisfaction and distortion are foundational issues for many individuals with eating disorders. These distorted perceptions can disturb self-esteem, affective regulation, and self-worth, often turning the pursuit of an idealized body image into an obsession. This internal conflict is further complicated by biological factors, including genetic predispositions, neurotransmitter imbalances, and hormonal fluctuations, all of which contribute to the physiological aspects of eating disorders.

Biological factors play a significant role in predisposing individuals to EDs, with genetic influences impacting metabolism, appetite regulation, and emotional responses. Neurotransmitter imbalances, particularly in serotonin and dopamine pathways, can disrupt mood, appetite, and stress regulation, contributing to disordered eating behaviors. Hormonal fluctuations also add complexity, such as amenorrhea associated with AN, insulin variations in BED, and the roles of ghrelin and leptin in appetite control and fat metabolism. Understanding these biological dimensions fosters a more comprehensive approach to addressing eating disorders, bridging the gap between biological and psychological perspectives.

A multidimensional approach to treatment and recovery

Effectively addressing EDs requires an integrative approach that combines psychological, medical, and nutritional interventions. Psychotherapy, support groups, and medical care are all essential in addressing the various facets of these conditions. A collaborative and multidisciplinary approach acknowledges the full complexity of eating disorders, promoting recovery in a way that considers everyone's psychological, biological, and social context.

Psychoanalysis, with its focus on unconscious conflicts, childhood experiences, and relational dynamics, offers a deep and enduring approach to treatment. By bringing unconscious conflicts into conscious awareness, individuals can gain insights into the root causes of their disordered behaviors and develop healthier coping strategies. This therapeutic process allows individuals to confront and resolve their internal conflicts, facilitating lasting recovery and promoting personal growth that extends beyond mere symptom management.

This overview serves as a foundation for exploring the multifaceted nature of eating disorders. By understanding the intricate interplay between psychological, biological, and societal factors, we can approach these conditions with empathy, depth, and a commitment to enhancing mental health care.

Importance of psychoanalysis in understanding and treating eating disorders

Uncovering the mind through psychoanalysis: A deep exploration of eating disorders

Psychoanalysis is a vital tool in understanding and treating EDs, offering a pathway into the unconscious mind and revealing the hidden emotional conflicts, unmet needs, and relational dynamics that often lie at the root of these complex conditions. Unlike approaches that focus primarily on behaviors and conscious beliefs, psychoanalysis delves into the deeper, often hidden, layers of the psyche, including unresolved issues from early childhood, familial relationships, and personal trauma. In doing so, psychoanalysis enables a more profound understanding of how and why eating disorders manifest, paving the way for lasting therapeutic change.

A central tenet of psychoanalytic theory is its emphasis on early childhood experiences, especially the powerful dynamics between parents and children. Early traumas, disrupted attachments, or dysfunctional family relationships during these formative years can profoundly shape an individual's relationship with food, body, and self-worth, often crystallizing during critical developmental periods such as puberty and adolescence. For example, children who grow up without a consistent caregiver may develop a sense of emotional insecurity, potentially seeking to fill this void later in life through disordered eating as a misguided attempt to meet these unmet needs.

In the case of EDs, psychoanalysis reveals how these unresolved needs can lead to deeply rooted conflicts between autonomy and dependence. Individuals with EDs often experience a struggle between a need for care and connection (dependency) and a desire for control and self-sufficiency (autonomy). This inner tension frequently expresses itself through disturbed eating behaviors. For instance, AN can be seen as an assertion of autonomy and control, while binge eating may represent a longing for comfort and nurturance.

Unconscious emotions such as guilt and shame are also common undercurrents in EDs. These emotions often stem from unresolved childhood conflicts or traumatic experiences, including abuse or neglect, and may drive disordered eating behaviors as a means of self-punishment or self-soothing. Psychoanalysis helps bring these hidden feelings to the surface, allowing individuals to confront and process the underlying sources of their guilt or shame. Some individuals with EDs may also repress traumatic memories, which remain buried in the unconscious yet continue to influence their thoughts, feelings, and behaviors. Through disordered eating, these individuals may unconsciously attempt to avoid or suppress the painful emotions associated with these repressed memories.

Sexuality and intimacy are other significant areas that psychoanalysis explores in relation to eating disorders. Issues of control and self-image in eating disorders often extend into intimate relationships, shaping how individuals relate to others. For some, the need to control food and body reflects a similar reluctance to relinquish control in intimate situations, which can lead to difficulties in forming close, meaningful connections. Others may avoid intimacy altogether due to feelings of inadequacy or fear of rejection, intensifying feelings of loneliness and disconnection. For instance, individuals with anorexia may display a tendency to reject intimacy, while those with bulimia may seek out frequent relationships, attempting to stabilize an unstable self-image through repeated relational experiences.

Psychoanalysis also introduces crucial concepts such as defense mechanisms, mental representations, and the symbolization process, all of which contribute to a deeper understanding of eating disorders. Defense mechanisms, for example, are unconscious strategies individuals use to cope with emotional distress. Behaviors like restricting, bingeing, or purging may be viewed as defense mechanisms that allow individuals to manage anxiety or fulfill unconscious needs. By identifying these defenses, therapists can guide individuals toward healthier coping mechanisms, gradually reducing the power of these disordered behaviors.

Moreover, psychoanalysis sheds light on distorted body image—a common feature in eating disorders. Through an exploration of internalized beliefs, social pressures, and emotional conflicts related to self-image, individuals can work toward developing a healthier perception of themselves. Unlike other approaches, psychoanalytic therapies emphasize the therapeutic relationship, particularly the dynamics of transference and countertransference between the patient and therapist. In this relational process, patients project unconscious emotions onto their therapist, creating a mirror through which they can explore and understand their own relational patterns. This dynamic offers invaluable insights into the patient's unconscious mind, illuminating the root causes of their ED and facilitating the healing process.

In addition to fostering insight, psychoanalysis plays a key role in the development of mentalization and embodiment within therapy. Mentalization, the ability to understand one's own and others' mental states, is crucial for individuals with eating disorders, who often struggle with self-awareness and emotional regulation. Through psychoanalytic exploration, patients learn to better understand and regulate their internal experiences, ultimately achieving a more stable and integrated sense of self. Embodiment, the process of reconnecting with one's physical self, is equally important, as individuals with EDs frequently experience a disconnection from their own bodies. By facilitating this reconnection, psychoanalysis helps patients establish a healthier relationship with their physical self.

While cognitive-behavioral therapy (CBT) and other short-term interventions are commonly used for treating eating disorders, psychoanalysis offers a unique, long-term approach that allows for a deeper exploration of the underlying issues driving these disorders. This approach promotes sustained personal growth that extends far beyond symptom management, potentially leading to long-lasting improvements in multiple areas of life. The benefits of this enduring approach are often seen in lasting changes to mental health, self-image, and relational patterns, not merely in the reduction of disordered eating behaviors.

In psychoanalytic therapy for EDs, uncovering unconscious conflicts is a transformative process that involves bringing buried psychological factors into conscious awareness. As individuals gain insight into the root causes of their behaviors, they become better equipped to replace destructive coping mechanisms with healthier strategies. This therapeutic journey enables them to confront, understand, and ultimately resolve their inner conflicts, paving the way for lasting recovery.

By guiding individuals toward self-discovery and personal growth, psychoanalysis plays an indispensable role in the treatment of EDs. It provides a framework for understanding these conditions as complex psychological phenomena rooted in the unconscious mind. Through psychoanalytic exploration, individuals can learn to integrate their emotional, relational, and physical selves, enabling them to find a path toward healing that resonates with the deepest layers of their psyche. In doing so, psychoanalysis not only addresses the symptoms of eating disorders but also promotes enduring transformation, offering hope and resilience to those grappling with these challenging conditions.

2 Historical context of eating disorders

Evolution of societal attitudes toward food and body image

Historical perspectives on eating disorders: From sacred fasting to modern clinical conditions

Fasting has historically held deep significance in various cultural, religious, and social contexts, often serving as a tool for purification, self-discipline, and spiritual transcendence. Across cultures, fasting has been woven into rituals and beliefs as a means of achieving piety, gaining forgiveness, or connecting with the divine. In many mystical traditions, fasting was believed to increase the efficacy of magical rites, as bodily purity was thought to enhance spiritual receptivity. Within these rituals, fasting transcended mere abstinence; it symbolized a triumph over bodily passions, framed by an idealized vision of purity and self-mastery.

The roots of fasting in ancient traditions can be traced to notions of self-discipline and well-being, as seen in practices among the Greeks, who viewed it as a method to attain physical and mental harmony. Fasting has also been employed as a form of peaceful protest and self-determination, as in Gandhi's protest fasts in India, where the act symbolized non-violent resistance and moral resolve. In these instances, fasting became a voluntary, internalized form of self-discipline, signifying strength and a powerful assertion of will.

Cultural patterns significantly influence the way fasting and food restriction are perceived, often shaping how eating disorders manifest. In many cultures, fasting has symbolic connotations, playing a role in mourning rituals or practices intended to ward off malevolent influences. Here, abstinence from food served to protect the body from contamination, aligning with beliefs that viewed the consumption of food as an invitation to unwanted forces. In these cultural contexts, fasting represents a complex, somewhat paradoxical form of self-violence: an act of deprivation that, while self-imposed, has powerful protective and purifying significance.

DOI: 10.4324/9781032724997-2

Religious traditions also employ fasting in both mystical and ritualistic dimensions, blending moral prescriptions with physical acts of self-denial. In "Catholicism", for instance, fasting before receiving the "Eucharist" symbolizes a state of purity, while abstaining from red meat during "Lent" signifies renouncing bodily pleasures in a display of mastery over instincts. Judaism similarly incorporates fasting in its rituals; "Yom Kippur" includes a fast that is both a physical abstention and a day devoted entirely to introspection and communion with God. Fasting thus becomes an instrument of spiritual refinement and societal connection, providing individuals with a framework for controlling bodily desires within a shared, collective experience.

One of the earliest documented links between fasting and what would later be recognized as an eating disorder appears in the life of St. Catherine of Siena (1347–1380). Renowned for her extreme fasting practices, Catherine subsisted on minimal food—consuming only bread, vegetables, and water—and eventually rejected even water (Baile Ayensa and González Calderón, 2012). Her self-imposed starvation was driven by a desire for spiritual purity and sanctity, aligning her suffering with religious ideals of holiness and immortality. In the context of the Middle Ages, this phenomenon of "holy anorexia" was celebrated as a testament to spiritual devotion, in stark contrast to the demonized image of witches, who were perceived as being consumed by bodily passions. These "anorexic saints" embodied an ideal of spiritual asceticism, serving as both an act of submission and a subtle resistance against a male-dominated ecclesiastical power structure (Behar, 2012). The historical link between female piety and self-denial underscores the gendered nature of this phenomenon, with fasting emerging as a distinctly feminine expression of spiritual purity and defiance.

As society shifted toward medical interpretations of mental health, the understanding of behaviors like fasting and extreme food restriction began to evolve. The "Enlightenment" era brought a new focus on "madness", marking the early stages of categorizing such behaviors as medical conditions rather than purely spiritual phenomena. With the emergence of psychoanalytic theory in the late 19th and early 20th centuries, pioneers like Freud introduced concepts of the unconscious, femininity, and identity formation that would provide new insights into the psychological roots of self-denial and disordered eating. Psychoanalysis reframed these behaviors as complex expressions of unconscious conflict, aggression, and identity struggles, marking a shift from moral or religious interpretations to a clinical understanding of eating disorders as manifestations of inner psychological turmoil.

The 20th century witnessed a profound transformation in societal attitudes toward the body, especially the female body, as mass media began to promote ideals of thinness and beauty. This period saw the rise of diet culture, with an increasing emphasis on calorie control, body sculpting, and aesthetic ideals that created a pervasive pressure to conform to unrealistic physical standards. Technological advancements reinforced this control, offering tools like calorie counting, body modification, and cosmetic surgery. Simultaneously, the feminist movement led to significant shifts in female autonomy and resistance to objectification, yet paradoxically, the female body became both a site of liberation and an object of societal control (Hepworth, 1999).

In the contemporary world, individuals find themselves caught in a paradoxical struggle: the desire to control their bodies through technology, the pressure to conform to idealized standards of beauty, and the need for self-acceptance. This complex cultural environment gives rise to identity-related issues, making disorders like anorexia and bulimia potent symbols of modern anxieties. In the case of anorexia nervosa (AN), fasting is not merely a social practice but a deeply personal and often isolating act of self-control. It can represent a rebellion against societal expectations, an act of self-determination that, while solitary, echoes the ascetic discipline of past eras. As noted by Bernard Brusset (1990), fasting in AN becomes a solitary ritual of self-mastery, with underlying opposition to external forces and a deep-seated intolerance for intrusion or interference. Brusset discusses the compulsive behaviors often observed in individuals with AN, particularly focusing on their addiction to running and excessive work. He notes that these activities serve as mechanisms for patients to exert control over their bodies and emotions, providing a sense of mastery and distraction from internal conflicts (Brusset, 1990).

Bulimia nervosa (BN) also reflects the imprint of contemporary cultural values, with its cycles of binge eating and purging embodying the tensions between indulgence and self-punishment. The act of "binging" mirrors modern ideals of speed and instant gratification, while purging represents an attempt to adhere to aesthetic standards. In the context of Zygmunt Bauman's concept of "liquid modernity" (Bauman, 2013), society's rapid pace and fluctuating expectations manifest in the bulimic cycle itself. This cyclical behavior captures society's ambivalence toward consumption and control, where indulgence is both encouraged and condemned.

In a world where appearance is frequently a measure of worth, purging can be seen as a means of countering the guilt and shame associated with straying from social ideals. The abundance of food stimuli is countered by equally prevalent "purging" methods, such as excessive exercise and strict dietary restrictions, which are widely accepted in modern culture. The pressures of the job market reinforce these ideals, compelling individuals to conform to physical standards to succeed professionally.

Thus, society perpetuates a sense of self-alienation, turning the body into a site of control and self-worth struggles, which often leads to a condition marked by a profound inner void.

Eating disorders today, therefore, exist at the intersection of historical, cultural, and psychological dimensions. They echo centuries-old practices of fasting as purification, yet reflect a distinctly modern obsession with image, identity, and control. Understanding the historical roots of fasting and self-denial allows for a richer, more comprehensive perspective on eating disorders, as they continue to mirror cultural ideals and individual struggles for identity and autonomy. In unraveling this complex history, we gain insights into how eating disorders represent not only a struggle with food but a profound, enduring conflict with self and society.

Cultural influences on eating disorders

The relationships between social frameworks, culture, and dietary habits are deeply interconnected, especially when considering the prevalence of eating disorders. In recent decades, eating disorders have become particularly common in Western or Westernized societies, including countries like Japan, and are most frequently observed in urban areas. However, this does not imply that such conditions are entirely absent in rural populations or other social settings. While initially described among middle- and upper-class individuals, eating disorders now appear across all social strata. Notably, these disorders are far less prevalent in societies where food is scarce, such as some indigenous African populations and non-Westernized societies, including Vietnam and Cuba. In these contexts, eating disorders are rarely observed, underscoring the cultural and social dimensions that influence their development.

The role of women within different social and cultural settings is crucial to understanding these dynamics. In contemporary Western societies, a slender female body is often viewed as a symbol of power and self-control. Conversely, in other societies where food is less abundant, a robust body is associated with strength and fertility, symbolizing a woman's ability to support a family and fulfill her social role. In cultures where food is scarce, corpulence is respected and considered a marker of social status and power. However, in food-abundant Western societies—though food distribution is not always equitable—corpulent figures are often viewed negatively, even comically, illustrating how aesthetic values are largely shaped by socio-cultural contexts.

Joel Paris (1996) suggests that social factors significantly contribute to the onset of certain disorders, including AN and personality disorders. His hypothesis posits that modern societies, characterized by rapid change and instability, create fertile ground for these conditions, while traditional societies, marked by stability and continuity, experience these disorders far less frequently. Building on the theories of Lerner (1958) and Inkeles and Smith (1974), Paris identifies a dichotomy between traditional and modern social structures. Traditional societies are characterized by low rates of change and strong intergenerational continuity, providing individuals with predictable social roles and expectations. In contrast, modern societies are defined by rapid change and intergenerational discontinuity, contributing to less predictable social frameworks.

The disruption of stable structures in modern societies and their replacement with more fluid, unstable frameworks create what Paris calls "rapid social change." This instability in the social fabric is a risk factor for psychopathologies, particularly for disorders related to identity and self-regulation, such as eating disorders (EDs), personality disorders, and addictive behaviors. In essence, the pressures and expectations of modern society shape contemporary forms of psychopathology, influencing the ways individuals perceive and interact with their bodies.

However, traditional societies are not without their own potential for creating psychological distress. These societies, with their relatively strict expectations and limited tolerance for deviation, may exert pressure on individuals to conform, often at the expense of personal expression. While traditional structures provide security and predictability, they can also stifle those whose traits or behaviors do not align with societal norms, leading to social inhibition and constriction. In contrast, modern societies, which prioritize autonomy and self-expression, encourage a more active, outwardly expressive personality style. Social structures in these settings reward behaviors aligned with independence and assertiveness, shaping the individual's sense of self in response to these values.

Moreover, cultural values play a powerful role in reinforcing certain behaviors while discouraging others. Through social reinforcement and modeling, societies increase the prevalence of traits that align with their expectations and suppress those that do not. As Paris (1996) notes, each culture establishes its own social tolerance levels for specific traits, thereby influencing how individuals within that society are shaped.

Psychoanalysis emphasizes early childhood experiences as formative imprints on personality development. In parallel, sociology considers extra-familial factors—such as social, peer, and community influences—as key in shaping personality traits. Research supporting the significance of non-shared environments in personality development highlights the importance of social factors. These findings underscore the impact of socialization outside the family, as culture influences family structures and affects social learning in broader contexts (Whiting and Edwards, 1988). Peer groups play a critical role in modifying personality traits, as do authority figures in community settings, including teachers and leaders of religious or ethnic organizations (Rutter and Rutter, 1993). Urie Bronfenbrenner's ecological systems theory emphasizes the profound impact of social context and community values on human development. He defined human development as:

> the scientific study of the progressive, mutual accommodation between an active, growing human being and the changing properties of the immediate settings in which the developing person lives, as this process is affected by relations between these settings, and by the larger contexts within which the settings are embedded
>
> (Bronfenbrenner, 1979)

This perspective underscores the importance of understanding the multiple environmental layers that influence an individual's growth, from immediate family and peers to broader societal and cultural contexts. The theory of social formation of certain psychopathologies is further supported by cases where low-prevalence disorders in traditional societies increase significantly among individuals who migrate to modernized environments. An example is AN, which is rare in traditional societies but becomes more common among individuals who move from traditional to modernized settings, as observed by DiNicola (1990). These differences underscore the impact of socio-cultural roles, particularly the evolving role of women, within each social and cultural framework.

Eating disorders exemplify the intricate relationship between the individual, their body, and the socio-cultural context within which their body is interpreted and valued. Within this framework, societal ideals and symbols associated with the body in contemporary society exert a powerful influence. Serge Moscovici (1961) introduced the concept of "social representations" to explain how societal views replace mere opinions or images, incorporating a complex weave of beliefs, thoughts, and attitudes about body image (Farr, 1994). These representations reflect society's values, creating a system of ideas and practices around body image. Individuals internalize these ideals, developing a personal theory of body image that aligns with their desire to integrate into their social fabric.

In this sense, the socio-cultural construction of the body shapes how individuals perceive and treat themselves, driven by the desire for social acceptance and inclusion. These cultural standards become a blueprint for self-evaluation, leading individuals to embrace or reject behaviors as they strive to align with societal expectations. Thus, EDs emerge as deeply embedded responses to the cultural, social, and psychological forces that shape identity and self-worth in a rapidly changing world.

Early clinical observations and conceptualizations

History of anorexia nervosa

Anorexia derives from Greek: An-orexia, where "an" is a negative prefix and "orexis" means to tend towards, desire something or someone, appetite. This word distinguishes hunger as an instinctual quality (biological fact) from appetite (driven by desire, seeking pleasure). Therefore, the concept of anorexia implies within its linguistic structure a lack of desire.

The earliest clinical descriptions of anorexia originated long ago. The oldest recorded description dated back to the 11th century in ancient Persia; Avicenna (980–1037) described a young prince suffering from symptoms of anorexia in a context of depressive symptomatology. The relationship between anorexia and depression will persist to our present day. Avicenna and his followers believed that the causes of *botlan-e-shahvat* (anorexia) and *noghsan-e-shahvat* (dysorexia) are the same (Nimrouzi and Zarshenas, 2018).

We can organize the history of anorexia in four different periods:

1 Preconceptual phase
2 Psychic phase
3 Clinical-Endocrinologic phase
4 Mental Disorders phase

First period: Preconceptual phase and first clinical descriptions

While Avicenna made early mentions of a condition resembling anorexia nervosa (AN), most historians attribute the first clinical description of this pathology to Richard Morton in 1694. In his seminal work, *Treatise on Consumption*, he referred to it as "Nervous Consumption," or "Phtisis Nervosa" (Albano, 1998). Earlier in the 17th century, figures such as Thomas Hobbes in 1668 (Benhabib, 2022) and John Reynolds in 1669 (Silverman, 1986) had made references to similar conditions, although these lacked detailed descriptions. Morton's account stood out for its clinical precision. He described the condition as a wasting of the "fleshy parts" of the body in the absence of fever, cough, or respiratory difficulties, resembling the wasting observed in tuberculosis. His description was notably comprehensive, including key symptoms such as loss of appetite, food refusal, hyperactivity, amenorrhea, constipation, and cachexia.

Morton recognized the severity of the condition, noting it could be "fatal" and "difficult to cure," especially when chronic. He observed that, initially, symptoms might seem mild to the patient, but by the time they sought medical intervention, it was often too late. He insightfully attributed the disorder to "violent passions of the mind" and speculated on contributing factors like "disorderly consumption of spirits and the air". In introducing these multifactorial causes, Morton highlighted the psychological aspects of the illness, emphasizing emotional and mental suffering—a perspective that resonates in today's understanding of the disorder. He also foreshadowed what Freud would later identify as the "secondary gain" of illness, whereby the condition could lead to lethargic and ultimately fatal outcomes. Notably, Morton described AN not only in women but also in an 18-year-old male, suggesting early recognition of its occurrence across genders.

In the 18th century, Robert Whytt (1767) reported on a 14-year-old male who experienced a significant loss of appetite and weight, followed by a recovery phase with weight gain that exceeded his previous baseline. Whytt's account is significant because it highlights a recurring challenge in treating eating disorders: the fear of losing control over-eating behaviors. This concern is often reflected in extreme weight fluctuations seen in some patients; a pattern documented in more recent studies (Blinder and Chao, 2019).

Around the same period, French physician Naudeau (1789) provided a clinical description of a 35-year-old woman presenting with epigastric discomfort, loss of appetite, and cachexia. He added to prior descriptions by observing the intense stomach ache often reported by severely malnourished patients with anorexia. He suggested this pain could be due to tension and stretching of the mesenteric pedicle—a consequence of the loss of intra-abdominal fat, which normally provides structural support to the organs (Aragona, 2021). Naudeau's observations offered a physiological perspective on the painful manifestations of extreme malnutrition, which had not been detailed in earlier accounts.

By the 19th century, anorexia was increasingly associated with hysteria, positioning it within the domain of psychological disorders. In 1859, Briquet's *Clinical and Therapeutic Treatise on Hysteria* documented cases of malnutrition linked to hysteria. He noted that some patients, despite having a normal appetite, refused to eat due to a fear of swallowing or an aversion to food. Briquet observed that these patients often experienced amenorrhea and noted fatal outcomes in two cases, underlining the life-threatening nature of severe anorexia. He also described a form of purging, where patients ate normally but induced vomiting—a precursor to current definitions of purging AN and BN (Briquet, 1859).

Briquet's descriptions set the stage for understanding the clinical forms of hysteria marked by food aversion and disgust, conditions that would later be seen as early expressions of purging anorexia and bulimia. His work foreshadowed contemporary classifications, as he identified both the physical symptoms and the psychological complexities involved, bridging early medical descriptions with later psychiatric interpretations.

Second period: Psychic phase

By the late 19th century, two prominent European physicians laid the foundation for the modern understanding of AN. In France Charles Lasègue (1873) and Sir William Gull in England (1874). These pioneers not only provided detailed clinical descriptions of the disorder but also introduced terms that have persisted in medical literature—Lasègue referred to it as "Hysterical Anorexia", while Gull used the term "Nervous Anorexia". Scholars of eating disorders often regard these two figures as inaugurating the "Psychic Phase" in the conceptualization of AN, focusing on the mental and emotional dimensions of the disorder.

Lasègue's 1873 description of "Hysterical Anorexia" outlined a condition primarily observed in young women aged 15 to 20, typically those experiencing emotional conflicts. He described initial symptoms of discomfort and epigastric pain, which led to a gradual reduction in food intake, constipation, and eventually amenorrhea accompanied by malnutrition. Lasègue referred to the condition as a "gastric focus of hysteria", illustrating his view of the illness as primarily psychological in nature, despite its digestive symptoms (Lanteri Laura, 1991). One illustrative case he detailed involved a young woman who experienced postprandial discomfort, progressively reduced her food intake, and eventually refused to eat entirely. Lasègue warned of the severity of the illness, noting that "the slightest medical error is irreparable" once the condition was established—a statement that underscores the critical importance of early intervention, a sentiment that remains relevant today.

Lasègue attributed the condition to disturbances within the digestive tract that triggered a larger mental illness, resulting in a distinctive clinical picture with specific symptoms and a predictable course. He grouped hysterical anorexia with other manifestations of hysteria, such as hysterical cough, transient catalepsy, and anesthesia. Lasègue was particularly insightful in recognizing the influence of intrapsychic and interpersonal factors, noting the family's role in the progression of the illness. He observed that family members often reacted to the patient's refusal to eat with pleas and threats, which only served to intensify the patient's resistance and draw more attention to their behavior. This dynamic of family interaction often made the patient the focal point of family interest, exacerbating the condition (Lanteri Laura, 1991).

Lasègue further described a pattern of hyperactivity at the onset of the disorder, followed by severe weakness as the illness progressed. This connection between physical activity and illness progression has become a hallmark observation in AN. He noted that initially, patients exhibited a state of heightened activity and even expressed satisfaction or contentment with their condition—an emotional state he identified as "truly pathological". As malnutrition progressed, however, this hyperactivity would transition to hypoactivity, driven by weakness and fatigue—symptoms now recognized as being associated with muscular atrophy in malnourished patients (Lanteri Laura, 1991).

In England, Sir William Gull published his findings on "Nervous Anorexia" around the same time, referring to it as "hysterical apepsia" or "hysterical anorexia" (Gull, 1888). Gull observed the condition primarily in young women aged 16 to 23, though he also documented cases in males. In fact, Gull is considered by some to be the first to describe the condition, as he had presented a case to the British Medical Association in 1868 of a young woman who became malnourished due to "hysterical apepsia". Gull attributed the disorder to a deficiency of gastric pepsin, focusing on symptoms like amenorrhea, constipation, slow pulse, emaciation, and hyperactivity. He noted specific physical signs in severe cases, such as bradycardia, which he interpreted as a homeostatic response to prolonged malnutrition.

Throughout the 19th century, numerous cases of AN were documented in France, reflecting Lasègue's influence and the growing medical interest in these disorders. French clinicians noted a variety of behaviors among these patients—some vomited, some avoided food due to fears of gastric pain, while others controlled their appetite out of a fear of obesity. These descriptions highlighted one of the disorder's defining characteristics: a distorted body image. Cases were reported across different age groups, including children and middle-aged individuals, allowing for the observation of various outcomes. Some patients recovered, while others progressed to severe malnutrition and death. In these cases, relationships with hysteria and compulsive behaviors were often identified, as well as occasional connections to psychotic disorders, with some anorexic patients later developing schizophrenia. Huchard coined the term "Mental Anorexia", a term still widely used today, particularly by Philippe Jeammet (1984) in France.

Building on Lasègue's observations regarding the family environment, French doctors began to recommend therapeutic approaches involving the patient's separation from their family to disrupt potentially harmful relational dynamics. Among these advocates was Charcot, who promoted isolation from the family as a beneficial treatment strategy (Fernández, 2015; Abínzano, 2019). King (1963) expanded upon earlier understandings of anorexia by distinguishing between "Primary Anorexias", characterized by a psychological refusal of food, and "Secondary Anorexias", where appetite loss was secondary to other medical or psychiatric conditions. Although some secondary sources have attributed similar advances to Gilles de la Tourette, historical records suggest that de la Tourette's contributions were primarily in the field of neuropsychiatry, particularly with the syndrome that bears his name. He did not formally articulate the symptomatic triad now associated with anorexia nervosa—self-starvation, distorted body image, and disordered eating behaviors. The modern understanding of AN, with its focus on body image distortion and disordered eating behaviors, emerged later, shaped by broader developments in psychiatric theory.

The modern conceptualization of AN, encompassing the triad of self-induced starvation, body image distortion, and disordered eating behaviors, was more precisely articulated in the late 19th century by physicians such as Sir William Gull and Charles Lasègue. Gull introduced the term "anorexia nervosa" and emphasized the psychological aspects of the disorder, while Lasègue highlighted the role of family dynamics and the patient's mental state in the development of the condition.

At the turn of the 20th century, Pierre Janet made further contributions to the understanding of AN, proposing a categorization of nervous anorexia into obsessive, psychasthenic, and hysterical forms (Aragona, 2021). Janet suggested that obsessive forms represented a struggle to control both appetite and body, while hysterical forms often involved spontaneous vomiting. He described hyperactivity as an attempt to combat fatigue, and he noted that such cases were frequently resistant to treatment.

Lastly, Andrée Thomas, in 1909, posited that AN should be viewed as an indeterminate syndrome, not strictly related to other conditions (Ruefli,

1993). This perspective reflects the evolving understanding of AN as a unique condition with complex interactions among psychological, familial, and cultural factors. Together, these early descriptions by Lasègue, Gull, Janet, and others laid the groundwork for the modern clinical understanding of AN, emphasizing the roles of mental distress, family dynamics, and body image in the development and progression of the disorder.

Third period: Clinical-endocrinological phase

In 1914, the German physician Simmonds introduced the concept of "pituitary cachexia", a condition characterized by anterior pituitary insufficiency that led to severe cachexia, or wasting syndrome. Simmonds's observations caused significant confusion regarding the etiology of AN, as his description shifted the focus from psychological factors to an endocrinological explanation. Many in the medical community began to question whether the psychogenic origins previously proposed were simply secondary reactions to primary glandular insufficiency. Simmonds's work marked a pivotal moment, sparking a wave of interest in the potential role of endocrine dysfunction, specifically panhypopituitarism, in the development of AN. This shift led to a widespread belief that AN was primarily an endocrine disorder that required purely endocrinological treatment (Simmonds, 1914).

During this period, the prevailing view was that AN resulted from deficiencies in pituitary function, believed to disrupt metabolic processes and lead to severe malnutrition. This interpretation heavily influenced clinical approaches, with endocrinologists advocating treatments focused on correcting hormonal imbalances rather than addressing psychological factors. As a result, medical professionals prioritized hormonal therapies aimed at restoring normal pituitary function as the primary treatment method. This perspective dominated for decades, shaping both diagnostic criteria and treatment protocols during that time.

However, in 1948, British pathologist Harold Sheehan challenged this interpretation. Sheehan pointed out that malnutrition was not a typical outcome of pituitary insufficiency, clarifying that severe malnutrition only occurred in terminal stages of pituitary disease and was not characteristic of anterior pituitary dysfunction itself. His work, published with W. J. Summers in 1949, argued that the pituitary gland's role in AN had been overstated and that the severe malnutrition seen in AN was not due to hormonal deficiencies. Sheehan's refutation effectively shifted the focus away from an exclusively endocrinological perspective and reopened the discussion of psychogenic and psychosocial factors (Sheehan and Summers, 1949).

Despite Sheehan's correction, the clinical-endocrinological phase left a lasting impact on the understanding, diagnosis, and treatment of EDs. The emphasis on endocrinological factors led to a more integrative approach to

AN, as researchers and clinicians recognized the potential for complex interactions between biological and psychological factors. This period of endocrinological focus also highlighted the importance of distinguishing between primary endocrine disorders and psychogenic conditions with secondary endocrine involvement.

Today, although the understanding of AN has largely returned to a focus on psychological and sociocultural factors, the insights from the clinical-endocrinological phase have contributed to a more nuanced view of the disorder. Modern research continues to investigate the biological underpinnings of AN, recognizing that, while psychological factors are central, endocrine imbalances may play a role in exacerbating symptoms or complicating recovery. The legacy of this period is evident in today's multifaceted treatment approaches, which integrate psychological therapy with medical monitoring of endocrine and metabolic health.

Fourth period: Mental phase and social construction of the concept

During this period, AN returned to its classification among mental health disorders, a shift that solidified its place within psychiatric nosography. It is now recognized as a specific clinical category in the field of psychiatry, as reflected in the last three editions of the American Psychiatric Association's *Diagnostic and Statistical Manual of Mental Disorders* (DSM) (1987, 1994, 2013). This reclassification underscores the evolution of AN from a condition once linked to physical, endocrinological origins back to its roots in mental and emotional disturbances, with a renewed emphasis on its complex psychosocial dimensions.

The historical evolution of AN as a concept has not followed a straightforward or progressive path; rather, it has adapted to reflect the prevailing medical, psychological, and social views of each era. Over time, the concept of AN has moved through phases influenced by clinical, psychological, and social science perspectives, integrating multiple approaches that collectively enrich our understanding of this disorder. As a result, contemporary views on AN do not view it solely as a mental disorder but recognize its development as influenced by cultural, social, and psychological factors. This phase not only reflects the contributions of medicine and psychology but also the role of social sciences in understanding and defining the disorder.

Significant contributions during this period expanded therapeutic approaches, clarified diagnostic definitions, and deepened our understanding of interpersonal relationships involved in the disorder's manifestation. In the United States, in 1939, psychoanalyst Frank Alexander's work on psychosomatic characteristics offered early insights into how psychological factors could influence physical health, marking an essential shift in understanding AN as a disorder with both mental and somatic dimensions (Nemiah, 1958). In France, Serge Lebovici explored the pathogenic maternal bond in 1948, proposing that early maternal-child relationships could play a critical role in the development of AN (Tezer-işir, 2023). In the 1950s, American psychiatrist Hilde Bruch further advanced the understanding of AN, suggesting that weight loss efforts were often distorted attempts at self-control in individuals experiencing profound feelings of helplessness and despair. She connected a deteriorating body image with a patient's compromised sense of internal control and self-worth, arguing that AN was, in part, a misguided attempt to exert control over one's life (Bruch, 1965, 1973).

In 1965, an international symposium held in Göttingen, Germany, marked a major milestone in the development of the concept of mental anorexia. This gathering brought together experts from the United States and Europe, including Eugene Bliss, Hilde Bruch, Helmut Thöma, and Mara Selvini Palazzoli, to discuss themes such as puberty, disturbances in body image, and the unique psychological structure of AN. Palazzoli emphasized the role of family dynamics in the development of AN. Her book *Self-Starvation* (Selvini Palazzoli, 1974) underscored the influence of family structures and interactions on the disorder, contributing to the foundation of systemic theory and illuminating how family roles and expectations shape the behavior and psyche of individuals with AN. This symposium was crucial in establishing the international significance of AN as a distinct mental health condition, recognizing its unique characteristics and the need for specialized therapeutic approaches.

Psychoanalysts in France, including Kestemberg and Decobert, further enriched this field in 1972 with their comprehensive study published in *"Le faim et le corps" (Hunger and the Body)*, which explored the intricate relationship between body image and eating disorders. Their work examined how body perception and self-image contribute to the development of AN, arguing that the disorder involves more than just issues with food—it is also a profound struggle with self-perception and body identity (Kestemberg, Kestemberg, and Decobert, 1972). This psychoanalytic approach highlighted the importance of understanding the symbolic meanings of starvation, body size, and control, all of which play into the anorexic experience.

In 1987, the American Psychiatric Association officially classified anorexia nervosa (AN) within the DSM-III-R under the category of "Childhood and Adolescent Disorders" (American Psychiatric Association, 1987), a categorization that persisted in the DSM-IV (American Psychiatric Association, 1994) and continues in the latest DSM-5 (American Psychiatric Association, 2013). This inclusion signifies the medical community's broad acceptance of AN as a distinct psychiatric condition, highlighting the critical role of psychological factors in its diagnosis and treatment. While this classification frames AN primarily as a mental health disorder, it also acknowledges the intricate interplay between its psychological, physical, and social dimensions.

In this phase, the social construction of AN has become an essential consideration in understanding the disorder. Contemporary perspectives recognize that AN does not develop in a vacuum; rather, it is shaped by cultural values, social expectations, and the symbolic significance attributed to body size and self-control. The concept of AN as both a mental disorder and a socially influenced phenomenon highlights the importance of cultural ideals of beauty, perfectionism, and discipline, particularly in Western societies, where thinness often symbolizes control, success, and desirability. Social and cultural constructs contribute to shaping individuals' perceptions of their bodies and their sense of self-worth, reinforcing behaviors associated with AN.

Overall, the *mental phase* and the social construction of AN represent a culmination of medical, psychological, and sociocultural insights. This period has led to a holistic approach to the disorder, emphasizing the integration of psychological therapy, medical management, and sociocultural understanding. With its recognition as a multifaceted psychiatric disorder, AN is now seen as a condition that transcends simple definitions, existing at the intersection of individual psychology, family dynamics, and broader cultural forces.

The historical development of the bulimia nervosa concept

The term "bulimia" originates from the Greek word βουλιμία (*boulīmia*), meaning "ravenous hunger," which is derived from βοῦς (*boûs*, "ox") and λῑμός (*līmós*, "hunger"). This etymology underscores the recognition of extreme eating behaviors in early cultures. The phrase translates to "hunger as intense as an ox" or "ravenous hunger," vividly capturing the concept of an uncontrollable appetite (Northville, 2024). While this ancient terminology reflects a longstanding awareness of episodes of extreme hunger, it was not until much later that such behaviors were formally classified as a distinct eating disorder, highlighting the evolution of understanding around bulimia nervosa (BN).

Initially, BN was regarded as an impulsive symptom rather than a distinct disorder, often linked to behaviors associated with restrictive dieting. It wasn't until 1979 that Gerard Russell, working in the United States, formally identified BN as a separate condition, categorizing it as a subgroup of AN (Russell, 1979). Russell's groundbreaking work highlighted BN as a psychological condition with distinct features, including cycles of binge eating followed by compensatory behaviors such as vomiting or excessive exercise. His definition marked a pivotal moment in the understanding of BN, transforming it from a dieting-related behavior into a recognized mental health disorder with its own diagnostic identity.

Historical perspectives on binge eating and purging behaviors

Although BN was only identified in recent history, behaviors associated with binge eating and purging can be traced back to antiquity, particularly in ancient Greece and Rome.

In ancient Greece, cultural and historical accounts suggest the existence of binge eating behaviors, particularly among the elite. Xenophon, in his work *"Anabasis"* (circa 370 BC), describes Greek soldiers consuming large quantities of food and subsequently inducing vomiting. This practice was often driven by a desire to continue feasting or alleviate the discomfort of overeating. The term *"opsophagos"* was used to describe individuals with an insatiable craving for delicacies, particularly fish. These individuals, often portrayed in Greek literature, were characterized by their uncontrollable desire for specific foods, leading to frequent overindulgence and earning a reputation for their excessive appetites.

Similarly, in the Roman Empire, historical records reveal comparable behaviors among notable figures. Emperors such as Claudius and Vitellius were infamous for their episodes of binge eating followed by purging. The *"Bacchanalian"* festivals of ancient Rome further exemplified this cultural tendency, celebrating excessive indulgence with feasting and drinking that often culminated in vomiting. This act, socially accepted and even expected during these festivals, reflected a cultural embrace of excess rather than an understanding of these behaviors as part of a psychological disorder.

While these historical examples highlight behaviors resembling what we now identify as BN, they were interpreted within the framework of their respective cultures. In both Greek and Roman societies, such actions were seen as expressions of luxury, indulgence, or social norms, rather than as symptoms of an underlying mental health condition. These accounts underscore the importance of contextualizing eating behaviors within their cultural and historical settings, illustrating how attitudes toward food and excess have evolved over time.

While these historical behaviors resemble aspects of modern bulimia nervosa, the cultural contexts and underlying motivations were fundamentally different. In ancient societies, such practices were often tied to social rituals, displays of wealth, or cultural traditions rather than the pathological self-perception and psychological distress characteristic of contemporary eating disorders.

Nonetheless, these accounts offer valuable insights into the long-standing complexity of human eating behaviors across different eras. They reveal how cultural frameworks have historically shaped the interpretation of behaviors that, centuries later, would be clinically recognized as core features of bulimia nervosa.

From hysteria to modern understanding

In the 19th century, bulimia-like behaviors began to appear in the broader diagnostic frameworks of the time, most notably within descriptions of hysteria. Hysteria, then considered a catch-all diagnosis for a wide range of symptoms primarily attributed to women, encompassed impulsive actions, emotional instability, and somatic complaints. Some of these behaviors bear a resemblance to contemporary understandings of BN, particularly in the realms of emotional dysregulation and impulsivity. Though binge eating and body image concerns were not universally highlighted in cases of hysteria, the impulsive behaviors described suggest a historical connection to disorders involving difficulties in regulating affect and impulses.

By the early 20th century, psychiatry began to develop a more refined understanding of behaviors that could now be linked to eating disorders. Early descriptions of AN, such as those by William Gull in the late 19th century, paved the way for more specific investigations into disordered eating behaviors. However, BN as a distinct entity remained under-recognized, with symptoms often dismissed as secondary manifestations of other psychological conditions.

The mid-20th century saw increasing interest in disordered eating as a psychological phenomenon, but it was not until the late 1970s that BN was formally recognized as a distinct clinical entity. Researchers like Cooper and Taylor (1988) contributed significantly to this development, emphasizing the role of body image disturbances and the complex interplay between binge eating and compensatory behaviors like purging. This marked a shift from viewing BN primarily as a behavioral issue to understanding it as a disorder deeply intertwined with self-perception, cultural ideals, and emotional regulation.

Cultural and psychological contexts of bulimia nervosa in the last two centuries

The evolving understanding of BN reflects broader societal changes in attitudes toward the body, indulgence, and control. In the Victorian era, for example, societal ideals of femininity emphasized restraint, modesty, and control over one's impulses, including those related to food and body shape. Overeating or exhibiting impulsivity was often pathologized, particularly in women, and seen as a moral failing or a sign of hysteria.

In the early 20th century, cultural shifts toward modernity and industrialization brought new pressures, including changing ideals of beauty and the commodification of the body. The burgeoning fields of psychology and psychoanalysis began to frame eating behaviors within the broader context of emotional conflict and unconscious drives. For instance, psychoanalytic theories often linked eating behaviors to unresolved oral-stage conflicts or to attempts to cope with unmet emotional needs.

The latter half of the 20th century saw a dramatic rise in the prevalence of EDs, coinciding with societal trends that placed increasing emphasis on thinness as a marker of success, discipline, and desirability. The advent of mass media and the proliferation of idealized body images played a crucial role in amplifying the pressures to conform to these unattainable standards. Within this context, BN emerged as a disorder that encapsulated the tension between indulgence and control—a reflection of the broader cultural paradox that simultaneously glorifies consumption and self-restraint.

Bulimia nervosa: A convergence of historical and modern perspectives

Although bulimia nervosa (BN) is a relatively recent addition to the catalog of psychological disorders, its roots stretch back through centuries of human behavior, blending ancient practices, evolving diagnostic frameworks, and contemporary psychological theories. BN reflects an enduring human struggle with the tension between restraint and indulgence, while simultaneously highlighting the profound impact of societal values on individual behavior and self-perception.

Historically, behaviors resembling BN can be traced to ancient cultures. In Greece and Rome, binge-purge cycles were part of ritualistic or hedonistic practices. Greek soldiers, as documented by Xenophon in *Anabasis*, indulged in overeating and induced vomiting to continue feasting, a behavior mirrored by Roman emperors such as Claudius and Vitellius. Similarly, the *Bacchanalian* festivals in Rome celebrated excess, with vomiting seen as a socially accepted extension of indulgence. These actions, however, were culturally sanctioned and tied to specific contexts of luxury and opulence, rather than recognized as pathological behaviors.

The 19th century brought new interpretations of such impulsive behaviors, particularly within the framework of hysteria, which was thought to reflect a loss of self-control rooted in psychological imbalance. This period set the stage for linking behaviors like overeating or purging with broader concepts of mental health and impulse regulation. It wasn't until the late 20th century that Gerard Russell formally defined BN as a distinct disorder in 1979, describing it as cycles of binge eating followed by compensatory behaviors such as vomiting, fasting, or excessive exercise. This marked a pivotal moment in understanding the disorder as more than a product of dieting but as a complex psychological condition intertwined with self-perception and societal influences.

In the modern era, BN has become a lens through which broader societal dynamics can be examined. The disorder not only reflects individual struggles with food and body image but also serves as a mirror of cultural attitudes toward consumption, discipline, and identity. The emphasis on thinness and self-control in contemporary society exacerbates these behaviors, as individuals attempt to reconcile internal vulnerabilities with external pressures. This cultural backdrop reinforces the notion that BN is both a deeply personal and socially constructed disorder, shaped by the intricate interplay of biology, psychology, and societal expectations.

Advancements in understanding BN as a distinct psychological disorder highlight the complexity of eating behaviors and their relationship to self-perception and cultural pressures. Yet, the historical context offers valuable insights into how these behaviors have evolved. From ancient practices tied to excess and indulgence to modern frameworks emphasizing psychological vulnerability, BN embodies the convergence of historical and modern perspectives. As researchers and clinicians continue to explore the disorder, integrating these historical narratives provides a richer understanding of the intricate relationship between human behavior, psychological resilience, and the cultural values that shape them.

Bibliography

Abínzano, R. V. (2019). El advenimiento de la anorexia como categoría psicopatológica: Discusión y delimitación entre Lasègue, Gull y Freud. *Perspectivas en Psicología*, 16(2): 90–97.

Albano, C. (1998). Richard Morton and nervous consumption. *Eating Disorders*, 6(1): 3–13.

Alexander-Mott, L. (2019). Anorexia nervosa: Definition, diagnostic criteria, and associated psychological problems. In L. Alexander-Mott and B. Lumsden (eds.) *Understanding Eating Disorders: Anorexia Nervosa, Bulimia Nervosa and Obesity.* London and New York: Routledge, 101–122.

American Psychiatric Association (1987). 3rd edition. *Diagnostic and Statistical Manual of Mental Disorders DSM-III-R.* Washington DC: American Psychiatric Association Publishing.

American Psychiatric Association (1994). 4th edition. *Diagnostic and Statistical Manual of Mental Disorders DSM-IV.* Washington DC: American Psychiatric Association Publishing.

American Psychiatric Association (2013). 5th edition. *Diagnostic and Statistical Manual of Mental Disorders DSM-5.* Washington DC: American Psychiatric Association Publishing.

Aragona, M. (2021). A conceptual history of Anorexia Nervosa: Specificity of the psychopathological perspectives. *Dialogues in Philosophy, Mental and Neuro Sciences*, 14(1): 21–29.

Baile Ayensa, J. I. and González Calderón, M. J. (2012). Anorexia nerviosa en el siglo XIV?: El caso de Santa Catalina de Siena. *Revista Mexicana de Trastornos Alimentarios*, 3(2), 80–88. doi:10.22201/fesi.20071523e.2012.2.225.

Bauman, Z. (2013). *Liquid Modernity.* New York: John Wiley & Sons.

Behar, R. (2012). Espiritualidad y ascetismo en la anorexia nerviosa. *Revista Chilenade Neuro-psiquiatría*, 50(2): 117–119.

Benhabib, S. (2022). Thomas Hobbes on my mind: Leviathan, Thomas Hobbes. *Social Research: An International Quarterly*, 89(2): 233–247.

Blinder, B. J. and Chao, K. H. (2019). Eating disorders: A historical perspective. In L. Alexander-Mott and B. Lumsden (eds.) *Understanding Eating Disorders: Anorexia Nervosa, Bulimia Nervosa and Obesity*. London and New York: Routledge, 3–35.

Briquet, P. (1859). Tratado clínico y terapéutico de la histeria. *La Histeria antes de Freud*, 43–50.

Bronfenbrenner, U. (1979). *The Ecology of Human Development: Experiments by Nature and Design*. Cambridge, MA: Harvard University Press.

Bruch, H. (1965). Anorexia nervosa and its differential diagnosis. *The Journal of Nervous and Mental Disease*, 141(5): 555–566.

Bruch, H. (1973). *Eating Disorders: Obesity, Anorexia Nervosa and the Person Within*. New York: Basic Books.

Brusset, B. (1990). Les vicissitudes d'une déambulation addictive (Essai métapsychologique). *Revue Française de Psychanalyse*, 54(3): 671–687.

Cooper, P. J. and Taylor, M. J. (1988). Body image disturbance in bulimia nervosa. *The British Journal of Psychiatry*, 153(S2): 32–36.

DiNicola, V. F. (1990). Anorexia Multiforme: Self-starvation in historical and cultural context: Part II: Anorexia Nervosa as a Culture-Reactive Syndrome. *Transcultural Psychiatric Research Review*, 27(4): 245–285.

Farr, R. (1994). *Papers on Social Representations*. Electronic Version ISSN: 1021–5573.

Fernández, A. M. (2015). Historia de la anorexia nerviosa. *MoleQla*, 20: 15–17.

Gull, W. (1888). Anorexia nervosa. *The Lancet*, 131(3368): 516–517. Original print: Gull, W. (1874). Anorexia nervosa (apepsia hysterical, anorexia hysteria). *Transactions of the Clinical Society of London*, 7: 22–28.

Hepworth, J. (1999). *The Social Construction of Anorexia Nervosa.*. London: Sage Publications.

Inkeles, A. and Smith, D. H. (1974). *Becoming Modern: Individual Change in Six Developing Countries*. Cambridge, MA: Harvard University Press.

Jeammet, P. (1984). L'anorexie mentale. *Encycl. Med. Chir. Psychiatrie 37350* A10 et A15, 2. Paris: Elsevier.

Kestemberg, E., Kestemberg, J., and Decobert, S. (1972). *La Faim et le Corps: Une Étude Psychanalytique de l'Anorexie Mentale*. Paris: Le Fil Rouge, PUF.

King, A. (1963). Primary and secondary anorexia nervosa syndromes. *The British Journal of Psychiatry*, 109(461), 470–479. doi:10.1192/bjp.109.461.470.

Lanteri Laura, G. (1991). Introducción al texto de Charles Lasège sobre la anorexia histérica. *Vertex Revista Argentina de Psiquiatría*, I(2): 55–57.

Lasègue, C. (1873). La anorexia histérica. *Vertex Revista Argentina de Psiquiatría*, I(2): 58–64. Original print; Lasègue, C. (1873). De l'anorexie hystérique. *Archives Générales de Médecine*, 1: 384–403.

Lerner, D. (1958). *The Passing of Traditional Society*. New York: Free Press.

Moscovici, S. (1961). *La Psychanalyse son Image et son Public: Etude sur la Représentation Sociale de la Psychanalyse*. Paris: Press Universitaires de France.

Nemiah, J. C. (1958). Anorexia nervosa: Fact and theory. *The American Journal of Digestive Diseases*, 3: 249–274.

Nimrouzi, M. and Zarshenas, M. M. (2018). Anorexia: Highlights in traditional Persian medicine and conventional medicine. *Avicenna Journal of Phytomedicine*, 8 (1): 1–13.

Northville, F. (2024). Where did the term bulimia come from? *Eating Disorder Resources*. https://eatingdisorderresources.com/where-did-the-term-bulimia-come-from.

Paris, J. (1996). *Social Factors in the Personality Disorders: A Biopsychosocial Approach to Etiology and Treatment*. Cambridge: Cambridge University Press.

Ruefli, E. L. (1993). *An Etiologic Model of Eating Disorders in Females*. Austin, TX: The University of Texas at Austin.

Russell, G. (1979). Bulimia nervosa: An ominous variant of anorexia nervosa. *Psychological Medicine*, 9(3): 429–448.

Rutter, M. and Rutter, M. (1993). *Developing Minds: Challenge and Continuity across the Life Span*. New York: Basic Books.

Selvini Palazzoli, M. (1974). *Self-Starvation: From Individual to Family Therapy in the Treatment of Anorexia Nervosa*. New York: Jason Aronson, (edition 1978).

Sheehan, H. L. and Summers, V. K. (1949). The syndrome of hypopituitarism. *QJM: An International Journal of Medicine*, 18(4): 319–378.

Silverman, J. A. (1986). Anorexia nervosa in seventeenth century England as viewed by physician, philosopher, and pedagogue an essay. *International Journal of Eating Disorders*, 5(5): 847–853.

Simmonds, M. (1914). Ueber embolische prozesse in der hypophysis. *Virchows Arch. Path Anat.* 217: 226–239.

Tezerişir, A. (2023). *Discourses of Daughters and Mothers: A Lacanian Study on Eating Problems* (master's thesis, Middle East Technical University).

Whiting, B. B. and Edwards, C. P.(1988). *Children of Different Worlds: The Formation of Social Behavior*. Cambridge, MA: Harvard University Press.

3 Clinical manifestations of eating disorders

Introduction

Individuals with eating disorders experience profound disruptions in eating behavior, primarily stemming from a distorted self-image. These disturbances reflect deep psychological conflicts that shape the clinical presentation of each disorder.

Patients diagnosed with anorexia nervosa (AN) often exhibit significant weight loss, an intense and pathological preoccupation with body image, and a distorted perception of their own bodies. This relentless pursuit of thinness and the altered self-view associated with AN drive restrictive eating behaviors and, in severe cases, may lead to life-threatening levels of malnutrition.

In contrast, individuals with bulimia nervosa (BN) experience episodes of binge eating, marked by consuming large quantities of food within a short time, followed by compensatory behaviors aimed at offsetting the caloric intake. These behaviors may include purging or extreme caloric restriction following binge episodes. Patients with BN also struggle with a distorted body image, often feeling intense shame about their eating habits, which may lead them to avoid eating in public or in the presence of others.

Patients with binge eating disorder (BED) engage in episodes of consuming unusually large amounts of food within a short period, often accompanied by a sense of loss of control over their eating. Unlike BN, individuals with BED do not typically engage in purging or other compensatory behaviors such as excessive exercise or fasting to counteract the caloric intake. As a result, BED is frequently associated with overweight or obesity, as the excess caloric intake is not offset by compensatory mechanisms.

The disorder is characterized not only by the quantity of food consumed but also by the emotional and psychological experiences accompanying these episodes. Patients often report feelings of guilt, shame, or distress following a binge episode, which can perpetuate a cycle of emotional eating. This emotional eating is frequently tied to underlying

DOI: 10.4324/9781032724997-3

psychological factors, such as low self-esteem, depression, or anxiety, which drive the urge to seek comfort or distraction through food.

The link between BED and overweight or obesity highlights the interplay between psychological and physiological factors. Repeated binge episodes can lead to significant weight gain over time, increasing the risk of obesity-related health conditions, such as type 2 diabetes, hypertension, and cardiovascular disease. However, it is important to note that not all individuals with BED are overweight or obese; the disorder can occur across a spectrum of body sizes and weights.

Understanding binge eating disorder (BED) requires a comprehensive approach that considers its psychological, behavioral, and biological dimensions. Effective treatment typically involves a combination of therapeutic strategies tailored to address the complex nature of the disorder.

Cognitive-behavioral therapy (CBT) is often a cornerstone of treatment, helping individuals recognize and break the binge cycle while addressing the emotional triggers that drive episodes of overeating. This therapeutic approach equips patients with practical tools to manage stress, regulate emotions, and develop healthier coping mechanisms.

Nutritional counseling and education play an essential role in treatment, guiding patients toward balanced eating patterns and helping them rebuild a positive relationship with food. In some cases, medication may be prescribed to address co-occurring conditions such as depression, anxiety, or impulsivity, further supporting the patient's progress.

An integrated treatment plan that combines these elements not only tackles the behavioral and emotional aspects of BED but also fosters long-term recovery by addressing the disorder's underlying causes and consequences.

BED is a significant mental health concern, not only because of its impact on physical health but also due to the profound psychological distress it causes. Recognizing and addressing this disorder is essential to improving the well-being of affected individuals and reducing the stigma often associated with disordered eating and weight-related issues.

Clinical manifestations of anorexia

Diagnostic criteria for anorexia nervosa (DSM-5)—(American Psychiatric Association, 2013).

Restriction of energy intake: A persistent restriction of energy intake relative to requirements, leading to significantly low body weight considering the individual's age, sex, developmental stage, and physical health. "Significantly low weight" is defined as a weight that is below the minimum normal range, or in the case of children and adolescents, below the expected minimum weight for their age and growth trajectory.

1   *Intense fear of gaining weight*: An intense fear of gaining weight or becoming fat, or persistent behavior that prevents weight gain, even though the individual is significantly underweight.
2   *Disturbance in self-perception*: A disturbance in the way one's body weight or shape is experienced, with an undue influence of body weight or shape on self-evaluation. There is often a persistent lack of recognition of the seriousness of the current low body weight.
3   *Subtype designations*:

- *Restrictive type*: During the past 3 months, the individual has not engaged in recurrent episodes of binge eating or purging (e.g., self-induced vomiting, misuse of laxatives, diuretics, or enemas). Weight loss is primarily achieved through severe dieting, fasting, excessive exercise, or a combination of these methods.
- *Binge-eating/Purging type*: During the past 3 months, the individual has engaged in recurrent episodes of binge eating or purging behaviors (e. g., self-induced vomiting, misuse of laxatives, diuretics, or enemas).

These criteria provide a structured framework to ensure consistent diagnosis and treatment planning for AN, focusing on both behavioral and perceptual disturbances central to the disorder.

Symptoms and associated disorders

Individuals with AN who undergo significant weight loss may exhibit a range of symptoms, including depressed mood, social withdrawal, irritability, insomnia, and decreased interest in sex. These symptoms can sometimes align with the criteria for major depressive disorder, especially in adolescents experiencing intense conflicts with their body image (Stice and Bearman, 2001). However, because similar symptoms are also seen in individuals experiencing starvation without AN, many of these depressive features may be secondary to the physiological effects of starvation. Therefore, it is crucial to reassess mood disorder symptoms once the individual's nutritional status has improved.

Obsessive-compulsive characteristics are also common in individuals with AN and may be related or unrelated to food. Many individuals become intensely preoccupied with thoughts about food, sometimes going so far as to collect recipes or hoard food items. Studies of starvation suggest that food-related obsessions and compulsions can occur or worsen with malnutrition. If obsessions and compulsions unrelated to food, body shape, or weight are present, an additional diagnosis of obsessive-compulsive disorder (OCD) may be appropriate.

Anorexia nervosa (AN) is also associated with other personality traits and behaviors, including a concern about eating in public, feelings of inadequacy, a need for control over one's environment, rigid thinking, reduced social spontaneity, and restricted emotional expressiveness and initiative.

Individuals with the binge-eating/purging type of AN may exhibit additional characteristics compared to those with the restrictive type. They are more likely to experience impulse control issues, engage in alcohol or substance abuse, display greater emotional volatility, and have a higher level of sexual activity. These behavioral and emotional differences highlight the complexity and variability within the clinical presentations of AN.

Course of anorexia nervosa

Anorexia nervosa (AN) typically begins in mid-adolescence, with an average onset age around 14 to 18 years. However, disturbances in body image, a key feature of the disorder, often appear earlier, during puberty. Some research suggests a bimodal pattern of onset, with peak incidence around ages 14 and 18. The onset of AN is frequently triggered by a stressful life event that causes significant psychological tension, such as parental separation or the end of a romantic relationship.

The progression and outcome of AN vary widely among individuals. Some patients experience a single episode and achieve full recovery, while others exhibit a cyclical pattern of recovery and relapse, marked by periods of weight gain followed by relapse. In the most severe cases, individuals may suffer from chronic deterioration, with a progressive decline over many years. This chronic course is the most dramatic and difficult to treat, whereas a single-episode recovery is relatively rare.

Hospitalization is often necessary to stabilize the patient's weight and restore electrolyte balance. According to the American Psychiatric Association (2022), anorexia nervosa (AN) has one of the highest mortality rates among psychiatric disorders, with long-term mortality estimated between 5% and 10%. Mortality is often due to severe malnutrition and medical complications related to starvation, such as electrolyte imbalances, which can lead to cardiac arrhythmias and sudden death. Additionally, individuals with AN have a significantly elevated risk of suicide, contributing to the overall mortality rate (Sullivan, 1995).

A notable aspect of anorexia nervosa's course is the frequent development of bulimic behaviors, with some patients transitioning to BN over time. This transition is often observed in individuals whose anorexia symptoms manifest early in adolescence and gradually shift toward bulimic behaviors as they mature. Conversely, it is also possible for individuals with BN to develop anorexic behaviors, reflecting the fluid and evolving nature of EDs across the lifespan.

Differential diagnosis

When evaluating AN, it is essential to consider other potential causes of anorexia and weight loss, especially if the presentation includes atypical features. Various medical conditions present significant weight loss or loss of appetite but are rooted in different etiologies. For example, disorders of the digestive tract, hidden neoplasms, and infectious diseases like brucellosis and tuberculosis may cause substantial weight loss, yet they do not involve the disturbances in body image characteristic of AN.

Similarly, in acquired immunodeficiency syndrome (AIDS), weight loss and loss of appetite are common; however, patients with AIDS do not typically experience body image distortion or a drive for further weight loss. In cases of wasting diseases, anorexia is typically accompanied by a marked decrease in appetite, without body image distortion, changes in movement or motor skills, and laboratory findings pointing to the underlying condition. In contrast, individuals with AN often retain a typical appetite but deny or resist it, coupled with characteristic laboratory findings that support the diagnosis of AN.

Certain conditions, such as superior mesenteric artery syndrome (characterized by postprandial pain and vomiting due to intermittent obstruction of gastric emptying), must be differentiated from AN, although they may occasionally appear in patients suffering from AN. This syndrome can arise due to the absence of mesenteric adipose tissue, which places strain on the vasculo-nervous pedicle and causes visceral discomfort like this syndrome.

Endocrine disorders, such as panhypopituitarism or tumors affecting the central nervous system (CNS), hypothalamus, or pituitary gland, can result in appetite disturbances but do not typically present with body image distortions. Certain cases of amenorrhea due to endocrine disorders should also be ruled out before diagnosing AN.

In the realm of mental health, it is important to recognize potential comorbidities while distinguishing AN from other conditions. Anxiety disorders are common among patients with EDs, and obsessive-compulsive disorder (OCD) and social phobia frequently appear in those with AN. The preoccupation with food, obsession with nutritional and caloric values, and rigid eating rituals observed in AN often contribute to social isolation and an avoidant attitude toward social interactions.

Some features of AN overlap with social phobia, OCD, and body dysmorphic disorder (BDD). Individuals with AN may experience significant distress and humiliation around eating in public, alongside obsessive thoughts or compulsive behaviors related to food or a strong preoccupation with perceived bodily imperfections. If social fears extend beyond eating behaviors, a separate diagnosis of social phobia is warranted, indicating comorbid social anxiety. Similarly, if obsessions and compulsions unrelated to food or body image are present, an additional diagnosis of OCD is appropriate. BDD, however, should only be diagnosed if the bodily concern is unrelated to body size or weight.

In major depressive disorder, significant weight loss can occur due to a secondary decrease in appetite; however, these patients generally lack the desire to lose weight or the fear of gaining weight that is central to AN.

Differential diagnosis is more complex due to frequent comorbidity with AN. In a major depressive episode without eating disturbances, there is typically no body image distortion, and reduced appetite is secondary to melancholic symptoms.

Schizophrenia may also involve unusual eating behaviors and weight loss, yet patients rarely exhibit fear of weight gain or body image disturbance. Weight loss in schizophrenia may be due to a lack of interest in eating, often related to psychotic symptoms rather than intentional weight control. Anorexia in psychotic patients is generally associated with delusions of poisoning or contamination, which become apparent in clinical interviews, aiding in differential diagnosis. Anorexia in catatonic patients is distinct due to marked immobility and the inability to eat without assistance, differentiating it from AN.

Clinical complications of anorexia nervosa

Anorexia nervosa (AN) presents a wide range of clinical complications due to malnutrition and electrolyte imbalances, affecting multiple organ systems.

- *Electrolyte imbalances*: Electrolyte imbalances are common, with hypokalemia (very low potassium levels) being particularly frequent. This imbalance can lead to cardiac issues such as arrhythmias and ECG abnormalities. Chronic hypokalemia may also cause constipation, skeletal muscle myopathies, and nephropathy. Hypomagnesemia (low magnesium levels) is another complication that can lead to muscle weakness, decreased concentration, fasciculations, paresthesias, arrhythmias, and memory loss. Hyponatremia, often due to excess water intake or inappropriate antidiuretic hormone regulation, may lead to further complications, including the risk of diabetes insipidus. Additionally, "Refeeding Syndrome" can occur when phosphate levels drop dangerously low during refeeding, manifesting as respiratory distress, cardiomyopathy, and neuropathies, all of which are potentially life-threatening.
- *Gastrointestinal complications*: AN commonly affects gastrointestinal motility, leading to delayed gastric emptying, constipation, loss of peristalsis, and irritable bowel syndrome. Steatorrhea and melanosis coli (dark pigmentation of the colon from laxative abuse) are also seen. Rectal prolapse, gastric dilation, and even rupture may occur in severe cases. Liver function tests and serum amylase levels may deviate from normal values, indicating stress on the liver and pancreas. Pancreatitis can also develop due to refeeding or binge eating episodes, and pancreatic atrophy has been observed in cases of long-term AN, affecting pancreatic function and insulin regulation.

- *Renal complications*: AN can led to functional and structural renal changes. Chronic hypokalemia causes potassium loss through urine, coupled with extracellular fluid contraction, leading to hyponatremia. Chronic malnutrition often results in calcium loss through urine, contributing to hypocalcemia. Cases of nephrocalcinosis, urolithiasis, and chronic renal failure have also been reported. Rapid weight loss can induce rhabdomyolysis and, in severe cases, acute renal failure. Chronic malnutrition can cause decreased renal volume and ptosis due to reduced perirenal fat.

- *Neurological complications*: Malnutrition in AN is associated with peripheral neuropathies and metabolic encephalopathy, often evident through diffuse EEG abnormalities. Brain imaging often reveals an increased ventricle-to-brain ratio, signifying malnutrition-induced changes. Severe electrolyte imbalances can contribute to neurological symptoms, such as myoclonic spasms, headaches, and even seizures.

- *Cardiovascular complications*: Cardiovascular issues in AN are among the most serious, with bradycardia (heart rate < 60 bpm) being common due to increased vagal tone, which can reverse with weight restoration. Prolongation of the QT interval and bradycardia place patients at risk for severe ventricular arrhythmias, particularly polymorphic ventricular tachycardia (torsades de pointes), which is associated with a risk of sudden death. Hypotension, orthostatic hypotension, and acrocyanosis are also frequent. ECG abnormalities, including low QRS voltage, T-wave inversion, and ST segment depression, are commonly observed. Additionally, mitral valve prolapses, and pericardial effusion can arise, especially in cases with thyroid dysfunction (Oka et al. 1984); (Inagaki et al. 2003). Cardiac complications account for approximately one-third of deaths in AN patient, with sudden death being particularly prevalent (Isner et al. 1985); (Neumäker, 1997).

- *Nutritional deficiencies*: Nutritional deficiencies in AN involve multiple minerals and vitamins, including calcium, magnesium, phosphorus, potassium, iron, and vitamins B1, B2, B3, B12, folic acid, and vitamin D. Calcium and vitamin D deficiencies contribute to bone disorders such as osteoporosis and osteomalacia, where the bones become brittle or weakened. Magnesium deficiency can cause tremors, spasms, and other neurological symptoms. Iron deficiency, common in AN, results in microcytic, hypochromic anemia, leading to fatigue, pallor, and dyspnea. Copper deficiency can cause neutropenia, leukopenia, and bone demineralization, as well as anemia due to impaired iron absorption. Deficiencies of thiamine (B1) can lead to "beriberi," presenting with mental confusion, edema, and muscle weakness, while riboflavin (B2) and niacin (B3) deficiencies manifest with symptoms like dermatitis and gastrointestinal issues.

- *Dental complications*: AN, especially with vomiting behavior, often leads to dental issues, including rampant caries and enamel erosion. Reduced salivary flow and frequent vomiting can result in enamel demineralization, perimolysis (erosion of lingual surfaces of upper anterior teeth), sensitivity, and gingival bleeding. Additionally, patients may experience burning sensations in the mouth, thermal sensitivity, decreased salivary flow, and parotid gland enlargement.

In summary, anorexia nervosa's impact spans a wide array of body systems, with potentially life-threatening complications across cardiovascular, renal, gastrointestinal, and neurological domains. Understanding these clinical manifestations is essential to managing the disorder effectively and addressing its severe physiological consequences.

Clinical manifestations of bulimia nervosa

Bulimia nervosa (BN) can occur as a distinct disorder or appear as a symptom within other eating conditions, such as the binge-purge subtype of AN or BED (American Psychiatric Association, 2013).

Bulimia nervosa (BN) typically begins in early adolescence and is characterized by recurring episodes of excessive food intake within a short period, usually one to two hours, during which individuals experience a profound loss of control over their eating. This overwhelming sense of being "unable to stop eating" defines these episodes, clinically referred to as "binges".

The act of binging often takes on a ritualistic quality, with patients developing intricate and secretive routines around their episodes. This may include hoarding or hiding food, seeking opportunities to binge in solitude, such as late at night when others are asleep, or meticulously planning the acquisition and consumption of food. The types of food consumed during binges can vary widely, ranging from typical snacks or comfort foods to unconventional and, in some cases, surprising items, including pet food.

Many individuals with BN exhibit strong preferences or cravings for specific types of food, often favoring sweets or highly palatable, calorie-dense items. This compulsive and covert behavior reflects the complex psychological and emotional drivers behind BN, where feelings of guilt, shame, and anxiety frequently accompany the cycle of binging, further reinforcing the secrecy and ritualization of these episodes. Understanding these patterns is crucial for developing empathetic and effective treatment strategies.

A key feature of BN is the intense compulsion to eat, which once initiated, continues until the individual feels a sense of extreme fullness or abdominal discomfort. Patients often report eating "until they can't stand it anymore". Unlike AN, BN typically occurs in individuals of normal weight or those who are slightly overweight, as the recurrent binging episodes are counterbalanced by compensatory behaviors.

To prevent weight gain, individuals with BN often resort to various compensatory measures after bingeing. These behaviors, aimed at "evacuating" the consumed calories, can include self-induced vomiting, laxative or diuretic abuse, and excessive exercise. In severe cases, these episodes and compensatory actions can become a daily cycle, reflecting the challenging and compulsive nature of BN.

Diagnostic criteria for bulimia nervosa (DSM-5)—(American Psychiatric Association, 2013).

1 *Recurrent episodes of binge eating, defined by both of the following*:

- Eating, within a discrete 2-hour period, an amount of food that is larger than what most individuals would consume under similar circumstances.
- Experiencing a lack of control overeating during the episode, with a sense that one cannot stop or control what or how much is being consumed.

2 *Recurrent inappropriate compensatory behaviors to prevent weight gain, which may include*:

- Self-induced vomiting
- Misuse of laxatives, diuretics, or other medications
- Fasting or restrictive eating
- Excessive exercise

3 *Binge eating and compensatory behaviors occur, on average, at least once a week for 3 months.*
4 *Self-evaluation is excessively influenced by body shape and weight,* with a disproportionate emphasis on physical appearance affecting self-worth.
5 *The disturbance is not exclusive to anorexia nervosa episodes.*

Although the DSM-5 no longer distinguishes between purging and non-purging subtypes of BN, I consider it valuable to maintain the classification from the DSM-IV (American Psychiatric Association, 1994) and DSM-IV-TR (American Psychiatric Association, 2000). Under this earlier framework, BN was further classified into two subtypes based on the presence or absence of purging behaviors:

- *Purging type*: In this subtype, individuals engage in self-induced vomiting, which, when frequent and repetitive, poses severe health risks, particularly due to electrolyte imbalances. Other expulsive behaviors, such as the misuse of laxatives, diuretics, and enemas, are also common and contribute to various medical complications.

- *Non-purging type*: In this subtype, individuals do not engage in purging behaviors but instead rely on compensatory methods, such as physical activity, to prevent weight gain. This may include extensive walking, rigorous exercise, jogging, and other forms of extreme physical training.

These diagnostic criteria help clinicians distinguish bulimia nervosa from other EDs and guide treatment by identifying key behavioral patterns and associated risks.

A critical aspect of BN is its strong association with impulsivity. Impulsive behaviors significantly shape the clinical presentation of BN and are essential considerations in assessing the severity and prognosis of the condition. The presence of impulsive symptoms, such as purging, signals potential dangers and highlights the need for careful monitoring, as these behaviors can pose serious threats to both the continuity and effectiveness of treatment.

Impulsivity is almost universally present in BN, influencing the patient's psychic functioning such that actions often replace verbal expression. Conflicts that remain unspoken are instead acted upon, placing patients at risk for various hazardous behaviors, including self-harm, suicide attempts, substance abuse, and impulsive sexual encounters. These behaviors provide insight into the severity of BN and suggest a mode of coping that circumvents verbalization and insight, reinforcing the impulsive cycle.

Additionally, depressive symptoms are nearly always present in BN. While binge eating can feel egosyntonic—aligned with the patient's desires—during the act, it quickly turns egodystonic afterward, bringing feelings of shame, guilt, and self-reproach. For some patients struggling with depression, binge episodes may offer brief moments of happiness or relief, only to be followed by intense remorse and dissatisfaction.

Notably, there is little difference in the diagnostic criteria for BN between the two main diagnostic frameworks, the DSM-5 (American Psychiatric Association, 2013) and the ICD-11 (World Health Organization, 2019), underscoring the universally recognized features of impulsivity and associated depressive symptoms as integral to the disorder's clinical profile.

Differential diagnosis

When diagnosing BN, it is essential to distinguish it from several other conditions with overlapping or similar symptoms:

- *Binge eating disorder (BED)*: BED involves recurrent binge eating episodes but lacks the regular compensatory behaviors seen in BN. Although individuals with BED may feel significant distress about their eating habits, they do not attempt to counteract binge episodes with measures like purging or excessive exercise. This distinction is crucial as BED focuses on the psychological distress related to eating without the physical risks of compensatory behaviors.

- *Obesity*: In obesity, recurrent binge eating episodes and compensatory behaviors are generally absent. Concern about weight in individuals with obesity typically reflects a realistic understanding of body image, without the distortions seen in BN. Efforts to lose weight are commonly motivated by a desire for improved health, rather than the distorted self-evaluation related to weight and shape observed in bulimia nervosa.
- *Hyperphagia in Klüver-Bucy syndrome*: Klüver-Bucy syndrome is a rare neurological disorder characterized by hyperphagia (compulsive overeating), visual agnosia, hypersexuality, and a compulsion to explore objects orally. The syndrome's unique neurological symptoms—such as compulsive licking, biting, and examining objects with the mouth—set it apart clinically, making it unlikely to be confused with BN.
- *Kleine-Levin syndrome*: This neurological disorder, which primarily affects adolescent males, involves episodes of hyperphagia (excessive eating) alternating with periods of hypersomnia (excessive sleep), often lasting for two to three weeks. The cyclical nature of hyperphagia and prolonged sleep episodes distinguishes Kleine-Levin syndrome from BN, where binge eating is typically a more regular and frequent behavior.

Accurate differential diagnosis is vital for appropriate treatment planning, as each of these conditions requires a tailored approach based on its specific symptoms and underlying causes.

Clinical complications of bulimia nervosa

Bulimia nervosa (BN) presents a variety of serious complications, with cardiovascular and electrolyte imbalances being among the most frequent and severe.

- *Electrolyte and cardiovascular complications*: Hypokalemia (low potassium levels) is common in BN, primarily resulting from self-induced vomiting, diuretic abuse, or laxative use. Although serum potassium levels may sometimes appear normal, intracellular potassium may be dangerously low, leading to symptoms like muscle weakness and cardiac issues. Intracellular potassium levels can be inferred by assessing the QTc interval on an electrocardiogram. Hypokalemia often correlates with high blood bicarbonate levels, and in cases of laxative abuse, may lead to metabolic acidosis. Diuretic use disrupts blood volume and results in urinary losses of sodium, potassium, and calcium, potentially causing hypochloremic alkalosis. Self-induced vomiting also leads to reductions in plasma sodium, potassium, and hydrogen ions, resulting in metabolic alkalosis. Additionally, hypophosphatemia may arise due to vomiting, excessive exercise, or the use of diuretics, laxatives, and antacids. Laxative abuse is also implicated in the occurrence of metabolic acidosis. Frequent fluid loss or restriction in BN can lead to serious electrolyte imbalances, a common reason for hospitalization.

- *Gastrointestinal complications*: BN can lead to inflammation of the salivary glands (parotid and submaxillary) and the esophagus. Repeated vomiting can cause esophagitis, esophageal spasms, and even esophageal tears, including the potentially fatal Mallory-Weiss tear, with cases of pneumomediastinum (air in the chest cavity) also reported (Rey et al., 1994). Gastric dilation is another risk, which can be triggered by binge eating or rapid feeding in a clinical setting. Gastric and intestinal motility issues are common, such as delayed gastric emptying, increased transit time, constipation, loss of peristalsis, irritable bowel syndrome, steatorrhea, and melanosis coli (a darkening of the colon due to laxative abuse). Some individuals with BN also misuse ipecac syrup as an emetic, which can accumulate in cardiac tissue and lead to irreversible cardiomyopathy and, in severe cases, fatal cardiac complications. Chronic purging can cause hypovolemia, leading to hyperaldosteronism to retain body fluids; when purging stops, reflex edema (a temporary swelling) may occur. Additionally, frequent vomiting exposes teeth to stomach acids, which lower salivary pH, erode enamel, and lead to dental cavities.
- *Mental health complications*: BN often involves significant mental health struggles, with individuals frequently feeling ashamed and attempting to hide their behaviors. Binge eating episodes typically occur in secret and are characterized by rapid consumption of food until the individual feels excessively full or even in pain. These binges are often triggered by dysphoric moods, interpersonal stress, intense hunger from restrictive dieting, or preoccupations with weight and body shape. Although binge episodes may temporarily alleviate dysphoria, they are often followed by self-loathing, guilt, and depressive symptoms. A sense of loss of control is a defining feature of binges, with some individuals experiencing dissociation during or after the episode. Over time, binges may transition from an acute loss of control to subtler, chronic difficulties in resisting or avoiding these episodes. However, this lack of control is not absolute; individuals may respond to external cues (e.g., stopping if someone enters the room).
- Depressive symptoms are highly prevalent in BN, with common diagnoses including dysthymic disorder and major depressive disorder (Cooper and Fairburn, 1986). For some individuals, mood disturbances develop concurrently with BN, while for others, they precede the onset of bulimic behaviors. Anxiety symptoms, such as

social anxiety or generalized anxiety disorder, are also common. Substance abuse, particularly alcohol and stimulants, occurs frequently, often with impulsive usage patterns. Stimulants are commonly used to suppress appetite and control weight. There is also a high comorbidity between BN and personality disorders, particularly borderline personality disorder (BPD), which is associated with impulsivity, emotional instability, and difficulties in interpersonal relationships.

- PTSD and specific phobias are frequently seen in individuals with BN. The association between BN and PTSD is thought to relate to high rates of childhood trauma in this population. Patients may also present with complex, mixed symptom profiles where anxiety and trauma-related symptoms dominate the clinical presentation.

The complexity of bulimia nervosa requires an understanding of its diverse clinical complications, which span cardiovascular, gastrointestinal, neurological, dental, and mental health domains. These interconnected complications highlight the need for a multidisciplinary approach to treatment, addressing both the physical and psychological dimensions of the disorder to optimize outcomes and minimize long-term risks.

Difficult patients: The role of impulsivity, addictive, and self-harm behaviors in eating disorders

The presence of comorbidities in patients with EDs, particularly in those with BN and purging-type AN, complicates prognosis and presents substantial clinical challenges. These comorbidities include impulsivity, self-harm, depressive episodes, personality disorders, anxiety disorders, and substance abuse. Early detection of these factors is essential to inform treatment guidelines, minimize risks, and improve patient outcomes. The presence of such complex factors necessitates a more intensive, multifaceted treatment approach to support recovery (Dapelo et al., 2020).

Impulsivity and eating disorders

Impulsivity is a significant feature in EDs and has become increasingly prominent in clinical presentations, contributing to therapeutic challenges. Defined as the inability to resist urges, impulsivity often results in behaviors that bring immediate gratification yet pose long-term harm. In EDs, impulsive behaviors—such as binging or purging—are often used as a quick release from psychic tension, though they are frequently followed by feelings of shame and guilt. This pattern is particularly prevalent in BN, where binge-purge cycles mirror impulsivity-related traits commonly associated with borderline personality disorder (BPD), which is itself frequently comorbid with EDs.

Impulsivity in EDs patients manifests in various ways, including difficulty resisting urges, taking unnecessary risks, and expressing anger through self-harm or aggression. Such behaviors are often triggered by stress, boredom, or emotional distress and are closely linked to personality traits and cultural contexts. Moeller et al. (2001) describe impulsivity as the tendency to react rapidly, often without consideration of the consequences, to both internal and external stimuli, resulting in negative outcomes for the individual.

Frosch (1977) identified key characteristics of impulsive actions, noting that they are often egosyntonic, minimally distorted, and typically associated with a pleasurable component. This egosyntonic quality means that impulsive acts, such as purging or self-harm, are experienced as urgent needs, providing temporary relief while perpetuating a cycle of impulsivity. The ability to detect impulsivity early in treatment is critical, as it can inform intervention strategies, including the use of psychopharmacological support when necessary. Severe cases of uncontrollable impulsivity may warrant psychiatric hospitalization to ensure patient safety.

Research by Rosval et al. (2006) highlights the variability in impulsivity among EDs patients. Attention deficits and motor inhibition issues are commonly observed in BN and purging-type AN, with non-planning impulsivity especially pronounced in BN. This impulsivity is closely linked to other high-risk behaviors, such as substance abuse, self-harm, promiscuity, and suicidal tendencies.

Substance abuse disorder and eating disorders

Substance abuse is notably more prevalent among individuals with BN and purging-type AN than in those with restrictive-type AN. The substances most frequently misused include alcohol, stimulants (e.g., cocaine and amphetamines), and opioids (Baker et al., 2010). Substance use exacerbates impulsive tendencies and contributes to antisocial behaviors, such as theft or engaging in risky actions while intoxicated, and it can also increase suicidal tendencies (Stice, Shaw, and Nemeroff, 2004). Additionally, substance abuse disrupts cognitive functioning, undermining the effectiveness of psychotherapeutic interventions. To enhance therapeutic outcomes, a period of abstinence—typically six months—is often recommended before engaging in psychodynamic treatments, as sobriety improves patient engagement and receptiveness.

Studies reveal a strong association between BN, BPD, and substance use disorders (SUDs), with alcohol, cocaine, cannabis, and tobacco being the most used substances. The choice of substance often depends on the effects patients seek. Stimulants like cocaine and amphetamines may suppress appetite and are frequently misused in attempts to control weight, while depressants like alcohol and cannabis can reduce inhibitions yet also stimulate appetite. Alcohol is also likely used as an aid to induce vomiting in individuals with BN, which could explain findings from Dunn, Neighbors, Fossos, and Larimer (2009), and Krug et al. (2011), indicating that purging is more closely associated with alcohol use than with other substances. Moreover, alcohol's disinhibitory properties make it appealing to individuals with social difficulties (such as challenges in interpersonal relationships), who might engage in problematic drinking for this purpose.

Certain personality traits—such as a tendency to seek new sensations, depression or anxiety, low self-esteem, and especially impulsivity—are believed to be common factors among those with EDs, such as BN, and those who misuse psychoactive substances (Calero-Elvira et al., 2009); (Nøkleby, 2012). This pattern is particularly evident on weekends when binge drinking often occurs, as patients lack the structure provided by day hospital support and frequently feel lonely, heightening their vulnerability. For many adolescent female patients, binge drinking serves as a maladaptive coping mechanism, offering temporary relief from feelings of isolation or emotional pain but leading to increased guilt, shame, and a heightened risk of relapse (Cruz-Sáez et al., 2013); (Herzog et al., 2006).

A similar weekend pattern is observed with synthetic stimulants, such as MDMA or other "party drugs", which are popular among BN patients seeking temporary mood enhancement and social ease. However, these substances can amplify impulsive tendencies and result in a cycle of excessive intake followed by physical and psychological crashes, further complicating treatment. Recognizing the specific risks associated with weekend binge drinking and synthetic stimulant use is essential for developing targeted treatment interventions and providing strategies that address these patterns, supporting recovery and reducing the risk of substance-fueled impulsive behaviors.

Depression and eating disorders: A complex comorbidity

Depression is a frequent comorbidity in EDs, particularly in BN, where it often manifests as dysthymia, major depressive disorder, or other depressive forms such as introjective or anaclitic depression (Blatt, 2004). There is a bidirectional relationship between depression and BN: each condition can worsen the other (Stice et al., 1998). For some individuals, binge eating provides temporary relief from depressive symptoms, offering fleeting comfort or pleasure. However, this coping mechanism often leads to increased body image dissatisfaction, shame, and guilt, which in turn can deepen depressive symptoms, creating a self-perpetuating cycle.

In BN, depressive symptoms are frequently driven by intense body image concerns, failed attempts at dieting, and the shame associated with bingeing and purging behaviors. This shame is compounded by disruptions in self-esteem, as patients commonly experience feelings of worthlessness and pervasive guilt. Research indicates that these feelings are not only outcomes of disordered eating behaviors but also powerful drivers that reinforce the cycle of depression and bulimic behavior, making it difficult for patients to break free without targeted intervention.

The relationship between depression and BN is complex, as depressive states can lead to feelings of isolation and low motivation, which may increase the likelihood of engaging in binge-eating episodes as a maladaptive coping strategy. For some individuals, these episodes are a brief escape from depressive states, but they are soon followed by heightened self-criticism and despair. The cycle of binging and purging often undermines a person's sense of self-control, exacerbating feelings of helplessness that are closely tied to depressive symptoms.

Effective treatment requires addressing both EDs and depressive symptoms, as untreated depression can significantly impede progress in managing ED behaviors. Research underscores the importance of a comprehensive approach that includes both psychological and pharmacological therapies where appropriate. For instance, cognitive-behavioral therapy (CBT) and dialectical behavior therapy (DBT) have shown promise in helping patients reframe negative thought patterns, improve emotional regulation, and develop healthier coping mechanisms. In some cases, antidepressant medications can also play a crucial role, particularly when depression is severe or resistant to psychotherapy alone.

Addressing depression in ED patients is not only essential for improving overall psychological well-being but is also pivotal in reducing the frequency and severity of ED behaviors. Depression can create a significant barrier to treatment engagement and motivation, so recognizing and managing depressive symptoms early in the treatment process is critical. By targeting both depression and ED symptoms simultaneously, treatment providers can help break the cycle of depression and disordered eating, promoting sustained recovery and improving long-term outcomes.

Personality disorders and eating disorders: The complicating role of borderline personality disorder

Personality disorders, particularly BPD, significantly complicate the treatment of EDs. Patients with co-occurring BPD, EDs, and additional comorbidities such as depressive or substance use disorders face heightened risks of self-harm, suicide attempts, and frequent hospitalizations. BPD is characterized by pervasive emotional instability, impulsive actions, and self-destructive behaviors, all of which amplify the challenges in managing EDs. These traits often lead to repeated cycles of self-harm and psychiatric crises, resulting in frequent disruptions in the treatment process and a need for recurrent interventions.

The impact of BPD on EDs is multifaceted. Emotional instability in BPD can drive individuals toward impulsive eating behaviors, such as bingeing or purging, as maladaptive coping mechanisms. The cycle of intense mood swings, combined with body image issues central to many EDs, makes it challenging for patients to regulate their emotions and behaviors consistently. As a result, treatment providers often encounter significant obstacles in establishing therapeutic rapport and achieving stable progress, as the patient's impulsivity and mood volatility can lead to setbacks, resistance to treatment, or premature treatment termination.

Kernberg (2004) observed that many patients with EDs exhibit a borderline personality organization (BPO), a framework of psychological functioning marked by identity diffusion, primitive defense mechanisms, and impulsive tendencies. Identity diffusion, for instance, can manifest as an unstable or distorted self-image, which interacts with the body image disturbances commonly seen in EDs, compounding the patient's dissatisfaction with their appearance. Primitive defense mechanisms—such as splitting, where people and situations are seen in black-and-white terms—further complicate relationships, including the therapeutic alliance, making consistent engagement in treatment more difficult.

The impulsive behaviors characteristic of BPD exacerbates the cyclical nature of self-destructive tendencies, which may include not only ED behaviors but also substance use, self-injury, and suicidal ideation. This impulsivity creates an ever-present risk of relapse or escalation, often requiring intensive therapeutic interventions and, in severe cases, inpatient or residential treatment settings. Even within structured programs, BPD traits such as an intense fear of abandonment and sensitivity to perceived rejection can lead to conflicts with staff and other patients, potentially disrupting the therapeutic environment.

Long-term outcomes for ED patients with comorbid BPD tend to be poorer due to the interplay between identity instability, impulsivity, and self-destructive behaviors. BPD contributes to an enduring pattern of emotional dysregulation, making it difficult for patients to develop and maintain coping skills that are crucial for EDs recovery. Intensive therapies, such as transference focused psychotherapy (TFP) have shown good results in BPD patients (Yeomans et al., 2015).

DBT specifically addresses emotional regulation, distress tolerance, and interpersonal effectiveness—skills that are essential in managing both BPD and ED symptoms.

Furthermore, the chronic nature of BPD necessitates a long-term, consistent, and multi-modal approach to treatment, addressing both personality disorder and ED symptoms effectively. Combining individual and group therapies allows clinicians to help patients build resilience against impulsive urges, foster a more cohesive sense of self, and reduce reliance on maladaptive behaviors. This integrated approach is essential for mitigating the heightened risks associated with BPD, enhancing emotional stability, and ultimately supporting more successful outcomes in EDs recovery.

Self-harm and eating disorders

Self-harm is prevalent among ED patients, particularly those with impulsive traits or BPD. Self-harming behaviors, which can range from superficial cuts to serious suicide attempts, have become more visible and normalized in adolescents, partly due to social media. These behaviors provide temporary relief from intense psychic pain and offer a way to express feelings of worthlessness or self-loathing. Self-harm often reflects an unconscious rejection of femininity or sexuality in ED patients, where self-punishment and negative body image are pervasive (Persano, 2022).

In ED patients, self-harm is a maladaptive strategy for processing distress and converting emotional pain into physical pain. Many patients have histories of trauma or neglect, which predisposes them to self-injury as a means of coping with unresolved emotions. For these individuals, self-harm is not necessarily linked to suicidal intent but serves to discharge emotional tension and reduce psychic pain.

Suicide and eating disorders

Suicide is a significant risk in ED patients, especially those with co-occurring BPD or depression. Adolescents are particularly vulnerable, with suicide ranking as the second leading cause of death in this age group. Patients with AN are 18 times more likely, and those with BN seven times more likely, to die by suicide compared to their peers (Smith, Zuromski, and Dodd, 2018). Suicidal and parasuicidal behaviors in ED patients often reflect unconscious attempts to regulate feelings of hopelessness, loneliness, or worthlessness. This risk is heightened in patients with BPD, who frequently rely on primitive defense mechanisms and exhibit intense emotional dysregulation.

Suicidal tendencies in ED patients are often intertwined with impulsivity and self-destructive behavior. Repeated parasuicidal behaviors, such as non-lethal overdoses or intentional self-harm, may serve as unconscious efforts to cope with internalized despair or anger. Addressing these tendencies requires a multidisciplinary approach that can simultaneously manage the EDs and its associated comorbidities.

The necessity of a multidisciplinary approach

Managing comorbidities such as impulsivity, substance abuse, depression, personality disorders, self-harm, and suicidality in ED patients requires an interdisciplinary approach. Treatment involves collaboration among psychiatrists, psychologists, nutritionists, social workers, and other specialists. This team approach allows for comprehensive assessment and intervention, addressing both the immediate symptoms and the underlying psychological and social factors contributing to EDs.

Patients with EDs and co-occurring conditions, particularly those involving impulsivity, substance abuse, personality disorders, and self-harm, face unique therapeutic challenges. These cases necessitate early detection of comorbid factors and implementation of an integrated treatment approach that incorporates both medical and psychological interventions. Through interdisciplinary collaboration, the complex needs of these patients can be addressed more effectively, supporting better outcomes and improving the quality of life for individuals struggling with EDs and associated risk behaviors.

Clinical approach and conceptualizations of eating disorders: A psychodynamic and interdisciplinary perspective

Eating disorders (EDs) are often chronic, with a significant number of patients displaying resistance to standard treatments. For approximately 20% of individuals with AN and 23% with BN, these conditions evolve into enduring eating disorders (EED), marked by a persistent course and greater resistance to intervention (Dapelo et al., 2020). These cases demand a comprehensive approach, integrating psychodynamic insights with interdisciplinary support to address the complex psychological, social, and physiological aspects inherent in EDs.

The interdisciplinary and multidisciplinary treatment model

The intricate nature of EDs necessitates a collaborative, integrative approach, incorporating perspectives from psychodynamics, psychiatry, nutrition, social work, and medicine. This integration is essential for providing holistic care, as EDs affect not only physical health but also mental well-being, interpersonal relationships, and quality of life (Persano, 2021). A shared understanding of patients' psychological landscapes enables team members to address not just symptoms but also underlying conflicts and relational dynamics.

In treating EEDs, effective models include multidisciplinary teams and centralize the role of group therapy. Psychodynamic group therapy is especially valuable in helping patients explore and express unconscious conflicts in a supportive environment, where they can witness shared struggles and gain new insights into their behavior. Additionally, day hospital programs are crucial transitional structures, enabling patients to practice therapeutic insights in their daily lives. Such programs bridge the gap between intensive inpatient care and reintegration into the community, supporting patients as they gradually regain independence (Zipfel et al., 2002); (Persano, 2021).

Psychodynamic psychotherapy and the role of medication in treatment

Psychodynamic therapy is fundamental to addressing the deeper psychological roots of EDs. This approach views symptoms as expressions of unresolved conflicts and unconscious desires, often rooted in early attachment patterns and relational dynamics. By exploring these issues within therapy, patients gain awareness of their inner worlds and learn healthier ways to cope with emotions, thus reducing the need for self-destructive behaviors. Both mentalization-based psychotherapy (MBT) and transference focused psychotherapy (TFP) have shown good results in these patients (Bateman and Fonagy, 2004); (Kernberg et al., 2008).

While psychopharmacological treatment can manage acute symptoms like depression, anxiety, or impulsivity, it serves as an adjunct rather than the core of treatment. Medication can help stabilize patients, making them more receptive to psychodynamic work. However, it is within the therapeutic space that patients are encouraged to explore and understand the roots of their behaviors. The dynamic process of transference—where patients project feelings onto the therapist—allows for real-time exploration of these unconscious patterns and offers opportunities for therapeutic breakthroughs.

Specialized therapeutic components in psychodynamic day programs

In psychodynamic-oriented day programs, therapy extends beyond symptom management to explore the deeper meanings behind behaviors, aiming to foster emotional growth and autonomy. These programs (Persano, 2021) often include the following:

- *Food and mealtime therapy*: Meals become a therapeutic opportunity where patients confront fears and anxieties around food. Psychodynamic principles allow patients to explore the symbolic meanings they assign to food, such as control, nurturing, and punishment, while working toward balanced eating within a supportive environment.
- *Family therapy and conflict resolution*: Family dynamics often play a central role in the development and perpetuation of EDs. Psychodynamic family therapy enables patients to address unresolved relational issues and improves family communication patterns that may reinforce disordered behaviors.
- *Exploration of responsible sexuality and gender identity*: Issues related to sexuality and identity frequently emerge in EDs, as patients may project body-related anxieties onto concerns about self-worth and gender. Addressing these aspects within a psychodynamic framework allows patients to explore identity issues within a safe, non-judgmental space.
- *Emotion-focused interventions*: Using psychodynamic techniques, therapists help patients explore distorted beliefs about body image and food. Patients learn to identify, process, and regulate emotions tied to self-perception, thus developing healthier coping strategies and reducing reliance on ED behaviors.

The importance of integrated medical, nutritional, and psychological care

The integration of medical, nutritional, and psychological support is essential in ED treatment, particularly in cases of severe malnutrition or electrolyte imbalance. Psychodynamically informed nutritional counseling not only provides dietary education but also examines patients' relationships with food, addressing unconscious associations between food, control, and self-worth. Medical monitoring is equally crucial to ensure physical stability and safety, allowing psychological work to proceed on a stable foundation. By providing a multidisciplinary safety net, the treatment team collectively supports the patient's journey toward self-acceptance and emotional resilience.

Patient-centered and flexible approaches psychodynamic treatment

Effective psychodynamic care requires flexibility and a patient-centered approach, adapting interventions to each patient's evolving needs, challenges, and responses. Psychodynamic therapists maintain a stance of curiosity and openness, allowing patients to direct the process and gain a sense of agency. This autonomy is reinforced by giving patients a say in their treatment plans, which enhances motivation, commitment, and the therapeutic alliance. Flexibility within psychodynamic work allows for revisiting core conflicts as patients deepen their self-understanding, fostering sustainable change.

Conclusion: The role of psychodynamic and interdisciplinary approaches in lasting recovery

An interdisciplinary psychodynamic approach is essential for addressing the complex, layered nature of EDs, where symptoms often mask deeper issues related to identity, relationships, and self-worth. The collaborative framework created by mental health professionals, medical staff, nutritionists, social workers, and family members provides a comprehensive treatment system that meets the diverse needs of individuals with EEDs.

This approach not only stabilizes physical health but also addresses the root psychological conflicts, promoting resilience and integration. By fostering social reintegration and emotional growth, psychodynamic treatment offers patients tools for a transformative journey toward lasting recovery and self-empowerment.

Bibliography

American Psychiatric Association (1994) 4th edition. *Diagnostic and Statistical Manual of Mental Disorders*. Washington DC: American Psychiatric Association.
American Psychiatric Association (2000) 4th edition TX. *Diagnostic and Statistical Manual of Mental Disorders*. Washington DC: American Psychiatric Association.

American Psychiatric Association (2013) 5th edition. *Diagnostic and Statistical Manual of Mental Disorders*. Washington DC: American Psychiatric Association.

American Psychiatric Association (2022). *Diagnostic and Statistical Manual of Mental Disorders* (5th edition, text rev.; DSM-5-TR). Washington DC: American Psychiatric Association.

Baker, J. H., Mitchell, K. S., Neale, M. C., and Kendler, K. S. (2010). Eating disorder symptomatology and substance use disorders: Prevalence and shared risk in a population based twin sample. *International Journal of Eating Disorders*, 43(7): 648–658.

Bateman, A. W. and Fonagy, P. (2004). Mentalization-based treatment of BPD. *Journal of Personality Disorders*, 18(1): 36–51.

Blatt, S. J. (2004). *Experiences of Depression: Theoretical, Clinical, and Research Perspectives*. Washington DC: American Psychological Association.

Calero-Elvira, A., Krug, I., Davis, K., Lopez, C., Fernández-Aranda, F., and Treasure, J. (2009). Meta-analysis on drugs in people with eating disorders. *European Eating Disorders Review*, 17(4): 243–259.

Cooper, P. J. and Fairburn, C. G. (1986). The depressive symptoms of bulimia nervosa. *The British Journal of Psychiatry*, 148(3): 268–274.

Cruz-Sáez, M. S., Pascual, A., Etxebarria, I., and Echeburua, E. (2013). Risk of eating disorders, consumption of addictive substances and emotional difficulties in adolescent girls. *Anales de Psicología*, 29(3): 724–733.

Dapelo, M. M., Gil, A. A., Lacalle, L., and Vogel, M. (2020). Severity and endurance in eating disorders: An exploration of a clinical sample from Chile. *Frontiers in Psychiatry*, 11: 869.

Dunn, E. C., Neighbors, C., Fossos, N., and Larimer, M. E. (2009). A cross-lagged evaluation of eating disorder symptomatology and substance-use problems. *Journal of Studies on Alcohol and Drugs*, 70(1): 106–116.

Frosch, J. (1977). The relation between acting out and disorders of impulse control. *Psychiatry*, 40(4): 295–314.

Herzog, D. B., Franko, D. L., Dorer, D. J., Keel, P. K., Jackson, S., and Manzo, M. P. (2006). Drug abuse in women with eating disorders. *International Journal of Eating Disorders*, 39(5): 364–368.

Inagaki, T., Yamamoto, M., Tsubouchi, K., Miyaoka, T., Uegaki, J., Maeda, T., … and Kato, Y. (2003). Echocardiographic investigation of pericardial effusion in a case of anorexia nervosa. *International Journal of Eating Disorders*, 33(3): 364–366.

Isner, J. M., Roberts, W. C., Heymsfield, S. B., and Yager, J. (1985). Anorexia nervosa and sudden death. *Annals of Internal Medicine*, 102(1): 49–52.

Kernberg, O. (2004). A Technical approach to eating disorders in patients with Borderline Personality Organization. In *Aggressivity, Narcissism, and Self-destructiveness in the Psychotherapeutic Relationship: New Developments in the Psychopathology and Psychotherapy of Severe Personality Disorders*. New Haven, CT and London: Yale University Press, 205–219.

Kernberg, O. F., Yeomans, F. E., Clarkin, J. F., and Levy, K. N. (2008). Transference focused psychotherapy: Overview and update. *The International Journal of Psychoanalysis*, 89(3): 601–620.

Krug, I., Puccio, F., Potingale, J., and Dang, A. B. (2023). A narrative review on the dual pathway model of bulimic pathology. In V. B. Patel and V. R. Preedy (eds.) *Eating Disorders*. Cham: Springer, 887–922.

Moeller, F. G., Barratt, E. S., Dougherty, D. M., Schmitz, J. M., and Swann, A. C. (2001). Psychiatric aspects of impulsivity. *American Journal of Psychiatry*, 158(11), 1783–1793.

Neumärker, K. J. (1997). Mortality and sudden death in anorexia nervosa. *International Journal of Eating Disorders*, 21(3), 205–212.

Nøkleby, H. (2012). Comorbid drug use disorders and eating disorders—a review of prevalence studies. *Nordic Studies on Alcohol and Drugs*, 29(3), 303–314.

Oka, Y., Ito, T., Sekine, I., Sada, T., Okabe, F., Naito, A., ... and Nomura, S. (1984). Mitral valve prolapse in patients with anorexia nervosa. *Journal of Cardiography*, 14(3), 483–491.

Persano, H. L. (2021). Day hospital intensive care for patients with eating disorders. In H. Schwartz (ed.) *Applying Psychoanalysis in Medical Care*. Abingdon, Oxon: Routledge, 71–90.

Persano, H. L. (2022). Self-harm. *The International Journal of Psychoanalysis*, 103(6): 1089–1103.

Rey, C., Alvin, P., Pariente, D., and Courtecuisse, V. (1994). Pneumomediastinum in a young girl with anorexia nervosa. *Archives de Pédiatrie: Organe Officiel de la Societe Francaise de Pediatrie*, 1(7): 652–654.

Rosval, L., Steiger, H., Bruce, K., Israël, M., Richardson, J., and Aubut, M. (2006). Impulsivity in women with eating disorders: Problem of response inhibition, planning, or attention? *International Journal of Eating Disorders*, 39(7): 590–593.

Smith, A. R., Zuromski, K. L., and Dodd, D. R. (2018). Eating disorders and suicidality: What we know, what we don't know, and suggestions for future research. *Current Opinion in Psychology*, 22: 63–67.

Stice, E., Shaw, H., and Nemeroff, C. (1998). Dual pathway model of bulimia nervosa: Longitudinal support for dietary restraint and affect-regulation mechanisms. *Journal of Social and Clinical Psychology*, 17(2): 129–149.

Stice, E. and Bearman, S. K. (2001). Body-image and eating disturbances prospectively predict increases in depressive symptoms in adolescent girls: A growth curve analysis. *Developmental Psychology*, 37(5): 597–607.

Stice, E., Burton, E. M., and Shaw, H. (2004). Prospective relations between bulimic pathology, depression, and substance abuse: Unpacking comorbidity in adolescent girls. *Journal of Consulting and Clinical Psychology*, 72(1): 62–71.

Sullivan, P. F. (1995). Mortality in anorexia nervosa. *The American Journal of Psychiatry*, 152(7), 1073–1074.

World Health Organization (2019). *International classification of diseases for mortality and morbidity statistics* (11th ed.). Geneva: World Health Organization. https://icd.who.int/

Yeomans, F. E., Clarkin, J. F., and Kernberg, O. F. (2015). *Transference-focused Psychotherapy for Borderline Personality Disorder: A Clinical Guide*. Washington DC: American Psychiatric Publishing.

Zipfel, S., Reas, D. L., Thornton, C., Olmsted, M. P., Williamson, D. A., Gerlinghoff, M., ... and Beumont, P. J. (2002). Day hospitalization programs for eating disorders: A systematic review of the literature . *International Journal of Eating Disorders*, 31(2): 105–117.

4 Psychoanalytic theory and eating disorders

Introduction to psychoanalytic concepts and their relevance to eating disorders

Eating disorders represent a range of manifestations that share specific characteristics, allowing them to be viewed as a trans-structural condition within psychoanalytic psychopathology. With their predominantly narcissistic nature, these disorders are closely linked to pathological narcissism, particularly through the internal conflict between the "unconscious body image" and the actual body. This conflict generates a pathological relationship with food and body weight, embodying deeper psychoanalytic conflicts involving sexuality, ideals, identity, and early emotional bonds.

Philippe Jeammet (1984) posits that anorexia nervosa (AN) reflects not only a physical symptom but also an "anorexia" of mental investments, characterized by a lack of verbal and psychic transformation, often expressed through bodily actions. Similarly, Gianna Williams (2000) describes the psychic functioning of individuals with eating disorders as primitive. In AN, this appears as a "no-entry" mechanism that closes off mental processing, symbolizing an early, dominant object relationship. Conversely, bulimia nervosa (BN) manifests as a porous psychic apparatus, wherein individuals compulsively incorporate experiences, later expelling them through purging, mirroring cycles of consumption and rejection at the psychic level.

Sexuality, control, and the body in eating disorders

Freud proposed that unconscious conflicts around sexuality often underlie psychoneuroses, a theory that finds strong resonance in eating disorders (EDs). In these disorders, the relationship with food transforms into a symbolic and often sexualized experience, encapsulating both desire and prohibition. For individuals with AN, the restriction of food symbolizes an unconscious struggle with femininity and sexuality, reflecting a complex internal dialogue about control over one's body. This becomes significant given that around 90% of individuals with AN are female, a group often

DOI: 10.4324/9781032724997-4

socialized with conflicting ideals of desirability and objectification. Many young girls feel a natural desire to transition into womanhood, yet they simultaneously harbor fears around this passage, leading to an unconscious drive to reject bodily changes associated with femininity.

In BN, the relationship with sexuality is ambivalent and conflicted, marked by a compulsive cycle of indulgence followed by rejection. This dynamic mirrors the individual's conflicted relationship with sexuality itself, where intense cravings are succeeded by guilt and shame. Just as individuals may binge on food only to purge it later, they may experience similar cycles with desires related to sexuality, oscillating between indulgence and rejection. Thus, eating disorders like AN and BN serve as psychodynamic expressions of repressed desires and fears surrounding sexuality, where food becomes a substitute for these unresolved unconscious conflicts.

Narcissism and the pursuit of an idealized self-image

Narcissism in EDs is deeply tied to the relentless pursuit of an idealized self-image, pulling individuals into an intense fixation on their appearance and self-worth as defined by unrealistic standards. This fixation is not simply about vanity but rather involves a distorted self-image driven by profound psychological needs, often rooted in unmet developmental needs and early relational experiences. The obsessive focus on achieving an ideal body or appearance places individuals in a self-destructive cycle of perpetual striving and inevitable failure, as the standards they set for themselves are unattainable and ever shifting. In this way, narcissism in EDs is sustained by a combination of internalized societal ideals and the influence of the death instinct, wherein the individual's own self-destructiveness is masked by the pursuit of perfection.

Clinically, this narcissistic drive manifests as a profound devotion to unreachable ideals, particularly in individuals who equate their self-worth with the attainment of exaggerated beauty standards. For those with EDs, beauty and thinness become symbols of an idealized self, where maintaining rigid control over one's body represents a means of self-validation. However, these unattainable standards result in a constant sense of inadequacy and personal failure, which exacerbates depression, anxiety, and narcissistic wounds. Failures to reach these ideals reopen wounds of self-worth, driving individuals to extremes in their physical and emotional efforts to embody these images, even at the risk of physical health and psychological stability. This continual striving leads to fragile, often temporary validation that quickly collapses under the weight of further self-criticism and unattainable expectations.

As Janine Chasseguet-Smirgel (1976) describes in her concept of "pathologies of ideality", EDs can emerge from an excessive attachment to ideals that disrupt the core structure of the personality. This attachment fractures the individual's sense of self, making them vulnerable to deep psychological suffering and even life-threatening behaviors. For example, the pursuit of thinness may initially begin as a socially or personally motivated goal but quickly evolves into a rigid, tyrannical standard, where body size becomes the defining measure of self-worth. In this "pathology of ideality", the ideal-self overshadows the individual's true self, leading to a disintegration of the authentic self and replacing it with a fragmented and fragile identity focused solely on appearance.

This narcissistic fixation also involves a paradoxical form of self-centeredness: individuals may obsess over their appearance and how they are perceived by others, yet this focus often excludes genuine self-care, compassion, or personal well-being. Instead, the intense focus on meeting idealized beauty standards causes individuals to neglect or even punish their own bodies in pursuit of this distorted ideal. The concept of the death instinct, introduced by Freud, is relevant here, as it suggests a self-destructive force within that overrides the instinct to preserve one's health or life. For some with EDs, this manifests as a willingness to endure starvation, physical harm, or dangerous behaviors to sustain an image that ultimately harms them.

This narcissistic drive toward an idealized image is further compounded by the impact of social and cultural influences, where ideals of beauty, success, and self-worth are frequently defined by appearance. Social media, advertising, and cultural representations of beauty reinforce and magnify this pressure, embedding these ideals into the psyche of vulnerable individuals. The constant exposure to perfected images and unrealistic standards leaves individuals feeling inadequate, even as they intensify their efforts to meet these standards. This cultural reinforcement of narcissistic ideals strengthens the pathology, deepening the individual's attachment to an ideal self that is impossible to achieve.

In the broader context of treatment, understanding the narcissistic underpinnings of EDs is crucial, as it allows for a deeper exploration of the individual's need for validation and their relationship with self-worth. Addressing the narcissistic core of these disorders requires therapeutic approaches that can disrupt the cycle of unattainable ideals and cultivate a more compassionate, authentic sense of self. Treatment approaches such as psychodynamic therapy aim to help patients understand and challenge the internalized ideals and distorted self-image, fostering an awareness that self-worth does not depend on physical appearance. In cases where narcissistic features are prominent, interventions focusing on building self-esteem, emotional resilience, and healthy relational boundaries can be essential in weakening the grip of the idealized self-image and reducing self-destructive behaviors

Body image and the imaginary dimension

The concept of body image, developed extensively by Paul Schilder (1950), encompasses the mental representation of the body, integrating sensory, kinesthetic, and tactile experiences into a unified "body schema". This schema is dynamic, continually reconstructed through interactions with the external world, extending beyond the physical body to include elements like voice, breath, and fluids.

Recent advances in neuroscience have provided valuable insights into the relationship between interoception—our awareness of internal bodily states—and AN. This field examines interoceptive accuracy (the objective ability to detect internal signals), sensitivity (the subjective awareness of these signals), and metacognitive insight (the capacity to assess one's accuracy in perceiving these signals). Research has shown that disruptions in these areas are intricately linked to AN, influencing how individuals perceive and experience their bodies. For instance, Fotopoulou (2015) states that interoceptive impairments in anorexia nervosa (AN) contribute to altered body image perception, making it difficult for individuals to integrate their physical self with their mental representation of the body.

Interoception plays a significant role in both the pathology and recovery of AN, particularly in the context of emotional regulation. During recovery, the ability to regulate emotions becomes critical in modulating interoceptive sensitivity. Research by Crucianelli et al. (2016, 2021) underscores that improvements in emotional regulation during this phase enhance patients' capacity to accurately process internal bodily signals. This improved interoceptive awareness helps bridge the gap between bodily sensations and body image, which is often profoundly distorted in individuals with AN.

By fostering a more accurate connection between internal signals and self-perception, these improvements contribute to the development of a more cohesive and integrated sense of self, addressing a key psychological deficit in AN. This connection not only supports recovery but also lays the foundation for a healthier relationship with one's body and emotional experiences.

In addition, research by Saramandi et al. (2022) indicates that individuals with AN tend to hold more pessimistic thoughts not only about their body size but also about their emotional bodies—how they feel about themselves physically and emotionally. This distortion is further exacerbated by metacognitive disturbances, which impair patients' ability to evaluate the accuracy of their body perceptions. Such disruptions suggest that for those with AN, not only are the internal signals skewed, but their confidence in interpreting these signals is undermined, further complicating the recovery process.

Taken together, these findings underscore the importance of addressing both interoceptive and emotional dysregulation in AN treatment. Enhancing interoceptive awareness and metacognitive insight could be key in helping individuals achieve a more accurate and integrated sense of self, supporting a more sustainable recovery process.

Social construction of body image

Body image is not solely an internal construct; it is profoundly shaped by social dynamics, cultural standards, and ideals of beauty. Social interactions, norms, and aesthetic expectations continually shape how individuals perceive their bodies, particularly impacting those with EDs. These societal ideals often transform into rigid, dictatorial standards, pressuring individuals—especially young girls—to embody an idealized version of beauty, sometimes referred to as the "ideal future woman". This external influence fosters a strong internalized desire to achieve an ideal that is culturally defined and often unattainable.

In the psychoanalytic context, this dynamic is reflected in the "imaginary dimension" of body image, where the Ideal of the Ego serves as an aspirational model that motivates individuals to align their self-concept with societal ideals (Hanly, 1983). For some, however, this Ideal of the Ego distorts into an obsessive pursuit of a version of themselves that is beyond reach. In severe cases of AN, this relentless striving has been described as an "aesthetic of horror", where the drive for perfection leads to self-destruction rather than self-fulfillment. These distorted ideals leaves individuals caught in a cycle of perpetual inadequacy and extreme measures to meet an unrealistic standard of beauty, reinforcing a harmful body image perception that can contribute to the onset or maintenance of EDs.

Body image, emotional regulation, and eating disorders

For individuals with EDs, body image and appearance become central sources of self-worth and gratification, often tied to the Ideal of the Ego. This attachment leads to pathological behaviors, driven by an internalized need to align with an idealized self-concept. The social opinions and representations of others play a significant role in shaping this drive, embedding cycles of temporary gratification followed by inevitable disappointment. In AN, for example, achieving control over bodily desires aligns with the Ideal of the Ego, fostering a sense of omnipotence and increasing resistance to recovery. Conversely, in BN, cycles of indulgence and restraint become cycles of humiliation and disappointment, where giving in to instinctual needs is followed by control rituals that ultimately fail, leaving the individual feeling empty and defeated.

In both AN and BN, these disorders reflect an ethical conflict with the Ideal of the Ego. In AN, the pursuit of the ideal leads to somatic disorganization, with severe physical effects from striving toward an impossible image. For those with BN, failures to achieve the self-ideal result in life-threatening behaviors and intense emotional distress. In both cases, the unattainable standard creates an endless loop of striving, falling short, and self-punishment, exacerbating emotional instability and deepening the individual's identification with the disorder.

Emotional dysregulation in eating disorders

Emotion regulation difficulties are central to the experiences of those with EDs. Philippe Jeammet (1984) suggests that AN reflects a fundamental detachment from object relations, impairing emotional processing and often leading to alexithymia, or a difficulty in recognizing and articulating emotions. For individuals with AN, this detachment acts as both a defensive mechanism and a result of inadequate "verbal nurturing" in early childhood, making it challenging to recognize or express emotions. This inability to process emotions contributes to a reliance on controlling food intake as a substitute for emotional regulation.

In contrast, those with BN frequently "act out" their emotions, engaging in cycles of binging and purging as a maladaptive strategy for managing difficult feelings. Disordered eating behaviors provide temporary relief from emotional turmoil but lead to subsequent guilt, shame, and despair, perpetuating a cycle of relief followed by regret (MacDonald et al., 2023). This pattern of emotional dysregulation reinforces the pathological behaviors associated with EDs, making recovery even more challenging without addressing underlying emotional needs.

Interplay between self-perception, social influence, and emotional needs

In sum, EDs reveal a complex interplay between internalized ideals, socially constructed body image, and challenges in emotional regulation. These disorders are not simply about achieving thinness or beauty; they reflect a fractured sense of self-worth, rigid ideals, and an intense struggle for validation and control. For individuals with EDs, the pursuit of an ideal body image becomes a psychological and emotional battleground, often obscuring or overriding their own needs and well-being.

Understanding body image within this multifaceted framework underscores the need for comprehensive treatment approaches that address psychological, social, and emotional dimensions simultaneously. Effective interventions must not only help individuals build a healthier body image but also work to dismantle internalized ideals, improve emotional regulation, and encourage self-compassion. By addressing these interconnected factors, treatment can help break the self-destructive cycles that characterize EDs, supporting individuals in reclaiming their self-worth and sense of identity outside of appearance-based standards.

Freudian perspective: Psychosexual development

Freud's early writings on hysteria and its connection to eating disorders

The relationship between hysteria and EDs was noted early in psychoanalytic literature. In his studies at the end of the 19th century, Freud observed that symptoms such as anorexia and vomiting could emerge as hysterical expressions. His initial theories on symptom formation emphasized that these physical manifestations were linked to unresolved emotional or traumatic events. Freud described cases where patients exhibited eating-related symptoms in response to emotional distress, noting how "anorexia and vomiting" could appear as common hysterical symptoms (Freud, 1893, p. 32).

For example, Freud described the case of Frau Emmy von N., whose vomiting began after reading a humiliating letter just before a meal. This reaction, as Freud observed, reflected a primitive, disgust-driven response rooted in her underlying emotional turmoil, rather than being merely a hysterical symptom (Breuer and Freud, 1893a). This case exemplifies Freud's view that somatic symptoms often stem from past experiences, functioning as symbolic expressions of repressed emotions.

In some cases, Freud noted that disgust for food was tied to unconscious processes. He suggested that aversion could transfer from a disliked individual sharing a meal to the food itself, a process Freud described as "transference" (Freud, 1893, p. 32). This mechanism illustrates two key aspects of symptom formation in hysteria: the unconscious shift of emotion from one source to another and the compromise created by the symptom, allowing the individual to direct their aversion at food rather than confronting the disliked person directly.

Psychosexual development and trauma's impact on eating behaviors

Freud's observations in *"The Aetiology of Hysteria"* (1896) explored how traumatic childhood events—often with a sexual dimension—could lead to hysterical symptoms later in life, sometimes coexisting with other life experiences. He posited that ED-related symptoms often stemmed from early traumas, particularly of a sexual nature. Freud and Breuer identified a phenomenon they called "retention hysteria", which arose when emotional tension could not be released, causing the emotional energy to redirect into the body, manifesting as physical symptoms. In one case, Freud described a 12-year-old boy who developed anorexia and vomiting following an incident of sexual trauma. His symptoms disappeared after he disclosed the traumatic experience, illustrating how the release of repressed emotions could alleviate physical symptoms (Breuer and Freud, 1893b, pp. 211–212).

Freud and Breuer's concept of overdetermination also plays a role in ED symptoms. They suggested that hysterical symptoms often arise from multiple, overlapping factors, including personality traits, traumatic experiences, and intense emotions. For example, in cases where patients experienced both early traumatic incidents and repeated exposure to distressing experiences, such as fear or disgust, their symptoms (like anorexia or vomiting) reflected a consolidation of these factors. The concept of overdetermination highlights how various life events can contribute to the formation of a single affective response, with the individual often only consciously remembering the most recent trigger.

Hysteria and conversion symptoms in eating disorders

Freud's work with hysterical patients led to the development of "hypnoid hysteria", a condition where psychic trauma disrupts consciousness, producing symptoms that appear as dissociated states. In the case of Katharina, a young girl who developed symptoms of vomiting after witnessing her father's inappropriate sexual behavior, Freud explored her trauma using free association. This method revealed deeper layers of parental abuse and suppressed emotions, which later manifested as physical symptoms. Katharina's case highlights how trauma, particularly involving sexual dynamics, can disrupt normal psychological development, leading to psychosomatic symptoms such as disordered eating (Breuer and Freud, 1893c).

This early work remains relevant today, as studies on EDs show a frequent association with childhood trauma, including sexual abuse, neglect, and emotional maltreatment. For individuals with EDs, these traumatic experiences can manifest in maladaptive coping mechanisms, such as restrictive eating or purging, as means to regain control, alleviate anxiety, or numb emotional pain. Freud's insights on the lasting impact of childhood sexual abuse continue to inform our understanding of EDs, emphasizing the importance of exploring these early experiences to address both psychological and physical symptoms.

Differentiating hysteria from trauma-related psychopathologies in EDs

In the clinical setting, it is essential to differentiate between symptoms arising from hysteria and those rooted in trauma-related psychopathologies. Freud's concept of hysteria involved repressed emotions or memories that surface through somatic symptoms, symbolizing unresolved psychological conflicts. Trauma-related psychopathologies, however, are direct consequences of traumatic experiences and can involve symptoms like hyperarousal, dissociation, intrusive memories, and distorted self-image. This distinction is crucial, as trauma-related symptoms often require therapeutic approaches that focus on trauma resolution, emotional regulation, and establishing a sense of safety.

For individuals with EDs who have a history of trauma, symptoms such as dissociation, body image distortion, and emotional numbing may overlap with features traditionally associated with hysteria, complicating diagnosis. These patients might exhibit somatic symptoms deeply rooted in trauma, yet if these symptoms are misinterpreted as purely hysterical or unrelated to trauma, therapeutic approaches may miss the underlying issue, risking continued psychological distress.

Incorporating Freud's foundational understanding of childhood trauma alongside modern trauma theory enhances clinicians' ability to navigate complex patient presentations. By recognizing how early abuse or neglect shapes the psyche and manifests in EDs, clinicians can adopt a holistic view of the patient. This approach fosters empathy, allowing clinicians to appreciate how traumatic experiences influence body image, self-worth, and interpersonal relationships, often creating challenges around boundaries, trust, and self-acceptance.

Psychic trauma and the sexualization of the digestive tract in EDs

Freud's concept of psychic trauma also highlights the digestive tract's early sexualization in relational interactions. As a primary area of symbolic exchange, the digestive system becomes central in expressing conflicts when trauma occurs. Libidinal interest in the digestive tract reflects its role in early relationships, making it a site where disruptions can lead to various psychopathologies. Many individuals with EDs report histories of childhood trauma, with disordered eating to manage the associated pain, fear, or shame. In some cases, restrictive eating serves to desexualize the self, protecting individuals from unwanted attention or sexual advances.

In the psychoanalytic understanding of hysteria, sexuality, and conversion symptoms, distressing emotions often "convert" into physical symptoms. Joyce McDougall illustrated this concept with a patient who said, "I wanted to vomit because I felt disgusting myself" (McDougall, 2013). Here, vomiting symbolized the patient's internal disgust, demonstrating how the body becomes a symbolic space for expressing unresolved inner conflicts.

Body image, sexuality, and self-worth in EDs

Body image distortion significantly impacts individuals' sense of sexual attractiveness and self-worth. Many people with EDs experience feelings of unattractiveness or shame regarding their bodies, leading to diminished sexual desire or avoidance of intimacy. For some, controlling food intake becomes intertwined with controlling sexuality, offering a way to cope with feelings of inadequacy or anxiety around intimacy. The body, in this context, serves as a battleground for conflicting needs for control, validation, and self-protection.

In summary, Freud's early observations on hysteria, trauma, and sexuality provide a foundational understanding of the complex psychological underpinnings of EDs (Freud, 1893). The relationship between EDs and sexuality involves not only body image and trauma, but also deeper conflicts related to sexual identity, cultural pressures, and symbolic roles of the body. By differentiating between hysterical and trauma-related symptoms and integrating trauma-informed approaches, clinicians can more effectively address the psychological, social, and emotional dimensions driving these disorders, ultimately fostering a more comprehensive and compassionate treatment process.

Object relations theory and its application to eating disorders

From birth, the human body begins to form perceptions of itself in relation to others. These early relationships are shaped by attractions to and connections with other bodies, which are experienced as either satisfying or painful. Through interactions with primary caregivers, the body develops an "erotic quality", gaining meaning through its experiences of contact, comfort, and care (Persano, 2019). These experiences are foundational, as they begin to shape the body's sense of itself and its role in relational exchanges.

During infancy, sensations from touch, holding, and caressing by caregivers imprint an erogenous dimension onto the body, forming initial layers of self-representation. This erogeneity flows through different parts of the body, particularly the areas Freud (1905) termed "erogenous zones", which gain significance at various developmental stages. Freud noted that bodily libidinization is guided rather than random, with specific areas receiving focused attention and care. For example, drawing on Linder's 1879 study on children's sucking habits, Freud observed that the infant's mouth becomes a focal point, soothing the child and often helping them fall asleep (Abraham, 1916). Nourishment and the pleasure of contact with the caregiver, especially during breastfeeding and skin-to-skin moments, intertwine, leading the infant to seek and mentally replay these experiences of comfort. When these experiences are negative or invasive, they evoke frustration and pain, which become embedded in the body's memory.

Thus, erogenous zones are not merely areas of heightened physical sensitivity; they are spaces of emotional and relational exchange. Ronald Fairbairn (1946) suggested that libido seeks more than just the release of tension; it seeks objects of attachment, highlighting the body's role as an instrument of relational connection. Extending this idea, we could say that the individual searches for the specific object that can offer the sought-after satisfaction (Persano, 2019). Additionally, the body's erogenous experiences are not limited to physical touch—they can be stimulated by sound, language, and gaze. Houzel (1990) further elaborates on this concept with his notion of the "psychic envelope", which refers to a sense of belonging to certain spaces and the fluidity of bodily boundaries between oneself and others.

Early relational disturbances and their impact on feeding and emotional regulation

Disruptions in early relational experiences profoundly impact both mother and child. For the mother, the child may become an object of desire, a presence within her emotional landscape that fulfills a part of her psychic needs. For the infant, however, the mother serves as a containing object, essential for developing a coherent sense of self. The infant clings to the mother for psychic development, and early object losses or failures in caregiving can result in internalized aggression that disrupts the child's narcissistic investment. This internalized aggression, as André Green (1980) describes, leads to "essential depression" or "dead mother syndrome", where the child experiences a pervasive absence of a structured presence, creating a chronic deficiency in emotional regulation.

Feeding, as an interaction embedded in culture, requires the mother to adapt to her child's unique needs. Without this individualized care, the mother may rely on ancestral or cultural caregiving patterns, which are applied mechanically without sensitivity to the child's specific desires. Such stereotyped caregiving disrupts emotional regulation, which often surfaces through the feeding process. The infant may respond defensively, rejecting food altogether—a pattern Williams (1997) termed the defensive "no-entry" style, often seen in restrictive AN. Conversely, in BN, the infant may initially accept food only to later reject it, suggesting a porous interaction with food intake and expulsion, where boundaries are less defined.

Insecure attachments and self-fragility in eating disorders

Intense and often volatile interpersonal relationships in individuals with EDs frequently expose deep-seated challenges in maintaining a stable, internalized image of attachment figures. These individuals may struggle with forming a reliable internal sense of others, which can lead to a continual need to recreate attachment bonds externally. As Jeammet (1992) posits, bulimic behaviors often serve as attempts to forge external attachment connections to achieve internal stability, reflecting a fundamental drive for relational security and the internal unrest that arises in its absence. A similar dynamic appears in those with AN, where a pervasive fear of losing control over-eating symbolizes a fear of engulfment, rooted in early relational insecurities and unmet attachment needs. This dread of overwhelming emotions mirrors the vulnerability associated with insecure attachment.

The ability to mentalize—understanding and interpreting one's own and others' mental states—develops within nurturing, secure relationships, where caregivers provide essential emotional mirroring and recognition (Fonagy et al., 2004). Such a relational environment fosters intersubjectivity, laying the foundation for infants to develop emotional self-regulation and a stable sense of self (Persano, 2022). When these early bonds are disrupted, however, the consequences extend beyond mere neglect. They may expose the child to passive aggression, which becomes internalized through identification with the aggressor. This process establishes a foundation for self-directed aggression, as the child begins to treat themselves with the same criticism and rejection, they experienced from early attachment figures (Kernberg, 1992). Over time, this internalized aggression may manifest as self-criticism and disordered eating behaviors, signaling unresolved attachment-related insecurities and a fragile sense of self-regulation.

Disordered eating behaviors are frequently responses to insecure attachment styles and efforts to manage self-fragility. Those with insecure attachments may struggle with emotional regulation and self-perception, adopting maladaptive coping mechanisms, such as disordered eating, to assert control over their inner experiences. Research underscores that insecure attachment styles are disproportionately common among individuals with eating disorders. Studies indicate that those with eating disorders exhibit higher levels of attachment insecurity and disorganized mental states than controls. Lower reflective functioning is associated with AN, and attachment anxiety correlates with eating disorder severity, potentially mediated by perfectionism and affect regulation strategies (Tasca and Balfour, 2014).

The link between attachment insecurity and EDs is further clarified through the role of emotional dysregulation. Individuals with insecure attachments often face difficulties in managing their emotions, leading them to employ disordered eating as a coping strategy. For example, those with anxious attachment might binge eat to soothe feelings of abandonment, whereas individuals with avoidant attachment may restrict food intake to retain a sense of control (Tasca et al., 2009).

Moreover, mentalization is often impaired in individuals with insecure attachments. This deficit can foster a fragile sense of self, leaving individuals struggling to interpret and regulate their emotions effectively. Consequently, disordered eating behaviors can arise as attempts to manage this internal instability.

In summary, disordered eating behaviors can be understood as expressions of insecure attachment and efforts to manage a fragile sense of self. Addressing attachment-related issues and fostering emotional regulation skills are essential components of effective treatment and recovery for individuals with eating disorders.

Psychic pain and self-directed aggression in eating disorders

Psychic pain, or profound suffering, is frequently rooted in traumatic childhood experiences where the infant's sense of self becomes dominated by aggression rather than loving or erotic energy. This self-directed aggression, as Persano notes, often serves as a defense against painful memories, especially those tied to unrepresentable emotional states. These states frequently manifest in repetitive actions, such as restrictive eating or purging, that symbolize a need to purge the self of painful feelings (Persano, 2022).

Kernberg (2004) describes this self-directed aggression as a relentless, sadistic assault on the body, symbolizing four main dynamics. First, it attacks the pleasure of eating, which represents the "good object" that supports survival and body enjoyment. This aggression reflects early frustrations and unmet needs in the mother-infant relationship. Second, it represents a hatred of the body as an extension of hatred toward the mother, symbolizing difficulties in the separation-individuation process. Third, it manifests as an assault on femininity, often emerging in the context of gendered expectations and conflicts around sexual identity. Lastly, in BN, binge eating denies dependency or expresses rage at real or imagined abandonment. In AN, struggles with the mother reflect a complex mix of intrapsychic conflict and maternal invasiveness, where the mother views the child as an extension of herself (Kernberg, 2004, pp. 212–214). Bion (1959) further observes that self-directed attacks may extend to cognitive and perceptual functions, attacking the capacity for thought as a form of aggression against relational bonds and mental coherence.

Early object relations and narcissistic vulnerabilities

Object relations can be marked by early interactions with a mother who seems perpetually dissatisfied, projecting messages like, "I cannot be enchanted by you, for others are more beautiful than you". For daughters, instead of feeling cherished, they internalize a sense of inadequacy and strive desperately to please, yet ultimately experience a deep sense of failure. By adolescence, these early relational breakdowns may manifest as damaged self-image and self-worth.

The tale of *Snow White* poignantly illustrates themes of self-worth and identity, depicting a young girl subjected to envious attacks from a "bad mother" figure—the witch—whose obsession with her own reflection drives the narrative. The witch's mirror continually reminds her that someone else, "Snow White", is "more beautiful", fueling her jealousy and resentment. In her envy, the witch seeks to eliminate Snow White, ultimately tempting her with poisoned food.

This story serves as a powerful metaphor for a fractured mother-child relationship, where the critical process of affective mirroring is disrupted. Such disruptions hinder the development of a cohesive sense of self-worth and stable identity in the child. The poisoned food, central to the witch's scheme, can also be interpreted symbolically as the transmission of negativity and emotional toxicity in the feeding relationship, further destabilizing the child's psychological development (Persano, 2005).

In this context, *Snow White* transcends its fairy tale origins to reflect deeper psychological dynamics, highlighting how disturbances in early relational experiences can shape self-perception and emotional well-being.

The "clinic of the gaze" and the mirror as mother

The theme of mirroring plays a crucial role in understanding the "clinic of the gaze", as explored by psychoanalysts. Paulina Kernberg (1984, 1987) observed that the mirror reflects not only the child's image but also the mother's projected view, with the child relating to this reflection as an equivalent object. For patients fixated on their mirror image, seeking validation often leads to disappointment, as they encounter a displeasing or distorted reflection. Rather than providing reassurance, the mirror suggests an unachievable standard, reinforcing the belief that they can never see themselves as beautiful. This pursuit of an idealized reflection alienates them from their bodies, reducing their self-image to a fragmented visual rather than a whole self. Resentment, initially directed at the distorted image, often turns inward, manifesting as self-hatred, which was initially directed outward but is internalized to protect others from their anger. In modern society, this "mirror" has expanded to include idealized media images, which perpetuate the belief that others are inherently more attractive.

Object relations theory further sheds light on the emotional and psychological underpinnings of EDs, revealing how early relational patterns, self-worth, and the need for validation converge in these conditions. Early bodily experiences of satisfaction or frustration shape the psyche, with the mother serving as an object of desire or disappointment. These foundational relational dynamics establish perceptions of self and others, which, when dysfunctional, contribute to a distorted self-image. By examining how attachment, aggression, and validation intersect in the psyche, clinicians can address the symbolic and relational dimensions of eating disorders, fostering empathy and effective therapeutic intervention.

Philosophical perspectives on the "gaze" resonate with these psychoanalytic insights. Sartre (1943) introduced the concept of the "lived body-for-others", emphasizing that our bodies are not merely personal experiences (body-subject) or objects of our observation (body-object); they are also entities that exist in the eyes of others, to be seen and judged. This awareness of being seen is both a primary human experience and a compensatory means of self-perception through the gaze of others (Stanghellini and Mancini, 2020).

For most individuals, identity forms through balancing their first-person experience of the body with an awareness of how they appear to others. However, in individuals with eating disorders, this integration often breaks down. They may struggle to inhabit their bodies from a first-person perspective, relying instead on external validation to connect to their bodily sense. Consequently, they experience their body primarily as an object viewed by others, which can deepen their detachment from a cohesive self-experience.

The role of Ego functioning in eating disorders and identity in eating disorder patients

The Ego is a complex mental structure central to managing drives and instincts in relation to reality. It enables reality testing, allowing individuals to distinguish between internal experiences—such as fantasies, dreams, and thoughts—and external reality. The Ego also provides a foundation for defense mechanisms and coping strategies, helping individuals process and respond to psychological stressors.

Ego functioning is shaped from early life through interactions with caregivers and external realities, forming lasting traces in both brain and mind that influence perception, behavior, and emotional regulation. These experiences create the foundation of self-concept and interpersonal dynamics, impacting how individuals relate to themselves and others.

According to Freud's structural model, the Ego functions as a mediator, constantly balancing the instinctual drives of the Id and the moral imperatives of the Superego (Freud, 1923). This dynamic is further complicated by the *Ideal of the Ego*, a concept introduced by later theorists (Abadi, 1983; Hanly, 1983; Winograd, 1983; Yampey, 1983). The *Ideal of the Ego* represents an internalized standard of perfection that individuals strive to achieve, serving as a benchmark against which they continuously evaluate themselves.

In addition to mediating these internal forces, the Ego also plays a critical role in regulating access to consciousness. During sleep, however, this regulatory function is temporarily relaxed, allowing unconscious material to emerge in dreams. Similarly, in dissociative processes, unconscious content can manifest indirectly, often revealing itself through symptoms. These symptoms serve as symbolic expressions of repressed conflicts, offering a glimpse into the unconscious dynamics that shape behavior and self-perception.

By navigating the tensions between the Id, Superego, and the aspirational demands of the *Ideal of the Ego*, the Ego plays a central role in maintaining psychological equilibrium, while also revealing the profound interplay between conscious and unconscious processes.

Ego functioning in eating disorders

In eating disorder (ED) patients, the functioning of the Ego varies considerably depending on their level of personality organization, influencing how symptoms manifest and progress. EDs are considered *transnosographic*, meaning they can span multiple structural diagnoses and levels of personality organization.

When ED symptoms are grounded in a neurotic level of organization, the individual generally maintains intact reality testing, distinguishing between internal experiences and external reality. In these cases, higher-level defense mechanisms such as repression are commonly used. Repression and its derivatives act to keep unacceptable desires and impulses from reaching conscious awareness. For example, individuals with hysterical traits may use dissociation, momentarily separating themselves from distressing emotions, while those with obsessive-compulsive tendencies might use reaction formation, converting unacceptable feelings into their opposites, thus masking underlying anxiety with compulsive behaviors.

In more severe or enduring eating disorders (EEDs) often associated with personality disorders, particularly narcissistic and BPD, Ego functioning is typically more impaired. In these cases, Ego functioning is often anchored in an archaic or early level of mental organization, resulting in less stable boundaries between self and others. This leads to the use of more primitive, less adaptive defense mechanisms. Narcissistic defenses—such as omnipotence, idealization, and devaluation—become prominent in the psychological structure of the individual, impacting self-perception, body image, and relationships with others. For instance, idealization may drive individuals to hold themselves to unrealistically high standards, while devaluation fosters feelings of inadequacy or self-loathing, often manifesting in extreme control over food and body weight.

In cases where EDs are linked to a BPO, Ego functioning is even more unstable, and primitive defenses such as splitting, acting out, and withdrawal are frequently observed. Splitting, characterized by a black-and-white view of self and others, can lead to alternating between idealization and devaluation. This binary perception often extends to body image, resulting in an inconsistent relationship with food and fluctuating self-worth. Acting out might manifest as impulsive behaviors, such as binge eating or purging, providing temporary emotional relief but ultimately reinforcing shame and inadequacy. Withdrawal serves as an emotional escape, distancing the individual from painful emotions and social interactions but also hindering recovery by isolating them from supportive relationships.

The role of body image and Ego functioning in eating disorders

Body image is a core component of self-concept, heavily influenced by Ego functioning, and plays a crucial role in the development and persistence of EDs. In patients with severe personality disorders, disturbances in Ego functioning often exacerbate body image distortions, impairing their ability to maintain stable reality testing in relation to themselves and others. For individuals with borderline or narcissistic personality disorders, self-perception often fluctuates, shaped by emotional states, interpersonal relationships, and external feedback. This instability in body image perception can lead to severe ED symptoms, where individuals may oscillate between extreme body criticism and fleeting satisfaction rooted in idealized body standards.

In cases where Ego functioning is severely compromised, body image distortions can create a profound disconnection between an individual's perception of themselves and their physical reality. Reality testing—a fundamental Ego function that differentiates internal from external reality—becomes increasingly unstable, further complicating the formation of a cohesive and stable body image. This weakened reality testing often results in heightened body dissatisfaction, impulsive behaviors, and drastic attempts to alter physical appearance, exacerbating both physical and psychological distress.

Impulse control and eating disorders

Impulse control is another critical function of the Ego that is often impaired in individuals with EDs. Many patients exhibit severe impulsivity across various domains, including substance dependency, aggression, impulsive sexual behavior, irritability, and volatile interpersonal relationships. These multi-impulsive behaviors are particularly common in BN and are associated with significant clinical complications.

Interestingly, some individuals with AN develop bulimic episodes over time, suggesting that anorexia may initially function as a defense mechanism against the fear of losing control and acting on impulsive urges. This progression highlights the complex interplay between control, impulsivity, and the evolving psychological dynamics of EDs.

Multi-impulsivity worsens the prognosis and complicates the therapeutic process. Studies from specialized ED treatment centers in Germany indicate that therapeutic outcomes are notably lower for patients with bulimic symptoms combined with multi-impulsive behaviors, anorexic symptoms, and multiple previous treatment attempts (Kächele et al., unpublished).

Consequently, some theorists classify BN within the addiction spectrum, viewing it as a dependency on specific behaviors for self-regulation (Jeammet, 1992). This addictive quality is often linked to early relational dynamics with caregivers, establishing psychic patterns dominated by dependency and repetitive compulsions. Bernard Brusset emphasizes that these addictive processes differ from neurotic, psychotic, borderline, or perverse organizations, existing within a multidimensional framework often observed in adolescent psychopathology (Brusset, 1998).

The addictive nature of bulimic behaviors, marked by cycles of repetition and dependency, reflects a need to fill an underlying void. Philippe Jeammet (1992) characterizes patients with BN as exhibiting "object hunger", a relational craving driven by a blend of drive-based needs and a particular narcissistic organization that relies on object relationships for self-regulation.

Identity formation and the role of the ideal of the Ego in eating disorders

Identity is a cornerstone of Ego functioning, and for individuals with EDs, identity often becomes inextricably entangled with the illness. This phenomenon is particularly prominent in cases where personality disturbances are present, leading individuals to build their identity around the disorder itself. Phrases like "I am anorexic" or "I am bulimic" exemplify how the disorder becomes a central lens through which they view themselves, relationships, and life. Such identification reflects more than a label; it compensates for a deeper psychic emptiness or fragmentation, effectively filling an otherwise unstable sense of self. This identity-based structure signifies a unique psychic organization, distinct from the symptomology seen in other conditions, such as hysterical neuroses, where symptoms are often more superficial and not deeply embedded within the individual's core sense of self.

In the case of EDs, the symptoms become woven into the very fabric of the individual's self-concept, influencing how they perceive themselves, relate to others, and navigate their daily lives. Unlike hysteria, where symptoms may arise temporarily as expressions of repressed conflict, ED symptoms become inseparable from the individual's self-image. They take on an existential dimension, forming a core part of the self-definition, which often complicates the therapeutic process. The disorder is not merely something they experience; it becomes an essential component of their identity. In turn, this deep identification with the disorder creates resistance to change, as any movement away from the ED can feel like a loss of self, making the journey toward a more autonomous and healthier identity more challenging.

This binding identity to the disorder reflects not only the presence of EDs but also underlying personality dynamics. In certain cases, the personality structure itself may lack a cohesive identity, resulting in a sense of self that is fragile and lacking in core stability. EDs then serve as a defense against this fragility, providing a rigid and dependable sense of self, albeit one that is maladaptive. This identity structure is reinforced through societal, familial, and cultural feedback, where the external validation of thinness, control, or restraint serves to solidify the disorder as a central part of who they are. For some, the disorder becomes a means of achieving validation, mastery, or self-worth, further embedding it within their self-concept.

The Ego's role in identity and the Ideal of the Ego

The Ideal of the Ego plays a particularly influential role in the development and maintenance of EDs. It acts as an internalized standard of perfection, dictating impossible standards of thinness, beauty, or self-control, which fuel the cycle of self-criticism, shame, and compulsive behavior characteristic of EDs. The Ideal of the Ego is not merely an aspiration but an unrelenting demand within the psyche. For individuals with EDs, this idealized standard exacerbates the internal conflicts between the Ego's role in managing reality, the Superego's moral constraints, and the Id's instinctual desires.

The Ideal of the Ego drives individuals to extreme behaviors by setting unachievable goals. The Ego, in its attempts to reconcile these demands, often resorts to defense mechanisms, such as denial, repression, and projection, to manage the pressure. Yet, these strategies frequently fail to alleviate the internal conflict, leading individuals into a spiral of self-criticism, perfectionism, and shame. They may internalize this unattainable ideal as a measure of self-worth, using the ED to feel they are fulfilling or approaching this ideal. Failure to meet these unrealistic standards deepens feelings of inadequacy and worthlessness, feeding back into the cycle of control and restriction over food and body image.

In the case of EDs, the Ideal of the Ego also plays a crucial role in reinforcing the patient's identification with the disorder. By striving toward these unattainable ideals, the Ego's efforts become bound to the disorder, making it a central part of the individual's self-concept. As a result, the path to recovery is not merely about managing symptoms but about dismantling the rigid ideals that support the disorder and building an identity that is independent of these ideals. This task requires a reorganization of the Ego's functioning, allowing it to adopt a more flexible, realistic self-image rather than one based on impossible standards.

Therapeutic work focused on these dynamics must address both the Ideal of the Ego and the underlying voids it seeks to fill. Effective interventions aim to help patients recognize and release the attachment to these rigid ideals while cultivating a more compassionate and forgiving self-concept. By confronting the dissonance between the Ideal of the Ego and the patient's reality, therapy can help patients redefine their sense of self-worth in ways that do not hinge on perfection or control. Through this process, patients can begin to build a cohesive and realistic identity that is not dependent on the disorder. This work can be challenging, as the Ideal of the Ego often provides the individual with a sense of purpose and structure. Yet, dismantling this idealistic foundation is essential to developing a healthy, integrated self-concept.

In essence, the Ideal of the Ego's role in EDs serves as a double-edged sword. While it provides the individual with a sense of striving and accomplishment, it also traps them in a relentless pursuit of an impossible standard. As long as their self-worth is dependent on meeting these ideals, the ego remains vulnerable, struggling to balance internal drives with a self-image that is constantly under siege. The therapeutic process, therefore, must not only challenge these ideals but also work to develop a more autonomous and self-compassionate identity that can exist outside of the disorder, paving the way toward a more integrated and stable sense of self.

The psychoanalytic exploration of Ego functioning and identity in EDs underscores the intricate interplay between self-perception, defense mechanisms, and internalized ideals. In patients with EDs, Ego functioning is often compromised, leading to significant challenges in impulse control, reality testing, and body image stability. The Ideal of the Ego, with its demand for perfection, further complicates this landscape by reinforcing the identification with the disorder, making recovery a profound reconstruction of self-identity.

For patients whose identities are bound to their disorder, the path to recovery involves dismantling rigid ideals, enhancing Ego stability, and fostering an autonomous sense of self. This multifaceted approach to therapy not only addresses the visible symptoms but also attends to the deep-seated conflicts and identity issues at the heart of EDs, paving the way toward a healthier, integrated self.

Affective regulation and the role of emotions and feelings

Human affect has evolved into an intricate system that integrates abstract representations and complex mental processes, accessible to conscious awareness. Emotions are central components of this system, exhibiting patterned, largely unconscious responses that are universal across cultures. Primarily expressed through facial expressions and body language, emotions communicate directly with others, rooted in specific chemical and neural processes. These patterned responses from within complex brain circuitry, serving a crucial regulatory role in maintaining life. Thus, the body acts as a primary medium through which emotions are expressed, contributing to survival.

While cultural factors shape how emotions are expressed and perceived, their fundamental structure is phylogenetically ingrained. Emotions are innate, shared universally, transcending sociocultural backgrounds. Babies are born with an automatic capacity to express emotions, which act as signals to caregivers and are essential for survival. Emotions are thus inherently communicative, as Paul Ekman and Wallace Friesen observed in their research on facial expressions (Ekman and Friesen, 1976). However, Tyson and Tyson (1990) noted that an infant's emotional expressions only become communicative if caregivers are responsive, transforming emotions into relational exchanges that support socio-emotional development.

Feelings and the translation of emotion into conscious experience

Feelings extend beyond basic emotional responses, encompassing perceptions that arise consciously through experience, sensory input, imagination, memory, and language. Language uniquely allows individuals to translate emotions into conscious experiences, leading to what we call feelings—a higher level of abstraction where emotions are not only felt but also recognized, interpreted, and reflected upon. This enables more nuanced emotional expression, allowing individuals to convey their internal experiences in ways influenced by cultural and personal factors.

In patients with EDs, this intricate affective process is often disrupted by alexithymia—a term introduced by Sifneos and Nemiah and later expanded by Taylor (2018). Alexithymia refers to a difficulty in recognizing, interpreting, and expressing emotions, which poses significant barriers to emotional awareness and complicates affect regulation. Alexithymia has been linked to the development and persistence of disordered eating behaviors. For example, Liberman noted that psychosomatic patients with alexithymia often lack emotional depth in their facial expressions, appearing rigid or as if their faces "say nothing" or display anger continuously (Liberman et al., 1986). Krause's research corroborates this, suggesting that these individuals suppress emotional expression to protect others from their feelings. Liberman proposed that such patients, having experienced emotional indifference early on, may treat others with similar emotional detachment, though they remain unaware of their own limited expressiveness.

The impact of alexithymia on affective processes in eating disorders

Following Philippe Jeammet's (1984) theories on AN as a disengagement from internalized object relations, we can infer that this process impacts basic and social emotions and higher-order feelings requiring symbolic connections. For patients with EDs, disengagement from emotions may function as a defense, shielding them from re-experiencing unresolved conflicts. However, alexithymia in these patients may stem from more than defensive processes; it may also result from a lack of early "bathing in words", where caregivers do not reinforce emotional states through language. Without this symbolic support, patients struggle to interpret and express their emotions, lacking the necessary framework for nuanced emotional understanding.

Thus, alexithymia reflects more than just limited emotional awareness; it signifies a deeper disruption in early relationships. When caregivers fail to validate or reflect an infant's emotions, the child may struggle to differentiate their emotions from those of others, creating blurred emotional boundaries and undifferentiated relationships. This lack of differentiation likely reflects the predominant relational style in the individual's early bonding experiences.

Substituting emotional expression with disordered eating behaviors

The inability to recognize, experience, and communicate emotions can exacerbate challenges for ED patients. Disordered eating behaviors often become substitutes for emotional expression, with actions like binging or restricting serving as outlets for unprocessed emotions. For example, bulimic behaviors often mirror addictive cycles, where patients turn to food as a substitute for the relational connections, they desire but find difficult to form. Philippe Jeammet (1992) described patients with BN as having "object hunger"—a relational need that combines drive-based urges with a particular narcissistic organization reliant on relationships to regulate emotions. Unfortunately, alexithymia prevents these patients from achieving the emotional fulfillment they seek, leading them toward compulsive eating behaviors rather than meaningful interpersonal connections.

In ED patients, the boundary between self and other can be blurred on an emotional level, leading to confusion not just in neurotic projections but also in "archaic projections", where self and external reality remain indistinct. This primitive projection, coupled with a limited emotional vocabulary, restricts patients' capacity to perceive, understand, and communicate their emotional states.

Affective regulation and the role of early attachment

Affective regulation develops within early infant-caregiver interactions, initially shaped by environmental factors and eventually fostering lasting structural changes. Secure attachment is vital for emotional regulation, allowing regulatory abilities to be transmitted from caregiver to infant. Initially, the caregiver regulates the infant's emotions, but over time, the infant internalizes these strategies, achieving greater emotional autonomy. Allan Schore highlighted this process, explaining that effective regulation within the caregiver-infant relationship leads to an "integration and restructuring of the infant's socio-emotional system on a higher level of complexity" (Schore, 1994, p. 32). As the socio-emotional system matures, regulation evolves from external reliance to internal management.

Self-esteem and its affective foundations

Self-esteem, often called the "affective picture of the self", is similarly shaped by early affective experiences. Positive self-esteem is generally tied to positive emotions, while low self-esteem often accompanies negative emotions. This dynamic is central to managing narcissistic affects, involving self-assessment through internal representations and sustaining structural cohesion in self-concept. High self-esteem fosters stability in these representations, promoting interest, engagement, and enjoyment. Conversely, low self-esteem destabilizes inner structures, diminishing positive affect and the ability to experience pleasure.

A caregiver's self-esteem and emotional stability also impact an infant's self-esteem. Schore (1994) explains that the caregiver's affective state shapes the infant's regulatory abilities and self-image, illustrating how early relationships profoundly influence emotional and self-regulatory development. When caregivers experience low self-esteem or emotional instability, the child's emotional stability may be compromised, increasing susceptibility to regulatory difficulties and affective disorders.

Affective dysregulation and eating disorders

Dysfunctional emotional processing and regulation are thought to underlie many psychological disorders, including EDs (Oldershaw, Startup, and Lavender, 2019). In BN, affect regulation challenges are particularly pronounced, making individuals vulnerable to intense emotional fluctuations—often referred to as "affective storms". These storms, marked by sudden, overwhelming emotional surges, can be triggered by minor stressors or interpersonal conflicts, leading to impulsive behaviors such as binge eating, purging, or self-harm as ways to alleviate distress.

Affective dysregulation in BN is often linked to early attachment disruptions or developmental experiences that undermine emotional self-soothing and trust. Consequently, individuals with BN may have few strategies to cope with intense feelings, frequently resorting to disordered eating behaviors as temporary escapes or reliefs. However, these behaviors often increase shame, guilt, and self-criticism, perpetuating a cycle of affective instability and disordered eating. Neurobiological factors, such as altered serotonin function, may further contribute to mood instability, impulsivity, and emotional reactivity in BN.

Therapeutic interventions for BN patients benefit from focusing on emotional awareness, enhancing self-regulation, and developing healthy coping strategies to manage affective storms. By fostering emotional literacy and regulation, therapy aims to help individuals break cycles of disordered behavior rooted in affective dysregulation and build resilience against emotional volatility.

The complexity of affect regulation and emotional processing in ED patients highlights the crucial role of early attachment experiences in shaping emotional stability and self-esteem. A secure caregiving environment fosters the infant's ability to internalize regulatory strategies, promoting emotional resilience and a stable self-concept. Conversely, disruptions in these foundational relationships can result in persistent difficulties in affect regulation, self-esteem, and emotional processing, often contributing to the development of EDs.

For ED patients, alexithymia reflects not only a lack of emotional awareness but a deeper disruption in early dyadic relationships. Their difficulties with affect regulation make them more vulnerable to emotional storms, fueling disordered behaviors as temporary coping mechanisms. Addressing these affective regulation challenges through therapeutic interventions that enhance emotional awareness, self-regulation, and interpersonal trust can facilitate recovery, breaking the cycle of dependence on disordered behaviors to manage unresolved emotional needs.

Bibliography

Abadi, M. (1983). Los precursores del Yo: El Yo Ideal, el Ideal del Yo y el Superyo en la constitución de la estructura yoica. *Revista de Psicoanálisis*, 40(3): 513–521.

Abraham, K. (1916). The pregenital stage of development. In *Selected Papers on Psychoanalysis*. Abingdon, Oxon and New York: Routledge. (2018 edition).

Bion, W. (1959). Attacks on linking. *The International Journal of Psychoanalysis*, 40: 308–315.

Breuer, J. and Freud, S. (1893a). Studies on hysteria: Case histories, Case 2: Frau Emmy von N. In *The Standard Edition of the Complete Psychological Works of Sigmund Freud, (2)*. London: The Hogarth Press, 48–105 (1991 edition).

Breuer, J. and Freud, S. (1893b). Studies on hysteria: Theoretical. Hysterical Conversion. *The Standard Edition of the Complete Psychological Works of Sigmund Freud, (2)*. London: The Hogarth Press, 203–214 (1991 edition).

Breuer, J., and Freud, S. (1893c). Studies on hysteria: Case histories, Case 4: Katharina. *The Standard Edition of the Complete Psychological Works of Sigmund Freud, (2)*. London: The Hogarth Press, 125–134 (1991 edition).

Brusset, B. (1998). *Psychopathologie de l'Anorexie Mentale*. Paris: Dunod.

Chasseguet-Smirgel, J. (1976). Some thoughts on the Ego Ideal: A contribution to the study of the 'Illness of Ideality'. *The Psychoanalytic Quarterly*, 45(3): 345–373.

Crucianelli, L., Cardi, V., Treasure, J., Jenkinson, P. M., and Fotopoulou, A. (2016). The perception of affective touch in anorexia nervosa. *Psychiatry Research*, 239: 72–78.

Crucianelli, L., Demartini, B., Goeta, D., Nisticò, V., Saramandi, A., Bertelli, S., ... and Fotopoulou, A. (2021). The anticipation and perception of affective touch in women with and recovered from anorexia nervosa. *Neuroscience*, 464: 143–155.

Ekman, P. and Friesen, W. (1976). Measuring facial movement. *Environmental Psychology and Nonverbal Behavior*, 1: 56–75.

Fairbain, W. R. D. (1946). Object relationships and dynamic structure. In *Psychoanalytic Studies of the Personality*. London: Routledge, 137–151. (1994 reprint).

Fonagy, P., Gergely, G., Jurist, E. L., and Target, M. (2004). *Affect Regulation, Mentalization, and the Development of the Self*. London: Routledge.

Fotopoulou, A. (2015). The neuroscience of body image: Insight from anorexia nervosa. *Cortex*, 72: 120–121.

Freud, S. (1893). On the psychical mechanism of hysterical phenomena. *The Standard Edition of the Complete Psychological Works of Sigmund Freud, (3)*. London: The Hogarth Press, 27–39 (1991 edition).

Freud, S. (1896). The aetiology of hysteria. *The Standard Edition of the Complete Psychological Works of Sigmund Freud, (3)*. London: The Hogarth Press, 189–221 (1991 edition).

Freud, S. (1905). Three essays on the theory of sexuality. Component instincts and erotogenic zones. *The Standard Edition of the Complete Psychological Works of Sigmund Freud, (7)*. London: The Hogarth Press, 167–169 (1991 edition).

Freud, S. (1923). The Ego and the Id. *The Standard Edition of the Complete Psychological Works of Sigmund Freud, (19)*. London: The Hogarth Press, 3–66 (1991 edition).

Green, A. (1980). La madre muerta. In *Narcisismo de Vida, Narcisismo de Muerte*. Buenos Aires: Amorrortu editors, 209–238 (1993 edition).

Hanly, C. M. T. (1983). Ideal del yo y yoideal. *Revista de Psicoanálisis*, 40(1): 191–203.

Houzel, D. (1990). El concepto de envoltura psíquica. In D. Anzieu, D. Houzel, J. Guillaumin, A. Missenard, M. Enriquez, A. Anziey, J. Doron, E. Lecourt, and T. Nathan (eds) *Las Envolturas Psíquicas*. Buenos Aires: Amorrortu editors, 38–67.

Jeammet, P. (1984). L'anorexie mentale. *Encyclo. Med. Chir. Psychiatrie Vol. 3, 37350*: A10 et A15; 2. Paris: Elsevier.

Jeammet, P. (1992). *La Boulimie, Monographies de la Revue Francoise de Psychanalyse*. Paris: PUF. Spanish versión: Las conductas bulímicas como modalidad de acomodamiento de las disregulaciones narcisistas y objetales. *Psicoanálisis con Niños y Adolescentes: n/A*, 1993, (5): 44–63.

Kächele, H., Kordy, H., Richard, M., and Research Group TR-EAT. *Outcome of Psychodynamic Therapy of Eating Disorders*. Stuttgart: Center for Psychotherapy Research, 1–39. (Unpublished).

Kernberg, O. F. (1992). *Aggression in Personality Disorders and Perversions*. New Haven, CT and London: Yale University Press.

Kernberg, O. F. (2004). A technical approach to eating disorders in patients with Borderline Personality Organization. In *Aggressivity, Narcissism, and Self-destructiveness in the Psychotherapeutic Relationship: New Developments in the Psychopathology and Psychotherapy of Severe Personality Disorders*. New Haven, CT and London: Yale University Press, 205–219.

Kernberg, P. F. (1984). Reflections in the mirror: Mother-child interactions, self-awareness, and self-recognition. *Frontiers of Infant Psychiatry*, 2: 101–110.

Kernberg, P. F. (1987). Mother-child interaction and mirror behavior. *Infant Mental Health Journal*, 8(4): 329–339.

Liberman, D., Grassanode Piccolo, E., Neborakde Dimant, S., Pistinerde Cortiñas, L., and Roitmande Woscoboinik, P. (1986). *Del Cuerpo al Símbolo: Sobreadaptación y Enfermedad Psicosomática*. Buenos Aires: Ed. Trieb, (2nd edition).

MacDonald, D. E., Solomon-Krakus, S., Jewett, R., Liebman, R. E., and Trottier, K. (2023). Emotion regulation in bulimia nervosa and purging disorder. In V. B. Patel and V. R. Preedy (eds.) *Eating Disorders*. Cham: Springer, 805–828. https://doi.org/10.1007/978-3-031-16691-4_44.

McDougall, J. (2013). *Plea for a Measure of Abnormality*. London: Routledge.

Oldershaw, A., Startup, H., and Lavender, T. (2019). Anorexia nervosa and a lost emotional self: A psychological formulation of the development, maintenance, and treatment of anorexia nervosa. *Frontiers in Psychology*, 10(219): 1–22.

Persano, H. L. (2005). Abordagem psicodinâmica do paciente com trastornos alimentares. In C. L. Eizirik, R. W. Aguiar, and S. S. Schestatsky (eds.) *Psicoterapia de Orientação Analítica: Fundamentos Teóricos e Clínicos*. Porto Alegre: Artmed Editora, 674–688 (chapter 49).

Persano, H. L. (2019). Las diferentes dimensiones del cuerpo humano. In H. L. Persano, et al. (eds.) *El Mundo de la Salud Mental en la Práctica Clínica,*. Buenos Aires: Akadia, 375–386 (chapter 32).

Persano, H. L. (2022). Self-harm. *The International Journal of Psychoanalysis*, 103(6): 1089–1103.

Saramandi, A., Crucianelli, L., Koukoutsakis, A., Nisticò, V., Baiza, A., Goeta, D., … and Fotopoulou, A. (2022). Belief updating about interoception and body size estimation in Anorexia Nervosa. https://doi.org/10.31234/osf.io/rntsf.

Sartre, J. P. (1943). *Being and Nothingness*. (H. E. Barnes, Trans.). New York: Philosophical library (1956 edition).

Schilder, P. (1950). *The Image and Appearance of the Human Body*. New York: International Universities Press. Spanish Edition (1958) *Imagen y Apariencia del Cuerpo Humano*. Buenos Aires: Paidós.

Schore, A. N. (1994). *Affect Regulation and the Origin of the Self: Neurobiology of Emotional Development*. New Jersey: LEA.

Stanghellini, G. and Mancini, M. (2020). Body experience, identity and the other's gaze in persons with feeding and eating disorders. *Phenomenology and Mind*, 18: 144–152.

Tasca, G. A., Szadkowski, L., Illing, V., Trinneer, A., Grenon, R., Demidenko, N., … and Bissada, H. (2009). Adult attachment, depression, and eating disorder symptoms: The mediating role of affect regulation strategies. *Personality and Individual Differences*, 47(6): 662–667.

Tasca, G. A. and Balfour, L. (2014). Attachment and eating disorders: A review of current research. *International Journal of Eating Disorders*, 47(7): 710–717.

Taylor, G. J. (2018). History of alexithymia: The contributions of psychoanalysis. In O. Luminet, R. M. Bagby, and G. J. Taylor (eds.) *Alexithymia: Advances in Research, Theory, and Clinical Practice*. Cambridge: Cambridge University Press, 1–16.

Tyson, P. and Tyson, R. (1990). La evolucióndel afecto durante el Desarrollo. In *Teorías Psicoanalíticas del Desarrollo: Una Integración*. Lima: Ed. Publicaciones Psicoanalíticas, 169–180 (chapter 9), (2000 edition).

Williams, G. (1997). Reflections on some dynamics of eating disorders "no entry" defences and foreign bodies. *International Journal of Psycho-Analysis*, 78: 927–941.

Williams, G. (2000). *Internal Landscapes and Foreign Bodies: Eating Disorders and Other Pathologies*. London: Duckworth, Tavistock Clinic Series.

Winograd, B. (1983). Las relaciones entre los conceptos Superyo e Ideal del Yo: Perspectivas en la articulación teórico-clínica. *Revistade Psicoanálisis*, 40(3): 505–512.

Yampey, N. (1983). El Superyo, el Ideal del Yo y el Yo Ideal en la clínica. *Revistade Psicoanálisis*, 40(3): 597–605.

5 Unconscious dynamics of eating disorders

Unconscious conflicts related to body image and self-esteem

Unconscious conflicts surrounding body image and self-esteem are powerful forces underlying the emotional and behavioral complexities observed in individuals with EDs. These dynamics often stem from early attachment patterns, unresolved internal conflicts, and the pervasive internalization of societal ideals around self-worth, control, and the dependence on external validation. From a psychoanalytic standpoint, EDs are not simply physical phenomena; they embody intricate psychological struggles encompassing identity, autonomy, and self-worth.

In psychoanalysis, EDs have been reframed from expressions of repressed drives or punitive mechanisms to manifestations of profound internal conflicts. This perspective highlights EDs as complex responses to cultural, familial, and psychological pressures. Adolescents, for example, experience a heightened struggle between their actual bodies and the idealized images they internalize from society's relentless narratives about aesthetic perfection. These impossible standards amplify self-criticism and diminish self-worth, further intensified by globalized media, which promotes narrow definitions of beauty, compelling individuals to conform to unrealistic ideals (Persano, 2005).

As individuals strive to meet unattainable ideals, they often adopt an intensely self-critical stance, evaluating their worth based on how closely they align with these images of perfection. This dynamic mirrors the myth of Narcissus, where individuals become fixated on an external reflection they can never fully embody, trapping them in an endless cycle of validation-seeking. The pursuit of this "excess of the ideal" creates a disconnection from one's authentic self, fostering a profound mind-body divide (Green, 1983).

This alienation echoes Cartesian dualism, where the body is perceived as separate from the self and is treated as an object to be reshaped, controlled, and even punished. Over time, the frustration and aggression originally directed at external standards of perfection become internalized. This inward turn manifests as severe self-criticism and self-loathing when

DOI: 10.4324/9781032724997-5

individuals inevitably fall short of these impossible ideals. The result is a perpetuating cycle of dissatisfaction and emotional suffering, deeply rooted in the conflict between societal pressures and personal identity.

Restrictive behaviors in EDs can serve as efforts to assert control. In AN, for example, restricting food intake symbolizes more than a dietary choice; it represents a disciplined resistance against external expectations and a method of carving out personal autonomy. Meanwhile, binge-eating and purging behaviors can function as forms of self-punishment or "cleansing", directed toward purging the body of perceived impurities. This "purification" parallels Freud's psychoanalytic concept of the "anal-sadistic phase", wherein individuals cleanse themselves symbolically, linking their bodies with sin or imperfection. In his 1917 work *"On Transformations of Instinct as Exemplified in Anal Erotism"*, Freud examines how this phase involves complex symbolic meanings. He explains that for the child, defecation represents not only a bodily function but a negotiation of control, purity, and morality: "The child looks upon its stools as a part of itself that it may either expel or retain... and that thus becomes a medium of exchange between itself and the adult" (Freud, 1917). This stage lays the foundation for the symbolic associations that later attach to the body, where attempts to expel impurities align with the self-punishment seen in purging behaviors. Here, purging reflects an unconscious drive to control and purify one's identity, underscoring a psychological struggle with self-worth and perceived imperfection.

In BN, the repetitive cycle of binging and purging serves not only as an attempt to control the body but as a coping mechanism for managing overwhelming emotions and unresolved feelings of inadequacy. Philippe Jeammet (1984) argues that these behaviors reflect a broader internal conflict, where food and body control become symbols for managing intense emotions that might otherwise feel unmanageable. For individuals with BN, binging may serve to "fill" an emotional void, temporarily soothing inner pain and satisfying an unconscious craving for comfort or validation. However, this sense of relief is short-lived, often leading to guilt, shame, and failure that subsequently trigger purging as an act of penance and self-purification.

In this way, purging becomes more than a mere physical act; it symbolizes an attempt to cleanse oneself of perceived impurities or failures, striving to eliminate the internalized negative feelings that often plague self-worth. The cycle itself reinforces these emotional patterns: each binge episode temporarily soothes the sense of inadequacy, while each purge provides a fleeting illusion of control, only to perpetuate a continuous struggle with self-criticism and self-loathing.

The psychoanalytic lens further interprets this binge-purge cycle as a defense against unmet emotional needs and unresolved dependency conflicts. Jeammet's concept of "object hunger" describes how individuals with BN may unconsciously use food as a surrogate for emotional needs that feel unfulfilled (Jeammet, 1992). In this way, food stands in for the love, support, or validation perceived as absent, while purging becomes not only a physical expulsion but a symbolic rejection of this dependency. This act reflects a deeper ambivalence about vulnerability and attachment, where individuals unconsciously grapple with their need for comfort while striving for autonomy.

Moreover, this binge-purge cycle illustrates the psychodynamic conflict between dependency and autonomy. Binging may symbolize acceptance of comfort and care, whereas purging acts as a rejection of these needs, striving instead for self-sufficiency. This oscillation between seeking connection and rejecting it as a weakness reflects an internal conflict, creating a repetitive pattern that obscures deeper psychological needs and anxieties about self-worth, intimacy, and control.

The societal obsession with unattainable body standards further compounds these conflicts, creating a cycle of self-alienation that heightens emotional distress. For many individuals with EDs, achieving culturally idealized thinness or perfection becomes the principal measure of self-worth. This drive often stems from early developmental experiences of conditional love, where self-worth was tied to external appearances or achievements. In such cases, self-worth divides into "acceptable" and "unacceptable" parts, reinforcing cycles of self-objectification and criticism.

Within the psychodynamic framework, EDs can also reflect unresolved dependency issues, where binge-eating serves as a surrogate for emotional nourishment. As Jeammet's "object hunger" highlights, food becomes a concrete substitute for missing emotional fulfillment. However, this object-centered focus fails to satisfy the deeper emotional emptiness it aims to resolve, perpetuating the cycle of dependency and rejection.

Research supports these psychoanalytic concepts, demonstrating that individuals with anorexia nervosa (AN) and bulimia nervosa (BN) often exhibit heightened sensitivity to both punishment and reward, which intensifies maladaptive behaviors and reinforces internal conflicts (Harrison et al., 2010); (Glashouwer et al., 2014). This heightened sensitivity, coupled with severe self-criticism, drives individuals toward unattainable standards, perpetuating feelings of inadequacy and failure.

In AN, for instance, restrictive behaviors may function as a symbolic rejection of dependency. The refusal of food becomes a metaphorical rejection of external influences, reflecting an attempt to assert self-sufficiency and autonomy (Von Wyl, 2000). These behaviors underscore the profound psychological struggles inherent in EDs, where the drive for control and perfection masks deeper conflicts surrounding identity, self-worth, and emotional vulnerability.

Agnes Von Wyl's research into patients with EDs sheds light on the intricate interplay between dependency and autonomy within their psychological framework. Individuals with AN often strive for independence and emotional distance, employing food restriction as a symbolic barrier against vulnerability and emotional dependence. This refusal to nourish the body can be interpreted as a rejection of external caretaking, reflecting a profound desire for self-sufficiency and control over their environment.

In contrast, individuals with BN may exhibit a more ambivalent dynamic, simultaneously seeking autonomy while maintaining a strong emotional connection to caregivers. Paulina Kernberg (2004) aptly descri- bed this phenomenon as the "Peter Pan Syndrome", referring to a reluc- tance to grow up and separate from familial ties. For patients with BN, the oscillation between binging and purging behaviors may reflect their inner conflict: the desire for autonomy juxtaposed with the fear of disconnection and abandonment. This dynamic underscores the core tension in BN, where individuals attempt to balance their need for emotional support with their yearning for independence.

Defense mechanisms such as projection, self-criticism, and self-directed aggression are commonly employed by individuals with EDs to navigate these emotional struggles. Through these mechanisms, fears of abandon- ment and rejection are often displaced onto the body, leading to a cycle of self-punishment and dissatisfaction. Schwartz (1986) further explored these dynamics, noting that patients with BN frequently internalize early object relations, which evolve into intrapsychic conflicts in adulthood. These conflicts are often accompanied by invasive and distressing fanta- sies, including unconscious fears or desires with incestuous connotations, such as fantasies of impregnation.

Such fantasies reveal the depth of unconscious anxieties that fuel the disorder's complex psychological landscape. They also highlight how unresolved early relational experiences shape the internal world of indi- viduals with BN, perpetuating cycles of dependency, fear, and self- destructive behavior. Together, these insights emphasize the need for a nuanced therapeutic approach that addresses the underlying emotional and relational conflicts, enabling patients to reconcile their desire for autonomy with their need for meaningful connection.

These findings underscore the profound interplay between early rela- tional experiences, defense mechanisms, and the symbolic use of the body in individuals with EDs, offering critical insights into their emotional and relational struggles.

Psychoanalytically, the behaviors exhibited in EDs are often deeply intertwined with defense mechanisms such as splitting and dissociation, which serve to manage overwhelming emotions and conflicts. Splitting involves dividing one's sense of self into "good" and "bad" aspects. For indi- viduals with EDs, this manifests as an extreme dichotomy in self-perception: success in adhering to restrictive behaviors or achieving an idealized body image is equated with being "good", while any perceived failure triggers intense self-loathing and feelings of worthlessness. This rigid division prevents the integration of positive and negative self-perceptions, exacerbating the internal conflict.

Dissociative defenses, on the other hand, allow individuals to detach from their emotions, often perceiving these feelings as alien or external to themselves. For those with neurotic personality structures, dissociation primarily serves to avoid confronting painful or distressing emotions, such as shame, guilt, or inadequacy. However, in individuals with borderline personality structures, splitting becomes more pervasive, stemming from blurred self-other boundaries. This leads to projective defenses, where internal emotions are attributed to others, further complicating the individual's ability to process and integrate their emotional experiences (Persano, 1997).

The interplay of splitting and dissociation not only disrupts emotional regulation but also hinders the development of a cohesive sense of self. In the case of splitting, the inability to reconcile conflicting aspects of the self, perpetuates cycles of self-criticism and punitive behaviors, often directed at the body. Dissociation, by severing the connection between emotions and self-awareness, reinforces feelings of alienation and detachment, making it difficult for individuals to address the underlying causes of their distress.

Moreover, these defenses operate in a relational context. For example, dissociation can lead to difficulty forming authentic connections with others, as emotional detachment prevents genuine engagement. Similarly, splitting may manifest in interpersonal relationships, where others are categorized as entirely "good" or "bad", mirroring the individual's internal divisions. This can create cycles of idealization and devaluation, further isolating individuals and reinforcing their reliance on maladaptive coping mechanisms.

Understanding these psychoanalytic dynamics is crucial for effective treatment. By helping patients recognize and integrate the fragmented aspects of their self-perception, therapeutic interventions can foster greater emotional resilience and self-acceptance. Addressing dissociative tendencies and teaching individuals to re-engage with their emotions in a constructive way are key steps in breaking the cycle of defense mechanisms that perpetuate eating disorder behaviors. This integrative approach can ultimately empower patients to develop a more balanced and compassionate view of themselves and their relationships.

Early attachment patterns strongly influence these dynamics, as insecure attachments foster unconscious fears of abandonment, rejection, and worthlessness. These anxieties are later expressed in disordered eating behaviors, where individuals project unresolved feelings onto their bodies, attempting to "discipline" and control their physical selves to manage deeper emotional turmoil. Through such projection, disordered eating becomes a symbolic expression of inner conflicts, transforming bodily control into an attempt to resolve psychological distress.

Understanding these psychoanalytic underpinnings offers critical insights into how unconscious conflicts around identity, autonomy, and self-worth manifest in body image and self-esteem struggles. Addressing these conflicts in therapeutic settings provides pathways toward self-acceptance, emotional integration, and a healthier relationship with both the body and the inner self.

Exploration of unconscious motivations behind disordered eating behaviors

Psychoanalytic perspectives on disordered eating reveal these behaviors as complex expressions of unresolved psychological conflicts, unmet emotional needs, and profound identity struggles. From this viewpoint, EDs are not merely about food or body image; they are closely intertwined with an individual's internal emotional landscape and self-concept. These unconscious motivations often reflect deeper issues related to control, self-worth, and autonomy.

One prominent psychoanalytic perspective suggests that EDs, particularly AN, arise from a "lost sense of emotional self". Individuals with AN may disconnect from their emotions, channeling their need for control into the body as a means of managing overwhelming feelings of vulnerability and dependency. Restrictive eating in this context is not simply a dietary choice but rather a way of exerting autonomy and creating distance from perceived inner chaos. By restricting food intake, individuals temporarily attain a sense of order and control, offering relief from psychological distress that may be too painful or confusing to confront (Oldershaw et al., 2019).

Lacanian theory offers a compelling perspective on EDs, linking their prevalence to the pressures of capitalist societies that idealize thinness, discipline, and bodily control. According to Lacanian psychoanalysts, societal standards compel individuals—particularly those vulnerable to EDs—to internalize ideals of self-regulation and perfection. Within this framework, the body becomes a project to be perfected, an object of constant scrutiny and self-management. This relentless pursuit of an unattainable ideal fosters intense self-criticism and emotional alienation from the physical self (Recalcati, 2013).

This alienation is emblematic of a deeper fragmentation of identity, as individuals struggle to reconcile their inner emotional needs with the external demands imposed by societal standards. Lacanian theory posits that the idealized body, shaped by cultural and capitalist imperatives, functions as an external object of control and desire. This objectification amplifies the individual's internal conflict, intensifying feelings of inadequacy and self-rejection when they inevitably fail to meet these impossible ideals.

The result is a vicious cycle: the more individuals perceive themselves as falling short, the more they attempt to compensate through extreme forms of bodily regulation. Restrictive eating, excessive exercise, and other disordered behaviors become misguided efforts to bridge the gap between the fragmented self and the unattainable societal ideal. Yet these behaviors only deepen the sense of alienation and exacerbate the internal conflict, as the body is treated as a separate entity to be controlled rather than an integral part of the self.

Lacanian theory illuminates how these struggles are not merely personal but also deeply rooted in cultural and ideological constructs. By framing the body as a site of societal control and the locus of internal conflict, this perspective underscores the broader systemic forces that fuel the development and perpetuation of EDs. Recognizing these dynamics is critical for both understanding and addressing the psychological and sociocultural dimensions of EDs, paving the way for more holistic and empathetic therapeutic approaches.

Disgust as emotion and defense

Massimo Recalcati offers a significant psychoanalytic insight by identifying disgust as a core emotional response in individuals with restrictive AN. For Recalcati, disgust is not merely an emotion; it acts as a relational force, binding individuals with AN to objects, food, and their own bodies. Disgust functions as a defense against vulnerability, enabling individuals to reject bodily needs and desires, which are seen as "impure" or "contaminated" (Recalcati, 2013). This aversion extends beyond simple distaste to become a powerful coping mechanism that distances individuals from perceived weaknesses, such as appetite or body fat. Through this lens, disgust fosters a purified self-image, one that appears free from physical and emotional vulnerabilities deemed unacceptable.

Thus, disgust becomes a strategy for controlling internal vulnerabilities and an unconscious attempt to achieve psychological "purity". By rejecting or purging what they perceive as impure or contaminated, individuals with EDs maintain a protective boundary against both internal and external threats. Yet, paradoxically, this defensive structure deepens emotional distress and alienation, preventing the integration of a cohesive self and reinforcing cycles of self-loathing. This fragmentation, which Lacan likens to a disruption in the "mirror stage", traps individuals in an endless pursuit of coherence through bodily control, as they struggle to reconcile their self-image with idealized societal standards (Roudinesco, 2003).

In psychoanalytic terms, disgust operates as both an emotion and a defense mechanism—a psychological boundary that shields individuals from confronting painful aspects of themselves. In the context of EDs, disgust extends beyond a mild aversion, embodying a complex rejection of perceived impurities within the self. This internalized disgust often targets specific body parts or foods, creating a "no entry" barrier that blocks experiences or emotions deemed too overwhelming to confront. Giana Williams (1997) describes these "no entry" defenses as symbolic walls designed to keep out "unacceptable" aspects of reality, including emotions, foods, or body parts that threaten the individual's sense of control and identity.

As Williams explains, this defense mechanism is rooted in a deep-seated fear of contamination or invasion, where the body is perceived as highly vulnerable to external intrusion. By creating rigid psychological and physical barriers, individuals gain a sense of control, enabling them to reject foods and emotions they associate with destabilization or vulnerability. In this framework, disgust functions as both a boundary and a defense, helping to create psychological distance from aspects of the self that evoke anxiety or self-loathing.

This dynamic often manifests as a cyclical need for "cleansing", reflecting an unconscious drive to shield oneself from perceived threats, both internal and external. In restrictive disorders like AN, the refusal of food becomes a symbolic and defensive act, guarding against experiences—whether emotional, relational, or physical—that are perceived as undesirable or overwhelming. The act of restricting not only enforces a sense of control but also reinforces a protective barrier, insulating the individual from anxiety and self-perceived flaws that feel too threatening to confront directly.

By understanding the role of disgust as a defensive mechanism, we can better appreciate how restrictive eating patterns function as an unconscious strategy to manage deeper psychological fears. This perspective highlights the complex interplay between emotions, self-perception, and behavior in EDs, offering valuable insights for therapeutic interventions aimed at addressing these underlying fears.

The concept of disgust in EDs is also closely related to the struggle with object constancy—the ability to maintain a stable and whole image of oneself or others, integrating both positive and negative qualities. In cases of AN, disgust often disrupts this constancy, leading to a fractured self-perception. Parts of the self, associated with perceived imperfections, are symbolically expelled, mirroring the rejection of a physically disgusting object. The "no entry" defense exacerbates this split, reinforcing a rigid self-image that prohibits undesirable aspects from entering consciousness. This creates an inflexible and divided self-concept, where individuals distance themselves from vulnerabilities to maintain an illusion of purity and control.

Constraint and frozen defenses in children: Precursors to eating disorders

In psychoanalytic theory, constraint and frozen defenses in children reflect a rigid psychological state where change feels impossible, and the world appears "frozen". Such defenses often stem from early traumatic experiences, where children create unchanging mental frameworks to keep reality static, even when this mental rigidity is limiting or uncomfortable. Selma Fraiberg and Paulina Kernberg, two influential figures in child psychoanalysis, describe how these defenses make a child's psychological landscape resistant to change. This "freezing" of the mind functions as a barrier against emotional turmoil, allowing the child to maintain a predictable world amid overwhelming feelings (Fraiberg, 1982).

Kernberg and colleagues explain that constraint, as a defense mechanism, significantly restricts a child's adaptability, compelling them to adopt rigid roles, routines, and behaviors. These patterns serve as a protective shield against emotional instability or perceived threats to their psychological equilibrium. Over time, such children become trapped in repetitive cycles, where the predictability of their behaviors provides a sense of safety but also limits their capacity for growth and change.

Within this defensive stance, their psychological world becomes static; any potential change is perceived as destabilizing and is therefore unconsciously blocked. By constructing these mental barriers, children create what Kernberg refers to as a "frozen" psychic landscape—a fixed psychological space where movement, flexibility, and emotional growth are arrested to keep overwhelming emotions at bay (Kernberg et al., 2000).

This frozen state, while offering temporary protection, comes at the cost of emotional adaptability and resilience. The rigidity of their internal world prevents them from engaging with new experiences or processing emotional challenges in a healthy manner, perpetuating a cycle of defensive withdrawal. Kernberg's insights illuminate how these mechanisms shape not only a child's emotional development but also their interactions with the external world, reinforcing patterns of avoidance and stagnation that can persist into adulthood.

At the core of these constraint defenses is a deep need for control, particularly in children who have experienced early trauma, unpredictability, or intense emotional overwhelm. For these children, rigid mental constructs provide a sense of security, allowing them to navigate the world without fear of encountering feelings they cannot manage. For instance, a child may develop strict routines around daily activities or take on inflexible roles in relationships, reinforcing a predictable environment that shields them from uncertainty and emotional upheaval. This rigid adherence to familiar patterns gives them a sense of safety, as they believe that preserving constancy will protect them from psychological vulnerability.

However, constraint defenses come at a significant cost to emotional development. By blocking new or potentially destabilizing experiences, children limit their capacity to explore and integrate new emotional and relational experiences. Paulina Kernberg notes that these children often exhibit repetitive, almost ritualistic behaviors that serve as a kind of "psychic armor". For example, a child may cling to a specific role within the family, resisting any actions or expressions that could disrupt that identity. This attachment to rigid roles and routines keeps the child in a static, self-restricted world where they are shielded from both positive and challenging experiences (Kernberg et al., 2000).

This defensive posture can also manifest as a refusal to engage with new people or ideas, as well as a rejection of their own evolving emotions. Because the child perceives change as a threat to their established stability, their emotional responses are often muted or suppressed, leaving them "stuck" and unable to form flexible, adaptive defenses. Such children may struggle to experience or express complex feelings, instead retreating into repetitive, shallow emotional responses that fit within their constrained psychological framework.

In Kernberg's view, constraint as a defense mechanism resembles a psychological fortress: the psyche remains guarded against threats but is also cut off from meaningful connections and personal growth. This rigidity stems from a fundamental fear of abandonment or emotional invasion, where any form of intimacy or vulnerability could expose them to feelings, they are unprepared to manage. Through these defenses, children effectively "freeze" their emotional development, keeping parts of themselves and their relationships in a fixed, unchanging state that feels safe but isolates them from deeper engagement (Kernberg et al., 2000).

The rigidity of constraint defenses also shows up in an aversion to ambiguity or fluidity in relationships and self-concept. Children with these defenses may adopt an "all-or-nothing" perspective, in which people, situations, or feelings are either entirely safe or entirely dangerous. This polarized worldview reinforces their psychological distance from anything that could introduce complexity or unpredictability. While this approach helps them maintain a sense of safety and control, it limits their capacity to adapt and engage with the nuances and changes inherent in emotional life.

In therapeutic settings, working with children who exhibit constraint defenses requires a careful, gradual approach that respects the protective function of these defenses. Therapy aims to gently introduce the possibility of change without directly threatening the child's sense of security. By creating a stable, consistent environment, therapists help children feel safe enough to start exploring new ways of thinking, feeling, and relating to others. Over time, therapeutic work seeks to "thaw" these rigid defenses, encouraging the child to adopt a more dynamic, flexible understanding of themselves and their world. As children begin to allow for change, they gradually develop healthier, more adaptable defenses, opening pathways to personal growth, resilience, and the integration of new emotional experiences.

While these constraints and frozen defenses can be protective, they also restrict emotional growth and adaptability. By maintaining a "frozen" psychic state, children are shielded from perceived dangers but are also deprived of the rich, evolving experiences that foster resilience and an integrated sense of self. Therapy offers a way forward, empowering children to explore and embrace change, allowing them to engage more deeply with themselves and others.

Connection to restrictive patterns in eating disorders

The impact of constraint and "frozen" defenses developed in early childhood often persists into adolescence and adulthood, manifesting as restrictive patterns commonly observed in eating disorders, particularly

AN. The need to control and maintain a "frozen" emotional landscape is reflected in the rigid and restrictive behaviors characteristic of AN. Similarly, individuals with avoidant/restrictive food intake disorder (ARFID) also exhibit an intense need for predictability and control over their food intake, routines, and body.

These restrictive behaviors serve as a psychological defense, offering a sense of safety and self-preservation amidst perceived chaos or vulnerability. Much like the child who seeks refuge in a predictable and controlled world to avoid emotional instability, individuals with restrictive eating disorders construct rigid barriers around their eating and daily lives. This defensive strategy mirrors the child's attempt to maintain a stable inner world by blocking out emotional and physical "intrusions" that feel overwhelming or threatening.

By imposing such control, these individuals temporarily alleviate their anxiety and maintain a sense of order, but at the cost of emotional flexibility and adaptability. Understanding these parallels between early developmental defenses and later restrictive behaviors in EDs provides valuable insight into the deeply rooted psychological mechanisms that sustain these disorders, highlighting the need for therapeutic approaches that address both the underlying emotional vulnerabilities and the behaviors themselves.

As these constrained defenses continue into adolescence, they can evolve into a full-blown restrictive eating pattern, where individuals feel compelled to control and limit their intake to preserve a sense of safety and predictability. For these individuals, the rigid structure around food and body image serves as a continuation of the frozen defenses developed in childhood. Restricting food intake becomes a way to maintain a "frozen" state, ensuring that feelings of vulnerability, fear, or unworthiness remain hidden and contained. The obsessive routines around food and the rejection of bodily needs reflect an unconscious drive to guard against potential emotional invasions, much like the child's fixed and predictable world.

Kernberg's concept of the "psychic armor" that shields individuals from overwhelming emotions is particularly relevant here (Kernberg et al., 2000).

In AN, the rigid adherence to dietary rules and the ritualistic aspects of food control serves as psychic armor, protecting the individual from the messiness and unpredictability of emotional life. This armor keeps the individual emotionally "safe" but, like the constraint defenses in children, also prevents meaningful engagement with both internal and external worlds. The result is a self-restricted existence, where the individual feels isolated, detached, and ultimately controlled by the very defenses meant to offer protection.

Ultimately, understanding constraint and frozen defenses in childhood provides critical insight into the unconscious dynamics of restrictive EDs. Psychoanalytic treatment can support individuals with EDs in exploring and understanding these early defense mechanisms, helping them move toward a more integrated, flexible sense of self that can tolerate vulnerability and change. Through therapy, individuals learn to replace the rigid defenses of control and restriction with more adaptive and emotionally fulfilling ways of engaging with themselves and their relationships. This process fosters a sense of safety that does not depend on extreme self-regulation but rather on a balanced and resilient self that can embrace life's inherent complexities and uncertainties.

Psychoanalytic insights into bulimia nervosa and binge-eating disorder

In psychoanalytic theory, BN and binge-eating disorder (BED) are seen not only as disturbances in eating behavior but as reflections of profound emotional and relational conflicts. Central to these disorders is the concept of "object hunger", a term introduced by Philippe Jeammet to describe how food becomes a substitute for unmet emotional needs and a temporary source of comfort (Jeammet, 1984). According to Jeammet, individuals with BN or BED experience an internal void—an emptiness often rooted in unfulfilled relational needs or unresolved emotional wounds. The binge-purge cycle, therefore, is more than a response to physical hunger; it is a psychological attempt to fill this emotional emptiness, providing a momentary sensation of satisfaction that, unfortunately, soon gives way to feelings of guilt, shame, and disconnection (Dicu et al., 2024).

In the context of BN, binging offers a fleeting escape from emotional pain, a symbolic effort to consume the care or comfort they feel is missing. The food represents not only physical sustenance but also emotional nourishment that the individual longs for but believes is unavailable from relationships. The temporary relief that binging provides, however, quickly turns into distress, leading to the compulsive act of purging. Through purging, the individual attempts to "cleanse" themselves of dependency, rejecting both the food and, symbolically, the relational need it represents. This ritualized cycle of binging and purging thus mirrors a deeper struggle with unmet needs for connection and support, followed by a strong desire to reject any sense of vulnerability or dependency associated with these needs (Jeammet, 1984).

This binge-purge cycle embodies an intense internal conflict between autonomy and connection. Individuals with BN or BED often oscillate between seeking emotional fulfillment and fiercely rejecting it, creating a "push-and-pull" dynamic that reflects their ambivalence toward intimacy and independence. Psychoanalytic theories suggest that these individuals are caught in a pattern of wanting closeness and care yet fearing the dependency and vulnerability that come with it. The act of binging symbolizes an unconscious attempt to receive love, care, or protection, while purging reflects an effort to regain autonomy and distance from the perceived threat of attachment. This ambivalence is often linked to early relational experiences, where dependency was associated with fear or disappointment, leading individuals to oscillate between seeking comfort and rejecting it as a defense against potential pain (Dicu et al., 2024).

Freud's concept of "oral fixation" provides additional insight into this dynamic, suggesting that unresolved needs from the oral stage of development can manifest in adulthood as compulsive behaviors related to the mouth, such as eating. According to Freud, the oral stage is associated with the need for nurturing and comfort, and unresolved issues during this phase can lead to difficulties with dependency and autonomy later in life. In BN and BED, this unresolved need for emotional sustenance reappears as a compulsion to binge, while purging represents an attempt to expel the dependency associated with that need.

This explanation suggests that Freud viewed EDs as more than just physical conditions; he believed they could be traced to early psychological conflicts involving dependency, nurturing, and emotional bonds. According to Freud, these issues originate in what he termed the "oral stage" of development, which is the first phase of psychological growth typically occurring in infancy. During this stage, a child experiences the world primarily through their mouth—through actions like feeding and sucking, they receive both physical nourishment and emotional comfort. This period is essential for forming bonds, establishing trust, and learning self-soothing. When the child's need for care and security is adequately met, they develop a sense of trust and a healthy foundation for relationships and self-regulation in the future.

However, if a child's needs for nurturing and consistency are disrupted—through experiences like emotional neglect, inconsistent caregiving, or early separation from caregivers—these early needs may remain unmet. Such disruptions can create deep, often unconscious, psychological scars, influencing how the child will handle dependency, self-soothing, and intimacy later in life. Freud proposed that these unresolved needs from the oral stage can lead to an "oral fixation". In adulthood, this fixation might manifest as compulsive, oral-based behaviors, such as overeating, smoking, or other actions that provide a temporary sense of relief or comfort through the mouth.

In cases of EDs, such as BN or BED, the act of binging can be seen as an unconscious attempt to satisfy unmet emotional needs left over from these early developmental experiences. Freud's theory interprets binging to symbolically "fill" an internal void, temporarily easing feelings of emptiness or emotional hunger. The act of purging, as in BN, may represent a different but related struggle. Here, the individual attempts to reject this need for comfort and dependency by "cleansing" themselves of the very thing that brings temporary relief. This cycle reflects a deeper internal conflict: on one hand, there is a longing for connection, comfort, and nurturing, while on the other, there is a fear of dependency and a strong drive for autonomy and control.

Freud's theory suggests that EDs can be understood as reenactments of early dependency conflicts, with food symbolizing unmet emotional needs from childhood. Binging and purging behaviors become symbolic mechanisms for managing these unresolved issues, enabling the individual to temporarily satisfy emotional needs while simultaneously striving for independence. Consequently, the eating disorder evolves into more than just a physical condition; it becomes a psychological response to early experiences of nurturing, loss, and dependency.

Moreover, the psychoanalytic concept of splitting—where individuals view themselves or others in rigid "all-or-nothing" terms—plays a significant role in the emotional experiences of those with BN and BED. For these individuals, the act of binging often provides a temporary "good" experience, a feeling of fullness or satisfaction that contrasts sharply with the feelings of shame and disgust that follow. This polarized view—where binging is seen as both satisfying and shameful—mirrors the internal struggle between self-soothing and self-rejection. After binging, the individual may experience intense self-loathing and guilt, which they seek to expel through purging. This process reflects an internal splitting, where individuals alternate between viewing themselves as "in control" during purging and "out of control" during binging, reinforcing a cycle of self-criticism and emotional volatility (Kernberg, 2004).

From a psychoanalytic perspective, the self-punishment observed in BN and BED can be understood as a manifestation of internalized aggression and frustration. Individuals with these disorders may direct anger inward, blaming themselves for their unmet needs and perceived dependency. The binge-purge cycle serves as a means of self-discipline, where purging functions as a punitive act aimed at "purifying" or "cleansing" oneself of shame and dependency. This dynamic is often rooted in experiences where individuals felt their needs were unacceptable or burdensome to others, leading to self-directed anger and attempts to control these needs through extreme behaviors. By engaging in the binge-purge cycle, they unconsciously seek to control and suppress these needs, reinforcing a belief that they are undeserving of care or compassion.

In BED, which lacks the purging aspect, the conflict manifests differently. Here, individuals experience a continuous struggle with emotional emptiness, leading to recurrent binging episodes without the act of purging as a form of control. This creates an ongoing pattern of self-soothing through food, yet leaves the individual feeling trapped and isolated. The absence of purging highlights an internalized sense of defeat, where the individual feels powerless to expel or control the dependency associated with binging. This leads to feelings of shame and self-criticism, reinforcing the cycle of emotional eating as a form of temporary comfort amid unresolved emotional pain.

Psychoanalytic treatment for BN and BED focuses on uncovering these underlying emotional conflicts and helping individuals explore the unconscious meanings of their binge-purge cycle. Through therapy, individuals are guided to recognize how their eating behaviors symbolize unmet relational needs and struggles with autonomy. By bringing these unconscious motivations to light, psychoanalytic therapy offers a pathway for individuals to confront and resolve the emotional issues they have previously managed through disordered eating. The therapeutic process allows them to develop healthier ways of seeking connection and nurturing, helping them break free from the cycle of self-punishment and dependency on food.

In conclusion, psychoanalytic insights into BN and BED emphasize that these disorders extend beyond issues of eating alone. They reveal a web of unconscious conflicts related to self-worth, autonomy, and relational needs, highlighting how the binge-purge cycle serves as an attempt to manage complex emotional experiences. By examining these underlying motivations, psychoanalytic therapy helps individuals move toward a more integrated, adaptive way of addressing their emotional needs, fostering resilience, and facilitating meaningful connections that do not rely on disordered eating behaviors.

Psychoanalytic treatment for eating disorders: Integrating the fragmented self

Psychoanalytic treatment for EDs focuses on uncovering unconscious motivations by exploring the emotional conflicts underlying disordered eating behaviors. Through therapy, individuals gain insight into the symbolic meanings behind their eating patterns, revealing how restrictive eating, binging, and purging express unmet needs, identity struggles, and internalized societal ideals. By examining these unconscious motivations, psychoanalytic therapy helps individuals confront the emotional issues they manage through disordered eating behaviors, facilitating resolution and integration.

The therapeutic goal is to heal the fragmented self, bridging the gap between body and mind to foster healthier relationships with food, body, and identity. This process involves delving into personal history, relationships, and emotional experiences to understand how early attachment patterns and societal expectations have shaped self-concept. Through this journey, individuals are empowered to cultivate a stable self-image not reliant on external validation, rigid control, or unrealistic body ideals.

Psychoanalytic perspectives thus reveal the multifaceted nature of EDs, emphasizing that they are not simply issues of food or body image but reflect a web of unconscious motivations and symbolic meanings. These insights underscore how restrictive eating, binging, and purging behaviors are intertwined with themes of self-worth, control, autonomy, and relational needs. By grounding therapeutic interventions in this understanding, psychoanalysis offers a path that goes beyond symptom management, guiding individuals toward self-acceptance, psychological resilience, and an integrated sense of identity and emotional well-being.

Symbolism and metaphors in eating disorder symptoms

Peter Fonagy introduces the concept of "reflective function" as the psychological mechanism that enables mentalization, effectively making the mental capacities required for understanding oneself and others operational (Fonagy et al., 1998). Reflective functioning, often synonymous with mentalization, is the active demonstration of this complex psychological capacity, deeply intertwined with self-representation and the comprehension of oneself in relation to others. As a multi-dimensional skill, reflective functioning encompasses both self-reflective and interpersonal components, allowing individuals to differentiate internal mental and emotional experiences from external reality and to distinguish between imaginary or "pretend" experiences and those that are "real". This ability enables individuals to separate intrapersonal processes, such as thoughts, feelings, and emotions, from interpersonal communications and behaviors. In this framework, the mind is conceptualized as an agency—a dynamic entity arising from developmental processes and constructed capacities formed through interaction with the external world, particularly with significant others (Fonagy et al., 2002).

The development of mentalization, however, is not immediate. It is a progressive process that unfolds as individuals mature and accumulate life experiences. This gradual acquisition implies that the ability to understand and represent mental states in oneself and others is a developmental milestone that varies across individuals, shaped by unique life circumstances, relational dynamics, and developmental stages. The capacity to mentalize is grounded in early mental representations formed in infancy, significantly influenced by interactions with primary caregivers. In these foundational exchanges, the caregiver's responsiveness to the infant's emotional states creates a "mirroring" effect, which is crucial for establishing a secure attachment. Secure attachment, in turn, forms a stable foundation for mentalization, fostering a relational environment that encourages exploration and understanding of both one's own and others' emotions and thoughts. According to Fonagy et al. (2002), children with secure attachments are more likely to develop sophisticated mentalization abilities, which, over time, enable individuals to manage and reflect on their emotions effectively, establishing a basis for empathy, self-awareness, and healthy relationships.

An advanced component of mentalization, known as "mentalized affectivity", represents a mature capacity for regulating and interpreting one's own emotional experiences. Mentalized affectivity refers to an individual's ability to identify, reflect on, and assign personal meaning to their emotional states, promoting greater self-awareness and emotional resilience. This reflective skill allows individuals to uncover the subjective meanings behind their emotional experiences, deepening their understanding of themselves and their reactions to the world. Developing this capacity not only aids in processing complex emotions but also enhances one's ability to respond adaptively to various social and emotional situations. Mentalized affectivity thus underscores the essential role of mentalization as a cornerstone of psychological resilience, relational competence, and the development of empathy and compassion (Fonagy et al., 2002).

For individuals with mental health challenges, particularly those diagnosed with EDs, the development of a stable self-representation and coherent understanding of objects, including body image, can be particularly complex. Patients with EDs often struggle to form an adequate mental representation of both the self and external objects, with body image frequently becoming a primary source of psychological distress. This deficit in the representational world has been termed "mental anorexia" (Jeammet, 1984), indicating an interruption in the ability to mentally symbolize the self and body. Jeammet posits that symptomatic behaviors seen in EDs reflect a disruption in mental representation—not only of the body but also of external objects and relationships. This lack of symbolic representation interferes with the broader symbolization process, creating profound challenges in certain areas of the mind and affecting the individual's ability to process and accept their physical form. Consequently, this symbolic deficit complicates the pathway to mentalization, impacting body image and broader aspects of self-perception and identity.

While most individuals with EDs experience difficulties in mentalization and symbolization, some reflective capacity may still emerge. Psychoanalytic theory interprets the symptoms of EDs as symbolic and metaphorical representations of unresolved psychological conflicts. These symptoms extend beyond surface behaviors related to food or body image, acting instead as expressions of deep-seated, often unconscious, emotional struggles. Each symptom—whether it involves restrictive eating, binging, purging, or obsessive focus on body weight—serves as a symbolic manifestation of hidden fears, unresolved relational issues, and unexpressed desires.

In this psychoanalytic framework, EDs are seen as indirect expressions of psychological tensions that cannot be consciously acknowledged or directly verbalized. Instead, these tensions are symbolized through behaviors associated with eating, weight, and self-perception, serving as metaphors for underlying emotional states. For instance, restrictive eating may represent a desire for control in individuals who feel powerless in other life areas, while binge eating might symbolize attempts to fill an emotional void or soothe anxiety. Purging behaviors, conversely, may be seen as attempts to "cleanse" oneself of painful emotions, guilt, or unresolved conflicts, reflecting an individual's effort to expel distressing internal experiences.

Eating disorders (EDs) also reveal underlying deficits in the ability to symbolize embodied experiences rooted in early relational patterns. In individuals with AN, for instance, symbolization deficits are often expressed through a concrete, literal approach to meaning making, which can hinder the development of more abstract or symbolic ways to process emotions and self-perception. This inclination toward concreteness prevents these individuals from interpreting or integrating complex emotional experiences, leading them to rely on rigid behaviors and thoughts related to food and body. In contrast, those with BN frequently experience significant challenges in self-regulation, struggling to process and manage their embodied experiences. In both disorders, these unprocessed embodied experiences tend to remain largely unsymbolized, reflecting an inability to integrate these experiences into a cohesive self-concept (Charles, 2021).

This symbolic deficit contributes to the persistence of disordered eating patterns, as individuals lack the internal resources to interpret and make sense of their emotions meaningfully, leaving them caught in cycles of behavior that externalize their unresolved inner conflicts.

Psychoanalytic theory thus interprets eating disorders as a "symbolic language" through which individuals communicate unresolved emotional tensions, both to themselves and, unconsciously, to others. This symbolic expression highlights the extent to which EDs intertwine with an individual's self-concept, identity, and relationships. The behaviors associated with EDs bridge conscious experience and unconscious conflict, allowing individuals to externalize struggles that might otherwise remain deeply repressed and inaccessible.

By acknowledging these behaviors as symbolic, psychoanalytic practitioners seek to help individuals uncover the hidden emotional and relational issues underlying their EDs. The therapeutic objective is not merely symptom reduction but also fostering a deeper understanding of the unresolved conflicts that drive these behaviors. Through therapeutic exploration and enhanced mentalization, individuals can gradually access, articulate, and address these hidden emotional struggles, ultimately finding healthier, more direct ways to manage their inner lives and achieve psychological stability and self-acceptance.

For example, in AN, food restriction often symbolizes a desire to control one's body and life. This control may represent an attempt to assert autonomy, especially when individuals feel overwhelmed by external pressures or an intrusive family environment (Oldershaw et al., 2019). The refusal to eat can also symbolize self-denial or self-punishment, reflecting internalized guilt or feelings of unworthiness. Lacanian psychoanalyst Darian Leader suggests that the thin body in AN act as a metaphor for self-sufficiency and resistance to desires or needs perceived as dangerous or destabilizing (Tolunay İşlek, 2020).

As discussed in Chapter 4, from a Freudian perspective, the body in EDs can become a battleground for expressing internal conflicts among the Id (wishes and drives), Ego (reality), and Superego (moral conscience). In this framework, individuals may use their bodies to communicate unspoken conflicts. For instance, the desire for a "perfect" body in AN reflects a struggle to achieve an idealized self-image, shaped by societal pressures and the Superego's critical judgments (Freud, 1923). This idealized self represents self-worth, where the "perfect" body signifies acceptance and validation.

Many psychoanalysts, drawing on the myth of Narcissus, interpret EDs as manifestations of an individual's search for self-validation through physical appearance. In the myth, Narcissus becomes entranced by his own reflection in the water, unable to look away, ultimately leading to his demise. This symbolic fixation serves as a powerful metaphor for the way individuals with EDs often seek worth and identity through their physical form. In her seminal 1978 work, *"Fat is a Feminist Issue"* psychoanalyst Susie Orbach (1978) explores how societal pressures and internalized ideals lead individuals, particularly women, to use their bodies as the main avenue for self-definition. Orbach argues that the body becomes a canvas upon which personal struggles, desires, and societal expectations are projected, often resulting in disordered eating behaviours as attempts to conform to these external standards. She emphasizes that this focus on the body as a primary site of self-definition can overshadow other aspects of identity, leading to a cycle of self-evaluation and dissatisfaction. By understanding this dynamic, Orbach (1978) advocates for a shift towards embracing the body as it is, rather than as a project to be constantly modified to meet external ideals.

In his 1990 work, *"Individuation and Narcissism: The Psychology of the Self in Jung and Kohut"*, Mario Jacoby introduces the concept of the "narcissistic trap", describing how individuals can become ensnared in a perpetual cycle of self-evaluation and dissatisfaction, seeking self-worth through external validation (Jacoby, 2016a). Jacoby explains that this trap creates a fragile self-esteem, heavily reliant on others' perceptions and approval. Individuals caught in this cycle often experience profound feelings of shame and inadequacy whenever they fail to meet their own idealized standards. This dynamic is particularly evident in EDs, where the mirror becomes a symbolic space reflecting the ongoing struggle with self-perception and self-worth. Jacoby emphasizes that escaping the narcissistic trap requires developing a more stable, internalized sense of self that is less dependent on external validation.

In this framework, individuals become trapped in a relentless loop of self-assessment, with their self-worth rooted in how they appear to others. This dependency on physical reflection as a source of value leads to an inherently unstable self-image, fostering shame and feelings of inadequacy whenever one fails to meet idealized standards. Jacoby's concept of the "narcissistic trap" reveals how individuals with EDs, particularly those grappling with body-image issues, frequently find themselves in a cycle of seeking self-esteem through approval of their appearance. However, as Jacoby notes, the "ideal" image is constantly shifting and ultimately unattainable, making any sense of self-worth fleeting and dependent on momentary satisfaction with their reflection.

In this cycle, the mirror becomes not a source of reassurance but a site of intense scrutiny and self-criticism. Rather than reinforcing confidence, the mirror's reflection becomes a trigger for self-judgment and shame, highlighting perceived flaws and deepening self-criticism. Jacoby (2016b) suggests that this shame arises as individuals repeatedly fail to measure up to their internalized ideals, leading to feelings of exposure and deficiency. This shame is compounded by the belief that one's worth is tied exclusively to physical appearance, fostering a sense of fundamental unworthiness whenever their image falls short of self-imposed standards. Here, the mirror serves as both judge and jury, deepening the emotional divide between the self and a more genuine, stable sense of self-acceptance.

Self-esteem within this narcissistic framework becomes nearly impossible to establish authentically, as it is anchored to unstable, often unrealistic, physical ideals. Instead of developing a consistent sense of self-worth, individuals caught in the narcissistic trap experience their self-esteem as transient and conditional, constantly undermined by moments of perceived failure. As Jacoby underscores, "the narcissistic trap is an unending chase for validation, where the individual's reflection is both comfort and condemnation". This cycle perpetuates a fragile self-esteem that oscillates between fleeting pride and profound shame, trapping the individual in a continuous, often painful, struggle with self-perception (Jacoby, 2016a).

In summary, Jacoby's concept of the narcissistic trap offers a powerful lens through which to understand the psychological struggle in EDs. The relentless pursuit of an idealized image leaves individuals feeling empty and unfulfilled, ensnared in a cycle that erodes both their self-worth and emotional resilience.

Within this framework, the mirror becomes a powerful and often punishing metaphor, symbolizing the individual's relentless cycle of self-evaluation and dissatisfaction. Each gaze in the mirror represents a momentary search for validation but frequently ends in disappointment or self-criticism. As McDougall (1989) notes, "The individual is entrapped in a loop of external appraisal, where the image they see determines how they feel about themselves", leading to a fragile sense of self-worth that depends on physical conformity to internalized ideals of perfection (McDougall, 1989).

However, this dependency on their reflection seldom fosters a stable sense of identity. Instead, it leaves individuals trapped in a persistent struggle with self-perception. According to Bruch (1973), individuals with EDs "live with a body they do not inhabit comfortably, always seeking but never fully grasping a sense of self that feels genuine or whole". This endless pursuit reflects the essence of the Narcissus myth, where self-worth is fleeting, conditional, and ultimately unattainable. The body becomes a "mirror prison", where one's sense of self is as transient as the reflection they see, offering only a momentary illusion of self-acceptance that quickly fades, compelling them to re-engage with the mirror in an endless, ultimately self-destructive cycle.

In therapy, psychoanalysts often use symbols and metaphors to delve into the unconscious meanings behind eating disorder behaviors, aiming to uncover deeper emotional conflicts and hidden motivations. This metaphorical framework enables both therapist and patient to explore symptoms as symbols, bringing repressed emotions to the surface. In this context, therapeutic goals are not merely symptom-focused; they center on helping patients integrate these symbols into a more cohesive and self-accepting concept of themselves. By doing so, patients can begin to understand the emotional roots of their eating disorder behaviors and how these actions may be unconscious expressions of unmet psychological needs or unresolved conflicts.

For instance, recognizing restrictive eating as a symbolic rejection of dependency needs can open the door to exploring early relational dynamics and how these experiences shaped the patient's sense of self (Bemporad, 1996). Through understanding restrictive behaviors to assert control or independence, patients can start to make connections between their symptoms and childhood experiences of dependency, autonomy, and validation. This process invites the individual to see how their need for control over their body might echo deeper fears about vulnerability, fear of engulfment, or a lack of agency in their early relationships. By externalizing these inner conflicts, psychoanalytic therapy helps individuals disentangle the need for restrictive eating from the underlying desire for emotional autonomy, facilitating more adaptive ways to assert control and self-worth.

Moreover, the psychoanalytic approach interprets eating disorder symptoms as complex symbolic expressions that often revolve around core themes, such as control, nourishment, self-image, and autonomy. Each symptom becomes a metaphor: restrictive eating may represent a desire to contain overwhelming emotions; binge eating could symbolize attempts to fill an inner void; purging may be seen as an effort to "cleanse" oneself of unresolved guilt or internalized shame. These interpretations form the foundation of therapeutic work, helping individuals understand that their symptoms are not simply about food or body image but rather convey profound, often unacknowledged psychological struggles.

In this therapeutic framework, eating disorders like AN and BN are not merely symptoms but are symbolic acts—manifestations of deeper conflicts involving self-worth, control, and autonomy. For instance, the need to achieve an idealized thin body in AN can be seen as an unconscious struggle to attain perfection and self-sufficiency, reflecting an attempt to suppress desires and emotions perceived as dangerous or destabilizing. This pursuit of an idealized self is frequently shaped by societal expectations and internalized critical standards, highlighting the tension between the individual's need for self-control and their struggle for self-acceptance.

Similarly, in BN, binging and purging behaviors symbolize a psychological cycle of seeking emotional nourishment and then rejecting it. Here, binging can represent the yearning for comfort and closeness, while purging symbolizes an attempt to regain control and autonomy. These symbolic behaviors mirror the push-and-pull dynamic in relational patterns, where individuals oscillate between longing for connection and the need for emotional independence. Understanding these behaviors as metaphors for unmet needs helps patients explore and address the unresolved issues that fuel their symptoms, creating a foundation for more meaningful change.

From a psychoanalytic perspective, the symbolic interpretation of EDs illuminates the ways in which these behaviors serve as a "language" for expressing unconscious conflicts. Through metaphors, patients can begin to articulate feelings they may not have had the words or awareness to express before. In therapy, helping individuals recognize and integrate these symbols into their understanding of themselves offers a path toward reconciling internal conflicts, ultimately fostering self-acceptance and psychological resilience.

Bibliography

Bemporad, J. R. (1996). Self-starvation through the ages: Reflections on the pre-history of anorexia nervosa. *International Journal of Eating Disorders*, 19(3): 217–237.

Bruch, H. (1973). *Eating Disorders: Obesity, Anorexia Nervosa and the Person Within*. New York: Basic Books.

Charles, M. (2021). Meaning, metaphor, and metabolization: The case of eating disorders. *The American Journal of Psychoanalysis*, 81(4): 444–466.

Dicu, A. M., Cuc, L. D., Rad, D., Rusu, A. I., Feher, A., Isac, F. L., ... and Barbu, F. S. (2024). Exploration of food attitudes and management of eating behavior from a psycho-nutritional perspective. *Healthcare*, 12(19): 1934.

Fonagy, P., Target, M., Steele, H., and Steele, M. (1998). *Reflective-functioning Manual Version 5 for Application to Adult Attachment Interviews*.

Fonagy, P., Gergely, G., Jurist, E. L., and Target, M. (2002). *Affect Regulation, Mentalization and the Development of the Self*. New York: Other Press.

Fraiberg, S. (1982). Pathological defenses in infancy. *The Psychoanalytic Quarterly*, 51 (4): 612–635.

Freud, S. (1917). On transformations of instinct as exemplified in anal erotism. *The Standard Edition of the Complete Psychological Works of Sigmund Freud, (17)*. London: The Hogarth Press, 125–133 (1986 edition).

Freud, S. (1923). The Ego and the Id. *The Standard Edition of the Complete Psychological Works of Sigmund Freud, (19)*. London: The Hogarth Press, 3–66 (1991 edition).

Glashouwer, K. A., Bloot, L., Veenstra, E. M., Franken, I. H., and de Jong, P. J. (2014). Heightened sensitivity to punishment and reward in anorexia nervosa. *Appetite*, 75: 97–102.

Green, A. (1983). El ideal: Mesura y desmesura. *Revista de Psicoanálisis*, 45(1): 9–39.

Harrison, A., O'Brien, N., Lopez, C., and Treasure, J. (2010). Sensitivity to reward and punishment in eating disorders. *Psychiatry Research*, 177(1–2): 1–11.

Jacoby, M. (2016a). *Individuation and Narcissism: The Psychology of Self in Jung and Kohut*. London: Routledge.

Jacoby, M. (2016b). *Shame and the Origins of Self-esteem: A Jungian Approach*. London: Routledge.

Jeammet, P. (1984). L'anorexie mentale. *Encyclo. Med. Chir. Psychiatrie Vol. 3, 37350*: A10 et A15; 2. París: Elsevier.

Jeammet, P. (1992). *La Boulimie, Monographies Revue Francoise de Psychanalyse*. PUF1992. Spanish version: Las conductas bulímicas como modalidad de acomodamiento de las disregulaciones narcisistas y objetales. *Psicoanálisis con Niños y Adolescentes*: n/A, 1993, (5): 44–63.

Kernberg, O. F. (2004). A technical approach to eating disorders in patients with borderline personality organization. *Aggressivity, Narcissism, and self-destructiveness in the psychotherapeutic Relationships: New developments in the psychopathology and psychotherapy of severe personality disorders*. New Haven, CT and London: Yale University Press, 205–219 (chapter 13).

Kernberg, P. F., Weiner, A. S. and Bardenstein, K. K. (2000). *Personality Disorders in Children and Adolescents*. New York: Basic Books.

McDougall, J. (1989). *Theaters of the Body*. London: Free Association.

Oldershaw, A., Startup, H., and Lavender, T. (2019). Anorexia nervosa and a lost emotional self: A psychological formulation of the development, maintenance, and treatment of anorexia nervosa. *Frontiers in Psychology*, 10(219): 1–22.

Orbach, S. (1978). *Fat is a Feminist Issue*. New York: Hamlyn.

Persano, H. L. (1997). Reflexiones en torno a los conceptos de Disociación y Escisión en la obra de Sigmund Freud. *Revista de Psicoanálisis*, 54(3): 773–791.

Persano, H. L. (2005). Abordagem psicodinâmica do paciente com trastornos alimentares. In C. L. Eizirik, R. W. Aguiar, and S. S. Schestatsky (eds.) *Psicoterapia de Orientação Analítica: Fundamentos Teóricos e Clínicos*. Porto Alegre: Artmed Editora, 674–688 (chapter 49).

Recalcati, M. (2013). *Escritos Sobre Anorexia*. Argentina: Editorial Los Robles.

Roudinesco, E. (2003). The mirror stage: An obliterated archive. *The Cambridge Companion to Lacan*. Cambridge: Cambridge University Press, 25–34.

Schwartz, H. J. (1986). Bulimia: Psychoanalytic perspectives. *Journal of the American Psychoanalytic Association*, 34(2): 439–462.

Tolunay İşlek, S. (2020). *Mutilated Bodies in Search for Perfection: A Psychoanalytic Analysis of Darren Aronofsky's Pi, Black Swan and Mother*. Istanbul: Istanbul Bilgi University, Institute of Social Sciences.

Von Wyl, A. (2000). What anorexic and bulimic patients have to tell: The analysis of patterns of unconscious conflict expressed in stories about everyday events. *European Journal of Psychotherapy, Counselling & Health*, 3(3): 375–388.

Williams, G. (1997). Reflections on some dynamics of eating disorders "no entry" defences and foreign bodies. *International Journal of Psychology*, 78: 927–941.

6 Early development and family dynamics

Impact of early attachment and family environment on eating disorder development

Protective shields and attachment

Freud underscores the importance of the nervous system in controlling impulses from the external world. He describes the psychic apparatus, governed by the pleasure-displeasure principle, as needing to expel unpleasant stimuli—a process foundational to the mechanism of projection. Projection, which Freud defines as an essential mental function that later evolves into a defense mechanism, allows individuals to rid themselves of overwhelming stimuli. Human mental functioning operates according to two primary principles: initially dominated by the pleasure-displeasure principle, later evolving to incorporate the reality principle (Freud, 1911). Functioning under the reality principle marks a developmental milestone, where the Ego sacrifices immediate gratification in favor of long-term satisfaction. In *"Beyond the Pleasure Principle"* (1920), Freud revisits this concept, emphasizing the need to progressively integrate elements of the external world to understand external stimuli's nature and fate better and to direct actions accordingly. Thus, reality becomes a core part of the individual's representational world. Freud underscores the necessity for living beings to shield themselves from intense stimuli. This protective function, which he describes as a "protective shield against stimuli" or an "anti-stimulus barrier", safeguards the individual from potentially overwhelming external forces (Freud, 1920). However, Freud's model predominantly focuses on intrapsychic metapsychology, leading us to question how environmental influences—particularly parental figures— play a role in this protective function.

Attachment theory: Expanding Freud's framework

Attachment theory, as originally developed by John Bowlby (1979) and expanded by others such as Mary Ainsworth (1989) expands Freud's

DOI: 10.4324/9781032724997-6

concept by emphasizing the significance of early attachment relationships in developing a child's capacity to manage and internalize experiences. The impact of early attachment and family environment on the development of EDs is profound and multifaceted, particularly when viewed through a psychoanalytic lens. Attachment theory suggests that the nature of early attachment relationships, particularly between parental caregiver (often mother) and child, forms the foundation for interpersonal dynamics, self-perception, and the ability to regulate emotions throughout life. In the context of EDs, disruptions or deficits in these early attachments are seen as significant contributors to pathology. Specifically, insecure or disorganized attachments may lead to internalized feelings of inadequacy, anxiety, and a heightened need for control, often manifesting in maladaptive coping mechanisms centered around food and body image.

Attachment theory stresses that a secure attachment with caregivers allows a child to process and modulate emotional and sensory experiences safely (Bowlby, 1979). The caregiver becomes an "external regulatory function", aiding the child in managing stimuli from both internal and external sources, thereby promoting psychological resilience. This secure attachment provides the foundation upon which the reality principle can develop, enabling the child to tolerate delayed gratification, frustration, and emotional regulation.

John Bowlby's seminal work, "Maternal Care and Mental Health", (Bowlby, 1951) underscores the critical role of a mother's presence in a child's emotional and psychological development. Bowlby posited that consistent maternal care is essential for healthy mental health outcomes in children, emphasizing that disruptions in this bond can lead to long-term cognitive, social, and emotional difficulties.

Bowlby's attachment theory further elaborates on the importance of the family unit in safeguarding children's well-being. He introduced the concept of monotropy, suggesting that infants form a primary attachment to one caregiver, typically the mother, which serves as a secure base for exploring the world and developing trust. This primary attachment is crucial for the child's sense of security and overall development.

The family environment, according to Bowlby, functions as a protective factor against potential psychological disturbances. A nurturing family setting provides the necessary support for children to form secure attachments, which are foundational for their emotional regulation and social competence. Conversely, a lack of maternal care or a disrupted family structure can lead to attachment issues, potentially resulting in behavioral problems and mental health challenges later in life.

In summary, Bowlby's research highlights the indispensable role of maternal care and a stable family environment in protecting and promoting children's mental health. His theories have significantly influenced contemporary understanding of child development and the importance of early relationships in shaping psychological well-being.

Under normal circumstances, the family structure acts as an anti-stimulus barrier for the infant, filtering external stimuli and regulating the release of impulses arising from within. This role, primarily fulfilled by parental figures but also reinforced by the extended family, as well as peers, assists the child in adapting to the reality principle, shaping their sense of reality, judgment, and emotional resilience. Parental figures, through stable and attuned caregiving, offer a "safe haven" and "secure base", buffering the child from excessive stimulation and helping the child navigate and integrate distressing experiences in a manageable way. In this framework, attachment is not only a developmental need but also a vital mechanism for emotional and sensory regulation, enabling the child to distinguish between self and other, internal and external (Persano and Goldberg, 1995).

Object relation theory

Psychoanalytic theory, particularly object relations theory, provides insight into how early family environments influence an individual's emotional life and sense of identity. In families where primary caregivers provide inconsistent emotional support or have a history of overprotection, critical communication, or enmeshment, children often struggle to develop a secure sense of self.

According to Donald Winnicott (1965), the absence of a stable and nurturing foundation during childhood can profoundly impact an individual's sense of self-worth and identity, leaving them vulnerable to psychological difficulties, including the development of EDs. Winnicott emphasized the critical role of the family in fostering a "holding environment", where the child feels safe and supported in their emotional and developmental growth. Without this secure foundation, children may struggle to form a cohesive sense of self, increasing the likelihood of maladaptive coping mechanisms later in life (Bollas, 1982).

From the perspective of Ego development, primary caregiving relationships significantly shape a child's ability to regulate emotions and establish self-worth. When these relationships fail to provide adequate support or attunement, children may resort to controlling behaviors—such as restrictive eating, binge eating, or purging—as compensatory strategies to manage emotional dysregulation and feelings of inadequacy (Bruch, 1973). These behaviors serve as substitutes for the emotional stability that was absent during their formative years, reflecting an attempt to reclaim a sense of control and agency in the face of internal turmoil.

Winnicott's (1960, 1971) concept of the "true self" versus the "false self" further illuminates this dynamic. In environments where the child's needs are consistently unmet or dismissed, they may develop a "false self", shaped by external expectations and defensive adaptations rather than authentic self-expression. For individuals with EDs, this disconnects between the true self and false self often manifests in the compulsion to regulate the body as a means of managing emotional chaos and external pressures. The family's role, therefore, becomes paramount in creating conditions that allow the true self to emerge and thrive, rather than retreating into restrictive and self-punitive behaviors.

This perspective highlights the intricate interplay between family dynamics, emotional development, and the emergence of EDs. By addressing these foundational disruptions in the therapeutic process, clinicians can help individuals rebuild a sense of self-worth and emotional regulation, ultimately facilitating a pathway to recovery.

Pathological identifications and eating disorders

Freud (1923) elaborates on the significance of identification processes within the family. He posits that early object investments—namely, the effects of early identifications formed in infancy—are universal and enduring. He emphasizes that the Ideal of the Ego, the most significant of these identifications, in patients with EDs, is deeply rooted in the primary caregivers of the individual's early history, making identification a group-based, shared process. Through attachment, the child internalizes parental figures as stable, nurturing presences, integrating aspects of them into their own Ego structure. This process fosters emotional regulation, trust, and an understanding of reality based on a sense of security and continuity provided by the family. The family, as the primary belonging group, thus functions as a filter for external stimuli, playing a central role for the infant who interacts with reality primarily through the family's lens. This "filtering" mechanism is reinforced through identification with primary caregivers, as each family transmits its values, ethics, and relational approaches. Embedded within a secondary social and cultural group—the surrounding societal—the family both identifies with this context and uses it to facilitate the projection and introjection of aggression, helping maintain family cohesion. Thus, each child has a primary belonging group (the family) and a secondary one (the broader social environment), both crucial in shaping personality development. Bowlby's attachment theory highlights that a secure attachment within the primary group fosters self-worth, confidence, and curiosity as well as autonomy, laying the foundation for healthy relationships with the secondary group and promoting adaptive ways of relating to external reality (Bowlby, 1979).

According to García Badaracco (1990), individuals acquire identifications that support the healthy structuring of the psychic apparatus. When the family and social environment foster what he terms "normogenic identifications" family members are better equipped to confront life's inevitable crises. Normogenic identifications, critical for healthy Ego development, contrast with pathological identifications, which result in psychic disintegration and have a pathogenic impact on the individual. When the family structure fails to operate as an anti-stimulus barrier, the child becomes exposed to potentially traumatic levels of psychological energy, hindering normal psychic development.

Psychoanalytic perspectives also emphasize the role of "introjection", a concept central to both Freud's theories and object relations theory. Introjection refers to the process by which individuals internalize the attitudes, beliefs, and anxieties of their caregivers, often forming the roots of a self-critical inner voice. For example, in families where there is a high focus on appearance, weight, or perfectionism, children may introject these ideals, leading to harsh self-judgments and the belief that self-worth is conditional upon physical appearance or the achievement of perfection (Espina et al., 2001). This internalized drive for extreme control over one's body often comes at the expense of physical and mental health, reinforcing the destructive cycle of eating disorder behaviors.

Family dynamics and the anti-stimulus function

In families of individuals with EDs, for example, this anti-stimulus function may be inadequate, failing to buffer the child from external pressures—particularly societal ideals regarding body image—that disrupt the development of a stable agency of Ideal of the Ego. These young individuals are thus left vulnerable to internal conflicts, often manifested in disorders centered around control and self-worth, rooted in unmet attachment needs and an internalized sense of inadequacy. Disruptions in attachment can result in a fragmented sense of self and reliance on maladaptive defenses, such as splitting or projection, to cope with anxiety and instability. In this view, the family's role is to provide both a physical and emotional "protective shield", offering the stability and predictability needed for healthy development. However, when the attachment bond is insecure due to an affective loss or dysfunctional families, children may develop hypersensitivity to external stimuli and struggle with impulse control, often compensating through control over their bodies or eating behaviors to manage internal distress (Bowlby, 1973).

Secure attachment fosters an environment where the child learns to navigate reality, balance internal impulses, and tolerate frustration. In contrast, an insecure attachment environment, lacking this protective function, leaves the child vulnerable to emotional dysregulation and maladaptive coping mechanisms that impact long-term mental health. For individuals with EDs, these attachment deficits often reveal themselves as struggles with self-control, worth, and an enduring need to impose order on a fragmented inner world.

Sociocultural influences on attachment and development

The concept of infants' secondary belonging groups (Persano and Ventura, 1994) highlights how cultural norms and values shape the development of the self. These influences, reflective of the era and environment, often become amplified during times of societal crisis or transformation. Such external pressures can introduce conflicting values, expectations, and ideals into the family system, placing significant strain on an individual's developing sense of identity.

Freud (1923) recognized that human development necessitates a prolonged period of dependency, which Margaret Mahler expanded upon by emphasizing its critical role in individuation. Mahler described the process of differentiation as one in which the child, initially enmeshed with the caregiver, gradually develops a separate and individuated self. It is within this dependency framework that initial object relations are formed, laying the foundation for the individual's relational style, emotional regulation, and coping mechanisms (Mahler, Pine, and Bergman, 1975).

Mahler further argued that without attachment, an infant would not survive, and severely insecure attachment places children at a heightened risk for developing serious psychological disorders. Development, therefore, relies on sustained attachment to a responsive and responsible caregiver. For Mahler, continued attachment to the primary object is intrinsic to the separation-individuation process, which fosters the emergence of autonomy, independence, and a cohesive identity (Mahler, Pine, and Bergman, 1975).

While attachment theory emphasizes the critical importance of secure bonds between infants and caregivers, it does not fully account for the essential development of separateness. As Blum (2004) points out, the separation-individuation process is equally crucial in promoting autonomy and individuality. The balance between attachment and the development of separateness is key to fostering a healthy sense of self, allowing individuals to navigate relationships and societal pressures with resilience and authenticity.

Modern family structures and evolving vulnerabilities

By offering consistent nurturing and boundaries, the family creates a stable environment that allows for healthy individuation. However, difficulties can arise when the family environment becomes destabilized due to crises such as parental loss, divorce, or the emergence of pathological factors within the parental dyad. Pathogenic circumstances—abandonment, neglect, or various forms of abuse (physical, psychological, or sexual)—can create lasting disruptions within the child's developing psyche, particularly during critical stages of identity formation. Such disruptions compromise the child's capacity to form a cohesive self, affecting their ability to navigate external reality with confidence and resilience. The significance of family stability is especially notable in the context of EDs, where identity and control issues are common. An unstable or traumatic family environment, lacking a consistent emotional "anti-stimulus barrier", can leave young individuals vulnerable to the pressures and ideals of the external world.

The role of family in eating disorders development

Eating disorders (EDs) often emerge in these environments as maladaptive responses to unprocessed distress or unmet attachment needs, with food and body image becoming substitutes for emotional regulation and identity control. Within these dynamics, the family may inadvertently reinforce distorted perceptions, especially when cultural ideals around beauty and achievement dominate familial values and expectations. The socio-cultural framework in which the family is embedded further complicates these dynamics. Prevailing societal trends—such as the idealization of thinness, success, and independence—can clash with the familial values that parents bring from their own histories. This inherited legacy, including ethical, aesthetic, and cultural ideals, must be reconfigured within each new generation, particularly during adolescence. This period of heightened vulnerability and self-exploration coincides with increased susceptibility to external influences, as adolescents struggle to balance familial expectations with broader societal messages around identity, appearance, and worth.

In the modern context, families of adolescents with EDs may unconsciously endorse or exacerbate societal ideals by placing high value on perfectionism, appearance, or control. In such cases, adolescents may internalize these ideals as components of their self-worth, equating their value with physical appearance or achievement, leading to a fragile Ego structure dependent on external validation. This focus can intensify a split between the adolescent's sense of self and their perceived "ideal self", heightening vulnerability to EDs as they seek to attain an unrealistic standard through control of their bodies. Attachment theory sheds further light on these dynamics, illustrating that when the primary caregivers can provide consistent, secure attachments, children develop a secure base from which to explore and a haven to return to. This attachment security allows for flexible exploration of external values and ideals, enabling adolescents to incorporate cultural influences without losing a core sense of self. However, when the attachment relationship is insecure, individuals may be more susceptible to the pressures of societal ideals, relying on external validation to feel a sense of worth.

Adolescents with insecure attachments, especially those in families lacking cohesion or stability, may be at heightened risk for depressive and anxiety disorders (Kerns and Brumariu, 2014); (Sund and Wichstrøm,

2002) as well as EDs (Tasca and Balfour, 2014). In these cases, adolescents often struggle to form a stable sense of self, turning to behaviors like controlling food intake or obsessing over body image as a means of establishing identity and control. When families do not provide the essential structure, validation, or support, the adolescent may develop a deep-seated sense of inadequacy. In response to these gaps, they attempt to manage their internal insecurities and anxieties through behaviors that seem to offer control over their circumstances—such as eating restrictions, weight obsession, or compulsive exercise. This control represents an unconscious effort to cope with conflicting internalized messages or to fill the void left by an absent or inconsistent parental presence.

The impact of modern societies in modern families and arising pathological conditions and eating disorders in their offspring

The pervasive influence of social media further compounds these challenges, exposing adolescents to idealized standards of beauty and success. This exposure often amplifies existing insecurities, reinforcing the need to seek validation through physical appearance or external approval. For families of adolescents with EDs, it becomes crucial to foster open communication and cultivate an environment where value-based identities—grounded in qualities beyond physical appearance—are encouraged. By supporting self-worth through achievements, personal values, and relational strengths rather than appearance alone, families can help adolescents develop a more resilient and stable self-image, reducing the compulsion to find control or validation through disordered eating behaviors.

Contemporary families are increasingly shaped by the crises inherent in the complex socio-cultural landscape of the late 20th and early 21st centuries. Mass media has become a pervasive force, infiltrating homes daily as a kind of "virtual family member", profoundly altering the dynamics of direct family communication. The depth and quality of emotional bonds are often eroded, replaced by a more superficial, image-based connection. Life is increasingly organized around visual immediacy and digital screens, where virtual reality often overshadows the warmth and intimacy of human interaction. This shift toward a visual and virtual culture weakens the meaningful exchanges essential for emotional depth, mutual understanding, and support within families.

Economic globalization, forced migrations, wars, and racial tensions continue to destabilize families, leaving them uprooted from familiar cultural practices and struggling to find stability. The loss of customs and traditions—exacerbated by these ongoing global crises—often leads to cultural clashes within families, where generational differences become pronounced, and shared values are no longer guaranteed (Persano and Ventura, 1994). This disruption significantly impacts attachment systems within families, as children and adolescents often feel disconnected from the stable, predictable environments they need for healthy emotional and psychological development.

The relevance of these insights, originally articulated 30 years ago, has only grown in the face of modern geopolitical crises. For instance, the Ukraine-Russia war has triggered one of the largest forced migrations in Europe since World War II, displacing millions of families. This displacement has fractured traditional familial and community ties, forcing parents and children to navigate new cultural contexts that challenge their sense of identity and belonging. Similarly, ongoing conflicts in the Middle East have created a prolonged refugee crisis, where families face the dual burden of escaping violence while adapting to often unwelcoming host countries, further straining their attachment systems and cultural identity.

In Africa, political instability, dictatorial regimes, and economic hardship have driven massive migrations, both internally and toward Europe. Migrants fleeing persecution or seeking better opportunities face not only physical risks but also the emotional toll of leaving behind cultural traditions and family support systems. For children, these journeys often mean interrupted education and the loss of foundational attachment figures, while parents grapple with providing stability in unfamiliar and often hostile environments.

In Latin America, the exodus from countries facing political and economic crises, such as Venezuela and Nicaragua, has disrupted millions of families. Many migrants head to neighboring countries, Europe, or the United States, often enduring perilous journeys. Children in these situations experience profound instability, as their parents struggle to rebuild lives amidst economic insecurity and cultural disorientation. The loss of extended family networks, coupled with exposure to xenophobia or systemic discrimination, deepens the cultural and psychological challenges faced by these families.

These modern dynamics reinforce the enduring relevance of Persano and Ventura's (1994) observations. The fragmentation of cultural identity and the destabilization of familial attachment systems are amplified by contemporary crises, leaving children and parents vulnerable to emotional and relational disconnection. Addressing these challenges requires a multifaceted approach that acknowledges the psychological toll of migration and displacement while fostering spaces for cultural continuity, integration, and emotional resilience.

In this global context, the role of mental health professionals, educators, and policymakers is critical. Interventions that strengthen family bonds, provide culturally sensitive support, and promote the preservation of traditions amidst change are essential for mitigating the long-term impacts of displacement. By bridging past insights with present realities, we can better understand and address the complex interplay between global crises, cultural identity, and family dynamics.

Attachment theory highlights the importance of a secure base, where caregivers provide consistency, safety, and a reliable emotional connection for the child. In these modern circumstances, however, traditional family roles have shifted dramatically. The image of the male as protector and primary provider—a central figure in Freud's early theories of family structure—is less prevalent as women increasingly participate in the workforce and share financial responsibilities. As both parents spend more time outside the home and engage in complex, individualized activities, individual achievements often overshadow shared family interests. This fragmentation reflects a postmodern influence on family dynamics, where the focus on personal accomplishment can detract from the collective support systems traditionally provided by the family.

This shift in family roles and priorities fosters relationships with a more narcissistic quality, characterized by a self-focused, image-driven interaction style. This development, particularly among adolescents, replaces the deeper, more complex, family-centered connections that Freud associated with oedipal and attachment bonds. The oedipal conflicts, once central to psychoanalytic theory and grounded in the structure of traditional family dynamics, are now weakened by the changing landscape of family roles. As traditional family structures transform, new and diverse family configurations emerge, reflecting an evolving socio-cultural backdrop where attachment patterns can become more fragile or insecure.

In today's culture, adolescents are increasingly drawn into a bidimensional mode of interaction, engaging more with visual media than with narratives, which are crucial for the development of fantasy, empathy, and complex thought. This reliance on the visual and immediate, compounded by sensory overload from media bombardment, can create a fragmented sense of self, impacting personality development and attachment formation. Instead of building a coherent internal narrative, young people often experience multiple and conflicting impressions of reality, influenced by idealized and sometimes unrealistic representations in media. As a result, the attachment process, which requires consistency, stability, and emotional presence, becomes more challenging, with adolescents experiencing relationships that are less about depth and more about image.

These contemporary family dynamics and media influences pose significant challenges to attachment formation and emotional security. Attachment theory posits that children require a "secure base" for healthy development—a dependable environment with emotionally available caregivers. However, the current socio-cultural environment, marked by economic pressures, fragmented family roles, and a pervasive media presence, can make it difficult for families to provide this base consistently. Without this foundation, adolescents may struggle to develop a stable sense of self, often compensating for emotional insecurities by turning to external validation and appearances, further heightening their vulnerability to issues such as low self-esteem, anxiety, and eating disorders.

In summary, the modern family faces profound socio-cultural challenges that impact attachment processes, altering how individuals relate to one another and how adolescents construct their sense of identity. The traditional family structures that once supported the development of secure attachments are giving way to new forms and values, where individual achievements and media-driven ideals replace shared values and deep, interpersonal connection. This cultural shift not only redefines family roles but also disrupts the consistency and stability required for secure attachments, leaving adolescents more susceptible to insecurity, self-esteem struggles, and mental health challenges.

A changing world from early 20th century to early 21st century in families

In *"The Ego and the Id"*, Freud (1923) observes that multiple, conflicting identifications within the Ego can lead to Ego fragmentation, and by extension, to a fragmented sense of self. Severe personality disorders have become increasingly prominent features of late 20th and early 21st-century society, shaped by social and economic crises that disrupt family stability and coherence. When families are destabilized in this way, they lose their capacity to support the developing child's ego amidst internal and external pressures, weakening their protective role in managing life crises, such as the onset of sexuality during puberty and adolescence. This disruption impedes the formation of a cohesive inner world, leading to a fragmented and often distorted perception of reality. In fractured family structures, the process of healthy identification is obstructed, resulting in increased clinical manifestations of risky behaviors among young people who may resort to extreme measures to escape psychic pain.

This fragmentation hinders the separation-individuation process essential for developing individuality, as outlined by Mahler, Pine, and Bergman, (1975). Without a stable family foundation, adolescents face challenges in establishing their identity, often leading to identity diffusion and compensatory over-adaptation. Parental constancy is crucial for transforming early libidinal investments into stable structural identifications within the psychic apparatus. However, postmodern family structures, with their limited contact and exchange among family members, complicate identification processes for children. Left vulnerable to influences beyond the primary and secondary identifications typically provided by intimate family groups, children struggle to build a stable identity foundation.

When the family ceases to function as a filtering system for external influences, the child's psychic apparatus encounters disturbances on three levels. First, from an economic perspective, the system becomes overwhelmed by excess tension, unable to process or release it adequately. Second, from a topical perspective, conflicting internal representations remain unintegrated, creating cognitive and emotional dissonance. Finally, from a structural perspective, these unresolved conflicts lead to splits within the Ego and Self.

The weakening of family structures and the resulting impact on a child's psychological development have contributed significantly to the rise in severe personality disorders, particularly those marked by identity diffusion—a defining feature of borderline personality organization (BPO), as noted by Kernberg (1984). When families are unable to provide a stable and cohesive environment, children often experience disruptions in their individuation process and fragile identity formation, creating vulnerabilities to both personality disorders and psychosomatic conditions, including EDs. These disorders frequently emerge in family contexts where the lack of secure connections leaves adolescents seeking control, validation, or emotional relief in maladaptive ways, with disordered eating patterns serving as symbolic expressions of their internal struggles with identity and autonomy.

This modern understanding of family dynamics contrasts sharply with the mid-20th-century observations of Mara Selvini Palazzoli (1974), who examined family patterns in patients with AN. Palazzoli's work identified families of AN patients as characterized by high levels of control, rigidity, and enmeshment, with strong expectations of compliance and loyalty among family members. In these families, conflicts often revolved around maintaining control and cohesion, with the family unit operating as a tightly bound system resistant to change or external influence.

Palazzoli's analysis (Selvini Palazzoli,1974), emphasized the restrictive and overly cohesive nature of these families, suggesting that such dynamics contributed to the development of AN by limiting the individual's autonomy and capacity for self-expression. However, issues such as emotional trauma, neglect, and abuse were notably less central to her profile. This focus on structural dynamics within the family reflected the prevailing psychoanalytic and systemic theories of the time, which emphasized family interactions as key determinants of psychological outcomes.

In contrast, contemporary research increasingly identifies attachment disruptions and emotional neglect as significant factors in the etiology of EDs. Today's studies underscore how a lack of emotional nurturance, coupled with insecure or disrupted attachment systems, profoundly impacts the development of self-worth, emotional regulation, and identity. This shift reflects broader changes in the understanding of psychological disorders, with greater emphasis on the interplay between emotional deprivation and relational trauma in shaping vulnerability to conditions like AN.

While Palazzoli's work provided valuable insights into the rigid and enmeshed structures of families affected by AN, modern perspectives offer a more nuanced understanding of the role of attachment and emotional care. Together, these viewpoints highlight the evolving nature of family dynamics in the study of EDs, from structural and behavioral patterns to the deeper emotional underpinnings that shape individual development.

Today's research offers a more nuanced understanding, showing a wider range of familial disruptions that predispose individuals to EDs. Factors such as trauma, emotional neglect, and a lack of secure, supportive relationships have become focal points, highlighting the role of early relational experiences and attachment dynamics in developing vulnerabilities to disordered eating. In contemporary families, marked by economic pressures, shifting parental roles, and the pervasive influence of media, there is often an erosion of the stability and emotional availability necessary for healthy child development. These conditions foster attachment insecurities, as children may lack the dependable emotional foundation required for secure self-concept formation.

This shift from rigid control to emotional neglect reflects broader socio-cultural changes impacting family dynamics. Where the families Palazzoli studied in the 1970s (Selvini Palazzoli, 1974) demonstrated tightly knit but overly controlled environments, today's families face fragmentation, where attachment-related issues and emotional instability have come to the forefront. The current emphasis on trauma and emotional neglect underscores the critical role that secure attachments, and emotionally supportive relationships play in healthy development. Insecure or disrupted attachments can lead to compensatory behaviors, as adolescents seek validation or autonomy through control over their physical self, resulting in disordered EDs as symbolic expressions of their need for stability and self-cohesion.

In sum, this evolution in understanding family dynamics—from Palazzoli's focus on control and rigidity to today's recognition of attachment insecurity and trauma—reflects a significant shift in how researchers and clinicians view the roots of EDs. As modern family structures change, so do the psychological landscapes of adolescents within them, making clear that supportive, secure relationships are crucial in buffering against identity diffusion and maladaptive coping mechanisms like disordered eating. This deeper awareness of attachment and emotional nurturance highlights the need for therapeutic approaches that address not only the symptoms but also the relational and emotional roots of these disorders.

The comparison between the two eras highlights a shift in understanding the family's role in EDs. In the 1970s, families of patients with AN were typically characterized as overprotective or excessively involved, often fostering enmeshed relationships. In contrast, contemporary research depicts families marked by emotional distance or disruption, where children may experience emotional neglect, lack of validation, or even trauma. This shift reflects the impact of modern socio-economic and cultural stressors on family dynamics, increasing children's vulnerability to attachment insecurities and emotional voids that may later manifest as EDs.

Insecure attachment and emotionally fraught family dynamics

Attachment theory sheds light on these findings, illustrating how early attachment experiences shape emotional regulation, self-perception, and coping mechanisms. Children raised in environments where caregivers fail to provide consistent emotional support and responsiveness are at higher risk of developing insecure attachments, which can manifest as difficulties in regulating emotions and developing a stable sense of self. Recent studies have highlighted a connection between anxious-insecure attachment patterns and poor self-esteem regulation. These findings suggest that when addressing body image concerns, clinicians should also consider insecure attachment patterns and their impact on affect regulation (Keating et al., 2013).

These vulnerabilities are particularly relevant to EDs, where maladaptive behaviors around food and body image often emerge as compensatory responses to unmet emotional needs and unresolved attachment conflicts. In cases where caregivers are neglectful or emotionally distant, children may struggle with feelings of worthlessness and an underlying sense of emotional deprivation, leading them to seek validation through external measures, including controlling their physical appearance.

Studies have shown a specific intergenerational transmission of disordered eating behaviors, indicating that children of mothers with EDs are at a higher risk of developing similar issues. For instance, research by Stein et al. (1994) reveals that mothers with ED diagnoses tend to be more intrusive with their infants during mealtimes and play. These mothers are also more likely to express negative emotions toward their infants during mealtimes, a setting that involves nourishment and bonding, but not necessarily during play. This pattern of intrusion and negative emotion around eating may contribute to an insecure attachment style in the child, where mealtimes are associated with emotional tension, control, and a lack of nurturance. This early relational experience can foster a disrupted relationship with food and self-regulation, laying a foundation for the development of eating disorder symptoms in later life.

Insecure attachment and emotionally fraught family dynamics also contribute to a predisposition for personality vulnerabilities that are often observed in individuals with EDs. From a psychoanalytic perspective, enmeshed or critical family environments create a context in which an adolescent or young adult may struggle with a fragmented sense of self and a lack of internal validation. As a result, behaviors surrounding food and body image become compensatory strategies for establishing control or self-worth in an otherwise uncontrollable or invalidating family context. Adolescents may attempt to create boundaries through restrictive eating or seek comfort and self-soothing through binge eating, unconsciously using these behaviors as ways to manage their emotional world when direct emotional support is lacking.

Eating disorder behaviors, therefore, can be understood as both a response to insecure attachment and as symbolic acts representing deeper unmet needs. Insecure attachments foster an internal experience of unworthiness or rejection, leading individuals to turn to external means, such as physical appearance or control over their bodies, to compensate for the perceived lack of inner value. These behaviors also function as a way of managing the psychic conflicts that arise from unresolved attachment needs. For instance, restrictive eating may represent a symbolic attempt to control or suppress vulnerability, while binging may be an unconscious effort to "fill" an internal void left by inadequate emotional connections in early life.

The psychoanalytic lens provides a nuanced understanding of these family dynamics and attachment-related vulnerabilities. It reveals how the early relational environment sets the stage for personality development, coping mechanisms, and self-perception. By examining these dynamics, psychoanalytic therapy can address the emotional and relational roots of EDs, enabling individuals to recognize and work through the underlying psychological issues that fuel their behaviors around food and body image. In this way, therapy offers the potential to transform eating disorder symptoms from expressions of unmet needs into opportunities for self-integration, healing, and the development of more adaptive ways of relating to oneself and others.

The role of trauma, neglect, and dysfunctional family dynamics

The role of trauma, neglect, and dysfunctional family dynamics is a central focus in the psychoanalytic understanding of EDs. Trauma, particularly in formative years, is viewed as a disruptor of an individual's ability to develop and sustain a stable sense of self. In psychoanalytic theory, early traumatic experiences—especially within the family setting—are seen as shaping one's inner world by creating internalized conflicts, unmet emotional needs, and impaired attachment patterns.

Paul Links (1990) compiled studies identifying key factors common in families of individuals with borderline personality disorder (BPD), such as real losses, emotional deprivation, neglect, abuse, and sexual trauma. Increasingly, these same dynamics are observed in families of patients with EDs, highlighting a significant overlap in family environments that create vulnerability to both conditions (Persano et al., 2005). These unresolved conflicts and deficits often manifest later as maladaptive coping mechanisms, with EDs representing a prominent expression of these underlying issues (Bruch, 1973).

Traumatic experiences and neglect during care: Dysfunctional families

Traumatic experiences, especially when paired with neglect or critical family dynamics, can leave individuals with a fragmented sense of identity and an impaired ability to regulate emotions, fostering conditions conducive to developing disordered eating behaviors. Studies indicate that adolescents with histories of self-harm or suicidal tendencies frequently endured childhood experiences of abuse, neglect, or mistreatment within the family setting, whether nuclear or extended. Such traumatic events form cumulative trauma (Kahn, 1964) within the individual's inner world, producing severe distortions of the emerging self. These impacts stem from a failure of the parental function to create a protective "stimulus barrier". This failure goes beyond a lack of loving care, imprinting an indelible mark of passive aggression endured during upbringing, often leading to self-directed aggression. As Kernberg (1992) and Persano (2022) note, once the individual becomes autonomous, the passively experienced aggression resurfaces, now directed inwardly toward the body and ultimately the self.

The punitive superego and internal saboteur

One of the significant concepts in psychoanalytic theory concerning trauma and EDs is the internalization of a "punitive Superego". When caregivers are harsh, critical, or neglectful, children may internalize this negativity, forming an overly punitive self-image that reinforces feelings of inadequacy and shame. The psychoanalytic concept of the Superego, which can become overly self-critical in response to unmet parental expectations or neglectful environments, is viewed as a driving force behind perfectionistic and self-destructive tendencies in individuals with EDs, Fairbairn denominated as the internal saboteur (Firestone, 1986). In this framework, restrictive eating, overexercising, or purging may serve as methods for achieving control or atoning for these deeply internalized, critical voices. This "punitive Superego" imposes unrealistic standards of self-control and perfection, amplifying the sense of guilt and shame that individuals with EDs often feel (Kernberg, 2008).

Emotional neglect and the fragile Ego

Neglect and lack of adequate emotional support within the family can reinforce a deeply internalized sense of unworthiness or insignificance, rendering individuals vulnerable to EDs as they seek to fill emotional voids or cope with feelings of inadequacy. From a psychoanalytic viewpoint, in a cold or inconsistent caregiving environment, the child may develop a fragile Ego structure that lacks resilience and becomes dependent on external validation for self-worth (Winnicott, 1971). Without sufficient mirroring or validation, many psychoanalysts contend, individuals may turn to controlling their bodies as a way of attaining a sense of stability or security. As Donald Winnicott emphasized, the need to exert control over one's environment, including one's own body, may originate from early "object-relational" failures, where primary caregivers fail to provide a stable and nurturing environment (Winnicott, 1971). This compromised sense of self may lead individuals to adopt food and body image control as mechanisms to compensate for the emotional void left by neglectful or unresponsive caregivers.

Introjection and dysfunctional family dynamics

Psychoanalytic theory also highlights "introjection" in families with dysfunctional dynamics, where children internalize the emotional turmoil and problematic communication patterns within the family system. In families characterized by enmeshment, over-control, or emotional neglect, children often internalize these maladaptive patterns, which manifest as self-punitive attitudes and perfectionistic behaviors that strive to meet unattainable standards (Minuchin, Rosman, and Baker, 1978). By "taking in" the voices and expectations of caregivers, individuals may be driven to extreme behaviors—such as restrictive dieting or excessive exercise—to reconcile or cope with the chaotic emotional environment of their upbringing (Birksted-Breen, 1989).

Ego splitting and fragmented self-concept

In cases of trauma, particularly experiences rooted in abuse, neglect, or abandonment, individuals may develop a fragmented self-concept consistent with the psychoanalytic notion of "Ego splitting". This fragmentation often leads to oscillations in self-perception, where individuals alternate between conflicting internalized views of self-worth and inadequacy. Melanie Klein (1946) described this phenomenon as *splitting*, a defense mechanism in which the self is divided into "good" and "bad" parts as a means of coping with unresolved trauma.

Klein's concept of splitting is particularly relevant in the context of EDs, where the body often becomes a battleground for managing internal conflicts surrounding worth, control, and guilt (Steiner, 2014). The division of the self into idealized and devalued aspects fosters a relentless preoccupation with eliminating perceived flaws and constructing a "perfect" version of oneself. This effort to achieve an unattainable ideal often serves as compensation for deeply ingrained feelings of inadequacy, shame, and self-loathing.

This dynamic manifests physically through restrictive eating, binging, or purging behaviors, which act as symbolic expressions of the psychological pain stemming from early traumatic experiences. Restrictive eating, for instance, may represent an attempt to assert control over the self and suppress emotional vulnerability, while binging or purging behaviors reflect a struggle to reconcile conflicting aspects of identity. These behaviors are not merely about food or body image but serve to manage the intense psychological distress rooted in early relational trauma.

Understanding the link between trauma, Ego splitting, and EDs provides valuable insights into the complex emotional dynamics underlying these conditions. Therapeutic interventions that address the fragmented self-concept, integrate conflicting aspects of identity, and foster self-compassion can help individuals navigate the deep psychological wounds that contribute to disordered eating behaviors.

Trauma and eating disorders as a coping mechanism

The impact of early trauma, especially within dysfunctional families where sexual abuse or neglect may occur, often deepens a child's fragmented self-concept. In such families, the lack of consistent, nurturing relationships deprives the child of a secure foundation for healthy identity development, leaving them vulnerable to severe psychological defenses. Psychoanalytic theory suggests that children who experience early sexual abuse or other forms of trauma may internalize profound feelings of shame, blame, and guilt, leading to a conflicted sense of self. These internalized feelings can drive them to seek control over their bodies as a coping mechanism, where bodily control becomes a symbolic way of managing the unresolved and overwhelming emotions associated with the trauma.

In this context, EDs often serve as a means for individuals to externalize and exert control over their inner turmoil. The body becomes a physical site through which they attempt to "process" and manage internal conflicts, expressing psychic pain and symbolically addressing feelings of violation and helplessness that were too overwhelming to confront in childhood. As Connors and Morse (1993) observed, approximately 30% of individuals with EDs report a history of childhood sexual abuse, highlighting a strong correlation between early trauma and the later development of disordered eating behaviors. For some patients, there is a direct link between sexual trauma and eating pathology, where bodily control becomes a way to cope with or even "erase" the memory of the traumatic experience through primitive defense mechanisms.

By using their bodies as a focal point for control, these individuals may be unconsciously attempting to reassert mastery over aspects of themselves that feel damaged or tainted by the trauma. This need for control is particularly significant in the wake of sexual abuse, where feelings of helplessness and violation disrupt the development of a stable self-concept. For these individuals, disordered eating behaviors offer a ritualistic and tangible way to address unresolved emotions, symbolizing an attempt to cleanse, punish, or protect the self from further vulnerability. This reliance on the body as a battleground for managing trauma reflects the profound psychological impact of early abuse and highlights the critical role of primitive defense mechanisms in navigating these unprocessed emotions.

This connection underscores how the absence of a secure, nurturing environment in early life can lead to profound disruptions in self-perception and coping. With their emotional pain unprocessed, individuals with a history of trauma may turn to EDs to channel these unresolved feelings, highlighting the critical role that early relational trauma plays in the development of disordered eating behaviors.

The concept of trauma as a trigger for "emotional numbing" also plays a significant role in the psychoanalytic understanding of EDs. Individuals with early trauma often adopt behaviors that either function as an escape from emotional pain or serve as a form of self-punishment, reflecting unresolved feelings related to trauma or chronic neglect. Psychoanalytic theory posits that restrictive eating, binge eating, or purging can be ways of dissociating from intense emotions; focusing on physical sensations like hunger, satiety, or physical discomfort becomes a mechanism for avoiding overwhelming internal experiences. Hilde Bruch observed that individuals with these disorders frequently report a sense of "numbness" or a lack of awareness about their own physical state. Bruch attributed this to a "blockage of feelings", suggesting that, in response to trauma, these individuals learned to dissociate from their emotions as a protective mechanism (Bruch, 1973).

Emotional numbing and disordered eating

This emotional numbness, reinforced through disordered eating behaviors, can become an ingrained way of managing trauma-related distress. For instance, restrictive eating may create a sense of calm or emotional detachment, reducing anxiety and helping the individual avoid the psychological pain associated with traumatic memories. Similarly, binge eating may serve as a temporary escape, a means of "filling" the void left by emotional deprivation or neglect. Conversely, purging behaviors may function as a ritualistic "cleansing", symbolizing an attempt to expel internalized shame or guilt stemming from unresolved trauma. By focusing on physical sensations, these individuals effectively create a barrier between themselves, and the emotional pain rooted in past experiences.

Perfectionism and symbolic use of the body

Trauma and dysfunctional family dynamics, especially those involving sexual abuse, also contribute to the development of perfectionistic and self-punitive tendencies. The desire to control body shape or achieve a "perfect" appearance can reflect an unconscious attempt to reclaim control lost during childhood trauma. The emphasis on bodily perfection is often a projection of the internal drive to "correct" or redeem oneself, thereby compensating for perceived personal flaws instilled through abusive or neglectful family interactions. As a result, EDs can become a way to symbolically transform and "purify" the self, offering a sense of autonomy and identity in the face of a fragmented self-concept shaped by early relational trauma (Madowitz, Matheson, and Liang, 2015).

From a psychoanalytic perspective, the symbolic use of the body in EDs highlights how unresolved trauma shapes both self-perception and coping mechanisms. Individuals with a history of trauma often direct their emotional distress inward, manifesting as self-destructive behaviors aimed at achieving unattainable ideals of perfection and purity. These behaviors, driven by a need to regulate internal conflict, reflect a psychological attempt to create coherence in a psyche fragmented by trauma, abuse, or neglect. As these individuals strive to manage their unresolved conflicts through bodily control, their eating disorder behaviors become physical expressions of internal psychic pain, embodying the split between the "good" and "bad" parts of the self.

Early trauma, dysfunctional family environments, and attachment disruptions contribute profoundly to the development of a divided and conflicted self. This fragmented self-concept often drives individuals to use eating disorder behaviors as coping strategies, creating a symbolic language through which they attempt to control, expel, or numb unresolved emotional pain. The psychoanalytic framework sheds light on the ways in which early relational trauma fuels the internal conflicts that lead to EDs, underscoring the importance of addressing these underlying issues in treatment to achieve meaningful, lasting recovery.

In sum, the psychoanalytic perspective on EDs reveals the critical impact of early trauma, neglect, and dysfunctional family dynamics on mental health. These factors create a foundation of fragmented self-worth, punitive self-judgment, and insecure attachment that can find expression in disordered eating behaviors. Through internalized familial messages, unprocessed trauma, and the need for control, psychoanalytic theory suggests that EDs function as complex coping mechanisms—means by which individuals navigate unresolved psychological pain by channeling it into the physical body. This understanding provides a foundation for therapeutic interventions that aim to address the emotional and relational origins of the disorder, allowing for healing that goes beyond mere symptom management to achieve deeper psychological integration.

Interactions between parents and children and their contribution to disordered eating patterns

The interactions between parents and children play a pivotal role in shaping the psychological landscape in which disordered eating patterns can emerge, as psychoanalytic theory emphasizes. Within the psychoanalytic framework, early family dynamics, especially those involving communication, boundaries, and expressions of emotion, contribute significantly to the development of an individual's self-concept, body image, and coping strategies, all of which are central to the formation of EDs. Interactions marked by enmeshment, criticism, or emotional neglect often leave children without the secure attachment needed for healthy emotional and identity development, leading them to seek control and validation through other avenues—often through controlling their body and food intake (Bruch, 1973).

Psychoanalytic theory underscores the concept of "object relations", where early relationships with primary caregivers profoundly shape the individual's inner world and sense of self. When parental interactions are fraught with tension, inconsistency, or over-control, children may develop distorted self-perceptions and struggle with self-worth, often turning to disordered eating to regain a sense of control or to cope with unmet emotional needs. For example, when a parent exhibits high levels of criticism or unrealistic expectations, the child may internalize a harsh self-critical voice, creating an internalized "Superego" that constantly pushes them to meet perfectionistic standards, often focused on body image and weight as symbols of achievement and worth. This internalized voice, reinforced by familial expectations or indirect messages, can drive the child toward obsessive control over food intake to achieve these perceived standards of perfection (Stein et al., 1994).

Maternal introjects in eating disorders

Moreover, the concept of "maternal introjects", in which children internalize their mothers' attitudes, anxieties, or perfectionism, is a central idea in psychoanalytic theory on EDs. Hilde Bruch observed that many individuals with EDs report feeling as though their self-worth is tied to their ability to meet their mothers' expectations, often leading them to strive for an idealized or overly controlled body to earn validation (Bruch, 1973). These maternal introjects become part of the child's psyche, driving the need to conform to family ideals that often revolve around body control and perfectionism. Children raised in environments where parents express explicit or implicit concerns about weight, appearance, or food may adopt these values, leading to behaviors such as restrictive eating or compulsive exercise as they attempt to live up to these internalized standards (Minuchin, Rosman, and Baker, 1978).

Control families, autonomy and independence

The dynamics of control within families, particularly around issues of autonomy and independence, are also highly relevant to the psychoanalytic view of EDs. In families where parents are overly controlling or enmeshed—meaning boundaries between parents and children are blurred—children may struggle to develop a separate identity. This can lead to a pattern of self-regulation through food to assert autonomy or to cope with feelings of entrapment (Selvini Palazzoli et al., 1998). AN, for instance, is frequently described in psychoanalytic literature as a symbolic rejection of nurturing, where food refusal represents an attempt to gain autonomy from parental control and an expression of unresolved ambivalence toward dependency (Selvini Palazzoli et al., 1998). In these cases, the act of controlling one's body through restriction becomes a way to symbolically reject the parental influence that the individual feels are overpowering or suffocating. Selvini Palazzoli and Viaro (1988) state that, in families with EDs, the primary difficulty lies in providing a nurturing space that offers reassurance, manages tension with empathy, and thus fosters the development of separate identities. Consequently, both parents and children may feel "starved" of emotional warmth, tenderness, and genuine, unconditional affection toward one another.

The psychoanalytic concept of "transference" also plays a role in understanding how disordered eating patterns can evolve within family interactions. Transference refers to the way individuals project past relationships, often with primary caregivers, onto new situations and people. For individuals with EDs, unresolved conflicts with parents may be projected onto their relationship with food and their bodies. If a child perceives parental approval as contingent upon physical appearance or achievement, they may project these feelings of conditional acceptance onto themselves, believing they must control their body or achieve thinness to earn love and validation. This unconscious projection can reinforce disordered eating behaviors as a means of fulfilling these perceived expectations.

Additionally, psychoanalytic theory emphasizes the importance of symbolic meanings attributed to food and the body within family interactions. In families where emotional expression is suppressed or discouraged, food can become a means of communication or a substitute for unexpressed feelings. For instance, compulsive eating may be seen to "fill" an emotional void, while restrictive eating may serve to deny unmet needs, reflecting a complex psychological negotiation with familial relationships (Winnicott, 1960). The psychoanalytic approach suggests that these patterns often arise from early experiences in which caregivers failed to attune to the child's emotional needs, leaving the child to turn to food as a source of comfort or control.

Father figures in eating disorder patients

Psychoanalysts have extensively examined the role of the paternal figure in family dynamics, particularly its impact on the development of EDs. Fathers who are distant, overly critical, or uninvolved in nurturing relationships can contribute to a dynamic where children feel emotionally unsupported, unworthy, or unseen. This lack of emotional connection often fosters a fragmented self-image, leading children to strive for perfection—especially in their physical appearance—to earn their father's approval and, by extension, societal validation.

In families where paternal figures adopt authoritarian or indifferent roles, the emotional distance can amplify vulnerability to internalizing unrealistic ideals. Children in these environments may equate achievement or physical perfection with the acceptance and love they crave. Disordered eating behaviors—such as restrictive eating or excessive exercise—become a means to construct an idealized version of themselves, one they believe will make them worthy of recognition or affection.

The paternal figure's influence is particularly significant because it often serves as a model for external authority and societal expectations. When fathers are overly critical or emotionally absent, the child's relationship with external validation becomes strained, leading to a cycle of striving for unattainable standards. This dynamic underscores how the paternal role, whether actively critical or passively indifferent, can shape the child's internal conflicts and drive the development of behaviors aimed at regaining a sense of control, worth, or belonging.

By understanding these dynamics, psychoanalytic perspectives highlight the critical need for interventions that address not only the individual's disordered behaviors but also the relational patterns within the family. Fostering open communication and nurturing connections between paternal figures and children can be instrumental in breaking cycles of perfectionism and self-criticism, paving the way for healthier self-perception and emotional well-being

Anorexia nervosa families

Families of patients with AN often exhibit distinct dynamics characterized by dysfunction and extreme closeness, creating significant internal tension. These families are marked by exaggerated overprotection, rigidity, and an intolerance of conflict, all of which hinder the development of autonomy in children. The family environment becomes a tightly controlled system where individuality is suppressed, and children are unable to explore their own identities or develop the emotional tools needed to navigate external challenges.

Marital conflicts often permeate parenting dynamics, resulting in alliances where children are drawn into coalitions with one parent against the other. This dynamic not only disrupts the family equilibrium but also undermines the child's ability to establish emotional independence and autonomy. As a result, the child may develop an intense dependency on the family of origin. Alternatively, in the absence of a supportive familial structure, they might seek substitute "families" through premature and often idealized romantic relationships, reflecting a longing for stability and belonging.

In such environments, open communication is typically minimal, and problems or conflicts are rarely addressed directly. Instead, unresolved tensions are expressed indirectly, often through somatic complaints, such as physical ailments or discomforts. These somatic manifestations can serve as a psychological outlet for unspoken emotions and conflicts, contributing to the development of pathological behaviors, including restrictive eating. This indirect expression of distress highlights the profound impact of disrupted family dynamics on the child's emotional and physical well-being, reinforcing the need for therapeutic approaches that address these relational patterns and their consequences.

The psychological health of family members, particularly mothers, also plays a significant role in the family dynamics of patients with AN. Research by Råstam and Gillberg (1991) highlights a high prevalence of depression and anxiety disorders among mothers of individuals with AN, with many family histories marked by unresolved grief and loss. Strober et al. (2000) found that mothers of patients with AN are often affected by EDs themselves, suggesting a possible intergenerational transmission of disordered eating patterns. Additionally, Lilenfeld et al. (1998) observed obsessive traits in some of these mothers, further contributing to the rigid and controlling atmosphere within the family.

These family dynamics, including overprotection, enmeshment, and poor conflict resolution, create fertile ground for the development and perpetuation of AN. The lack of open communication and the emphasis on perfection and control leave children ill-equipped to express their emotions or cope with stress in healthy ways. Understanding these familial patterns is essential for developing effective therapeutic interventions, not only for the patient but also for the family. Addressing these underlying dynamics can help create a more supportive and open environment, fostering both individual growth and familial healing.

Bulimia nervosa families

In contrast to the rigid and overly controlled dynamics often seen in families of patients with anorexia nervosa, families of patients with BN tend to exhibit a distinct and equally challenging set of dysfunctional characteristics. These families are frequently marked by chaos, lack of structure, and hostility, reflecting a deep "hunger" for affection and a pervasive sense of emotional emptiness. Weak or nonexistent boundaries within the family exacerbate this instability, creating an environment where control is absent, particularly around mealtimes, and family cohesion is difficult to maintain.

Emotional expression in these families is often unpredictable and disorganized, with impulsivity, outbursts, and, in some cases, violence shaping the relational dynamics. Histories of addiction, domestic violence, and neglect are common, further disrupting the emotional stability needed for healthy family functioning. This chaotic environment fosters insecure attachment patterns in children, as the lack of reliable emotional support leaves them feeling unsafe and unmoored during critical stages of development.

Parental behaviors significantly contribute to this instability. Mothers in these families frequently display insecurity, impulsivity, and mood disorders, which further undermine their ability to provide consistent emotional support (Hudson et al., 1987). Fathers may exhibit impulsive aggression, authoritarian tendencies, or a marked emotional distance. Histories involving child neglect or even sexual abuse are more prevalent in these families, compounding the relational trauma that children experience. Additionally, there is often an intergenerational transmission of disordered eating behaviors, with a history of BN observed among parents (Strober et al., 2000).

These patterns of dysfunction and instability leave children in these families particularly vulnerable to developing BN. The impulsivity and emotional volatility that characterize the family system mirror the binge-purge cycles of BN, where individuals oscillate between extremes of indulgence and expulsion, reflecting the emotional chaos of their upbringing. The lack of stable boundaries and emotional security in the family system undermines the child's ability to develop healthy coping mechanisms, leaving them reliant on disordered eating behaviors to manage overwhelming emotions and a deep sense of inadequacy.

Understanding the dynamics of these families provides critical insights into the relational and emotional factors that contribute to the development of BN. Interventions should address not only the individual's symptoms but also the broader family system, promoting healthier communication, emotional regulation, and the establishment of boundaries. By addressing these underlying familial dysfunctions, therapeutic approaches can help break the cycle of chaos and insecurity that perpetuates disordered eating behaviors across generations.

A comprehensive perspective on families of individuals with eating disorders

In families affected by EDs, there is often a noticeable lack of cohesion and flexibility, reduced emotional expression, and limited intrafamilial communication, paired with increased paternal overprotection and rejection. Autonomy and engagement in social or cultural activities are frequently undervalued, fostering an overall deteriorated family atmosphere marked by negative emotions toward one another. Many individuals with EDs report feeling ignored and unloved by their mothers, a profoundly challenging reality to process consciously. Consequently, symptoms of EDs may emerge as expressions of displaced emotional deprivation.

Feeding is a culturally mediated process transmitted intergenerationally. Each mother must discover her baby's unique needs and desires. When this process fails, the mother may default to ancestral identifications, mechanically repeating them without uncovering her child's genuine needs. This stereotyped care disrupts affect regulation, negatively impacting the feeding process (Persano, 2005).

The persistence and severity of EDs, endurance eating disorders (EEDs) are notably influenced by family dynamics, with higher levels of dysfunction correlating with more enduring and severe manifestations of these conditions. Research indicates that familial factors such as emotional neglect, abuse, and lack of cohesion significantly contribute to the development and maintenance of EDs. It was found that adverse childhood experiences, including familial dysfunction, are associated with increased morbidity and mortality in individuals with EDs (Brewerton, 2022).

Moreover, the intergenerational transmission of disordered eating behaviors underscores the impact of family environment. Mothers with EDs often exhibit intrusive behaviors and express negative emotions toward their infants during mealtimes, which can disrupt the child's relationship with food and contribute to the development of EDs (Marazi et al., 2023).

Addressing family dysfunction is therefore crucial in the treatment of EDs. Therapeutic approaches that involve family-based interventions have shown promise in improving outcomes by fostering healthier family dynamics and supporting the individual's recovery process.

Psychoanalytic theory offers valuable insights into how parental interactions and family dynamics contribute to the development of EDs. Mechanisms such as introjection, transference, symbolic uses of food, and dynamics of control play significant roles in shaping inner conflicts and unmet emotional needs. Through early family relationships, these dynamics imprint lasting psychological patterns, with disordered eating emerging not solely as a matter of food or body image but as complex, often unconscious responses to unresolved familial tensions and conflicts. The psychoanalytic perspective thus emphasizes that addressing these familial influences is essential to understanding and treating the deep-seated roots of eating disorders.

Bibliography

Ainsworth, M. S. (1989). Attachments beyond infancy. *American Psychologist*, 44(4): 709–716.

Birksted-Breen, D. (1989). Working with an anorexic patient. *The International Journal of Psychoanalysis*, 70(1): 29–40.

Blum, H. P. (2004). Separation-individuation theory and attachment theory. *Journal of the American Psychoanalytic Association*, 52(2): 535–553.

Bollas, C. (1982). On the relation to the self as an object. *The International Journal of Psychoanalysis*, 63(3): 347–359.

Bowlby, J. (1951). *Maternal Care and Mental Health.* Geneva: World Health Organization. Spanish version: *Los Cuidados Maternos y la Salud Mental.* Buenos Aires: Ed Humanitas (1964).

Bowlby, J. (1973).*Attachment and Loss: Volume 2: Separation: Anxiety and Anger.* New York: Basic Books.

Bowlby, J. (1979). The Bowlby-Ainsworth attachment theory. *Behavioral and Brain Sciences,* 2(4): 637–638.

Brewerton, T. D. (2022). Mechanisms by which adverse childhood experiences, other traumas and PTSD influence the health and well-being of individuals with eating disorders throughout the life span. *Journal of Eating Disorders,* 10(1): 162.

Bruch, H. (1973). *Eating Disorders: Obesity, Anorexia Nervosa and the Person Within.* New York: Basic Books.

Connors, M. E. and Morse, W. (1993). Sexual abuse and eating disorders: A review. *International Journal of Eating Disorders,* 13(1): 1–11.

Espina, A., Ortego, M. A., de Alda, Í. O., Yenes, F., and Alemán, A. (2001). La imagen corporal en los trastornos alimentarios. *Psicothema,* 13(4): 532–538.

Firestone, R. W. (1986). The "inner voice" and suicide. *Psychotherapy: Theory, Research, Practice, Training,* 23(3): 439–447.

Freud, S. (1911). Formulations on the Two Principles of Mental Functioning. *The Standard Edition of the Complete Psychological Works of Sigmund Freud, (12).* London: The Hogarth Press, 213–226 (1991 edition).

Freud, S. (1920). Beyond the Pleasure Principle. *The Standard Edition of the Complete Psychological Works of Sigmund Freud, (18).* London: The Hogarth Press, 3–64 (1991 edition).

Freud, S. (1923). The Ego and the Id. *The Standard Edition of the Complete Psychological Works of Sigmund Freud, (19).* London: The Hogarth Press, 3–66 (1991 edition).

García Badaracco, J. (1990). *Comunidad Terapéutica Psicoanalítica de Estructura Multifamiliar.* Madrid: Tecnipublicaciones, S.A.

Hudson, J. I., Pope, H. G., Jonas, J. M., Yurgelun-Todd, D., and Frankenburg, F. R. (1987). A controlled family history study of bulimia. *Psychological Medicine,* 17(4): 883–890.

Kahn, M. M. R. (1964). Ego distortion, cumulative trauma, and the role of reconstruction in the analytic situation. *The International Journal of Psychoanalysis,* 45: 272–279.

Keating, L., Tasca, G. A., and Hill, R. (2013). Structural relationships among attachment insecurity, alexithymia, and body esteem in women with eating disorders. *Eating Behaviors,* 14(3): 366–373.

Kernberg, O. F. (1984). *Severe Personality Disorders.* New Haven, CT and London: Yale University Press.

Kernberg, O. F. (1992). *Aggression in Personality Disorders and Perversions.* New Haven, CT and London: Yale University Press.

Kernberg, O. F. (2008). *Aggressivity, Narcissism, and Self-destructiveness in the Psychotherapeutic Relationship: New Developments in the Psychopathology and Psychotherapy of Severe Personality Disorders.* New Haven, CT and London: Yale University Press.

Kerns, K. A. and Brumariu, L. E. (2014). Is insecure parent–child attachment a risk factor for the development of anxiety in childhood or adolescence? *Child Development Perspectives,* 8(1): 12–17.

Klein, M. (1946). Notes on some schizoid mechanisms. *International Journal of Psycho-Analysis*, 27: 99–110.

Lilenfeld, L. R., Kaye, W. H., Greeno, C. G., Merikangas, K. R., Plotnicov, K., Pollice, C., Rao, R., Strober, M., Bulik, C. M., and Nagy, L. (1998). A controlled family study of anorexia nervosa and bulimia nervosa: Psychiatric disorders in first-degree relatives and effects of proband comorbidity. *Archives of General Psychiatry*, 55(7): 603–610.

Links, P. S. (1990). *Family Environment and Borderline Personality Disorder*. Washington DC: American Psychiatric Press.

Madowitz, J., Matheson, B. E., and Liang, J. (2015). The relationship between eating disorders and sexual trauma. *Eating and Weight Disorders*, 20(3): 281–293.

Mahler, M., Pine, F., and Bergman, A. (1975). *The Psychological Birth of the Human Infant*. New York: Basic Books.

Marazzi, F., Orlandi, M., De Giorgis, V., Borgatti, R., and Mensi, M. M. (2023). The impact of family alexithymia on the severity of restrictive eating disorders in adolescent patients. *Child and Adolescent Psychiatry and Mental Health*, 17(1): 139.

Minuchin, S., Rosman, B. L., and Baker, L. (1978). *Psychosomatic Families: Anorexia Nervosa in Context*. Cambridge, MA: Harvard University Press.

Persano, H. L. (2005). Abordagem psicodinâmica do paciente com trastornos alimentares. In C. L. Eizirik, R. W. Aguiar, and S. S. Schestatsky (eds.) *Psicoterapia de Orientação Analítica: Fundamentos Teóricos e Clínicos*, Porto Alegre: Artmed, 674–688 (chapter 49).

Persano, H. L. (2022). Self-harm. *The International Journal of Psychoanalysis*, 103(6): 1089–1103.

Persano, H. L. and Ventura, A. D. (1994). Un nuevo desafío para la psiquiatría: El auge de los trastornos de personalidad en las sociedades en crisis del siglo XX. *Sinopsis (Revista de A.P.S.A.)*, 10(27): 48–59.

Persano, H. L. and Goldberg, C. M. (1995). Internal world: Its configuration through the family. In *International Psychoanalytic Studies Organization: Proceedings of the XIIIth International Congress on July 29th, 30th & August 2nd*. San Francisco: International Psychoanalytic Studies Organization, 50–65.

Persano, H. L., Autelli, G., Sinay, M., Varese, A., and Zanon, P. (2005). Patrones Familiares y su Relación con los Trastornos de la Conducta Alimentaria, Poster XXICongreso Argentino de Psiquiatría de APSA 2005, Alianza Global en Adicciones y Trastornos de la Personalidad, Mar del Plata: APSA.

Rastam, M. and Gillberg, C. (1991). The family background in anorexia nervosa: A population-based study. *Journal of the American Academy of Child Adolescent Psychiatry*. 30(2): 283–289.

Selvini Palazzoli, M. (1974): *Self-starvation: From Individual to Family Therapy in the Treatment of Anorexia Nervosa*. New York: Jason Aronson.

Selvini Palazzoli, M. and Viaro, M. (1988). The anorectic process in the family: A six-stage model as a guide for individual therapy. *Family Process*, 27(2): 129–148.

Selvini Palazzoli, M., Cirillo, S., Selvini, M., and Sorrentino, A. M. (1998). *Ragazze Anoressiche e Bulimiche. La Terapia Familiare*. Milan: Raffaello Cortina Editore.

Stein, A., Woolley, H., Cooper, S. D., and Fairburn, C. G. (1994). An observational study of mothers with eating disorders and their infants. *Journal of Child Psychology and Psychiatry*, 35(4): 733–748.

Steiner, J. (2014). The equilibrium between the paranoid-schizoid and the depressive positions. In R. Anderson (ed.) *Clinical Lectures on Klein and Bion*. London: Routledge, 46–58.

Strober, M., Freeman, R., Lampert, C., Diamond, J., and Kaye, W. (2000). Controlled family study of anorexia nervosa and bulimia nervosa: Evidence of shared liability and transmission of partial syndromes. *American Journal of Psychiatry*, 157(3): 393–401.

Sund, A. M. and Wichstrøm, L. (2002). Insecure attachment as a risk factor for future depressive symptoms in early adolescence. *Journal of the American Academy of Child & Adolescent Psychiatry*, 41(12): 1478–1485.

Tasca, G. A. and Balfour, L. (2014). Attachment and eating disorders: A review of current research. *International Journal of Eating Disorders*, 47(7): 710–717.

Winnicott, D. W. (1960). Ego Distortion in Terms of True and False Self. In *The Maturational Processes and the Facilitating Environment: Studies in the Theory of Emotional Development*. New York: International Universities Press, 140–152.

Winnicott, D. W. (1965). *The Family and Individual Development*. London: Routledge.

Winnicott, D. W. (1971). *Playing and Reality*. London: Tavistock Publications.

7 Transference and countertransference

Understanding transference and countertransference in the context of eating disorder treatment

Freud's foundational work

Building on Freud's foundational work, the concept of transference has become integral to psychoanalytic understandings of psychopathology and therapeutic processes. Freud was the first to describe how shifts in unconscious affect and mental representations influence both symptom formation and the therapeutic relationship. In his early writings, particularly those addressing symptoms associated with anorexia, Freud introduced transference to explain how unconscious meanings shift across different mental representations. In his studies of cases such as Emmy von N. and Katharina, he observed that childhood experiences could reappear in adolescence, albeit in modified forms, through processes of displacement and transference onto new representations (Breuer and Freud, 1893a; Breuer and Freud, 1893b). This insight was crucial for understanding how unresolved conflicts persist across developmental stages, expressing themselves through transference and symptom formation. Freud noted that symptoms often serve as symbolic expressions of these unconscious conflicts, illustrating the continuity of psychic life across time. Thus, transference becomes more than a therapeutic phenomenon; it is a primary mechanism by which individuals internalize and reenact early relational patterns in new forms, sustaining these patterns across different phases of life.

In *"The Dynamics of Transference"* Freud further defined transference as the unconscious reenactment of early relationship patterns, often brought into the therapeutic context. He emphasized that transference acts as a "bridge" between past experiences and present behaviors, making it essential for understanding the development of neurotic symptoms. For neurotic individuals, Freud noted, transference tends to be particularly intense and forms a core resistance to therapeutic change. In these cases, transference goes beyond simple repetition, becoming a defensive process

DOI: 10.4324/9781032724997-7

that complicates patients' ability to engage adaptively with current relationships. Freud described this resistant transference as manifesting in forms such as negative transference and erotic transference (Freud, 1912).

Freud also explored how transference operates as a regressive process that serves as resistance to adaptation. He argued that this regression is driven by libido, or psychic energy, which retreats from present reality and reinvests in past experiences. This withdrawal of cathexis from current experience pulls the individual back into familiar but maladaptive relational patterns, reflecting an attachment to early emotional bonds. Freud posited that, to achieve therapeutic change, individuals must confront these unconscious attachments to integrate healthier, more adaptive ways of relating to themselves and others. Through this process, transference shifts from being a barrier to becoming an avenue for healing, as patients gain insight into unresolved conflicts (Freud, 1912).

Freud's exploration of transference laid the groundwork for understanding how unconscious processes and relational dynamics impact mental health. By recognizing transference as both an obstacle and a path to self-understanding, Freud highlighted the therapist's role in facilitating the patient's awareness of these patterns. Through this awareness, the repetitive, compulsive aspects of transference become opportunities for growth and transformation. This conceptualization has since become foundational in psychoanalytic theory, deepening our understanding of how unresolved unconscious conflicts shape human experience.

Historical perspectives on countertransference

Countertransference has become a valuable therapeutic tool in the treatment of complex and challenging patients, especially those with borderline personality disorder (BPD) and eating disorders (EDs). Adolph Stern, who first introduced the term "borderline" in 1938, described a group of patients whose symptoms straddled the realms of neurosis and psychosis. In his influential paper *"Psychoanalytic Investigation of and Therapy in the Border Line Group of Neuroses"* Stern noted that borderline patients often displayed significant emotional instability, impulsivity, and complex interpersonal issues, making them difficult to treat using traditional psychoanalytic approaches. His insights underscored the critical role of countertransference in therapy with borderline patients, as he recognized that their intense and unpredictable relational dynamics could provoke strong and challenging responses in therapists (Stern, 1938).

Heinrich Racker refined the understanding of countertransference by introducing the concepts of *concordant* and *complementary* countertransference. In *"Transference and Countertransference"* Racker (1959) explained that concordant countertransference occurs when therapists find themselves identifying with the patient's feelings, whereas complementary countertransference arises when therapists feel as if they are embodying a significant figure from the patient's life, such as a parent or former caregiver. In the treatment of BPD, both types of countertransference are highly relevant, as patients may unconsciously provoke complementary responses, leading therapists to occupy roles like those of rejecting or unavailable caregivers. Racker stressed the importance of therapist self-awareness to avoid unconsciously enacting dynamics that may reinforce the patient's relational trauma (Racker, 1948). Around the same time, Paula Heimann (1950) emphasized the role of countertransference as a window into the patient's inner world, highlighting how therapist's emotional responses could provide crucial insights into the patient's psyche (Stefana, Hinshelwood, and Borensztejn, 2021).

Countertransference in borderline personality disorders

Therapists working with BPD patients frequently encounter a range of countertransference responses, including frustration, helplessness, anger, boredom, and at times, an overwhelming urge to "rescue" the patient. The intensity and unpredictability of BPD patients' emotional states can challenge a therapist's objectivity, making it difficult to maintain therapeutic effectiveness. Otto Kernberg and Glen Gabbard expanded on these insights by emphasizing the importance of managing these reactions mindfully, understanding countertransference as both a potential therapeutic tool and a challenge requiring careful navigation. Kernberg has noted that countertransference often mirrors the patient's own intense internal conflicts, urging therapists to adopt a "firm yet empathetic stance" to avoid becoming entangled in the patient's emotional turbulence (Kernberg, 1965, 1990; Yeomans, Clarkin, and Kernberg, 2015). Gabbard similarly highlights that effectively managing countertransference is essential in BPD treatment to prevent therapists from unconsciously reenacting the patient's unresolved relational traumas, which frequently involve cycles of idealization and devaluation (Gabbard, 1995).

The therapeutic value of countertransference is not limited to BPD treatment but extends to the treatment of EDs, where similar dynamics can emerge. Patients with EDs often evoke strong emotional reactions in therapists, including feelings of maternal protectiveness, frustration, anxiety over self-harm, and even fear for the patient's survival. Like patients with BPD, individuals with EDs may unconsciously elicit these responses in ways that mirror their inner conflicts around control, self-worth, and dependency. Gabbard (2001) has pointed out that countertransference reactions can act as a mirror of the patient's internal world; the therapist may feel the very affects that the patient is unable to express consciously.

Countertransference in the psychodynamic treatment of EDs

Countertransference awareness is crucial in the psychodynamic treatment of EDs patients, as it allows therapists to distinguish between the patient's projections and their own emotional responses. This differentiation is essential in creating a therapeutic environment that is both compassionate and boundary, which, in turn, provides a safe space for patients to explore their underlying fears, conflicts, and unmet needs. In the context of EDs, where behaviors around food and body image often function as defenses against unresolved psychological pain, the therapist's ability to hold and reflect on countertransference reactions enables the patient to confront and process these core issues within a supportive framework (Persano, 2006).

In psychodynamic treatment, countertransference becomes a powerful diagnostic and therapeutic tool, offering insight into the unconscious dynamics that drive eating disorder symptoms. Many patients with EDs have histories of early relational trauma, attachment disruptions, or internalized feelings of inadequacy. These issues often manifest in their interactions with therapists, who may experience strong reactions such as protectiveness, frustration, or even anxiety about the patient's well-being. For instance, the therapist might feel compelled to "rescue" the patient, echoing the patient's own ambivalence about dependency and autonomy. As Gabbard (2001) notes, countertransference can serve as a "mirror" reflecting the patient's inner struggles, and by carefully examining these reactions, therapists can better understand the patient's unconscious needs and conflicts.

In the treatment of EDs, this understanding of countertransference aligns with Racker's distinctions between concordant and complementary countertransference. Concordant countertransference occurs when the therapist resonates with the patient's emotional experience, while complementary countertransference occurs when the therapist feels as though they are embodying someone significant in the patient's relational world, such as a caregiver. These dynamics can be especially pronounced in patients with EDs. For example, a therapist may unconsciously adopt a role reminiscent of a critical or controlling parent, reflecting the patient's own internalized self-criticism and perfectionism. Racker emphasized the need for therapists to be aware of these reactions to avoid unconsciously enacting dynamics that may reinforce the patient's relational trauma, a concern particularly relevant in eating disorder treatment (Racker, 1948).

The importance of managing countertransference in treating patients

Otto Kernberg and Glen Gabbard have both underscored the importance of managing countertransference in treating patients with intense emotional needs, such as those with EDs and BPD. Kernberg argues that countertransference often mirrors the patient's own intense internal conflicts, requiring therapists to adopt a "firm yet empathetic stance" to avoid being overwhelmed by the patient's emotional volatility (Kernberg, 1965, 1990). This stance is especially relevant in ED treatment, where patients may elicit strong feelings of protectiveness, frustration, or even helplessness in their therapists. As Gabbard emphasizes, these reactions, when carefully analyzed, can reveal important aspects of the patient's relational and emotional struggles, helping the therapist to avoid re-enacting the patient's traumas and instead facilitate a therapeutic process that encourages psychological resilience and self-integration (Gabbard, 1995).

Using countertransference in this way allows therapists to gain a deeper understanding of the patient's internal world and the relational patterns that sustain eating disorder behaviors. This approach recognizes that the behaviors associated with EDs, such as restrictive eating, binging, and purging, often serve as symbolic expressions of unmet emotional needs and unresolved conflicts. By carefully reflecting on their own emotional responses, therapists can gain insight into these underlying issues, helping the patient explore and address the complex relational dynamics that fuel their symptoms (Persano, 2006).

In clinical practice, countertransference-informed treatment can significantly enhance the psychodynamic approach to EDs. For example, a therapist who feels a strong desire to protect a patient with AN may be experiencing a form of complementary countertransference that reflects the patient's unconscious wish to be cared for, coupled with fears of dependency. By recognizing and interpreting this dynamic, the therapist can help the patient explore and articulate these ambivalent feelings, fostering a therapeutic environment in which the patient can address underlying attachment anxieties and develop healthier ways of relating to themselves and others.

In summary, countertransference is not merely an obstacle in the treatment of EDs but a powerful tool that, when skillfully managed, offers insight into the relational and emotional complexities of these patients. As Kernberg, Gabbard, and Racker have demonstrated, the therapist's emotional responses provide a pathway to understanding and addressing the unconscious conflicts driving eating disorder behaviors. By avoiding the re-enactment of the patient's traumas and facilitating a space for safe exploration, therapists can foster healing, self-integration, and resilience in patients with EDs, ultimately guiding them toward healthier ways of managing their internal conflicts and relational needs.

Object relations theory

Object relations theory explores how early relational experiences, or "objects", become internalized within the psyche and shape interpersonal patterns throughout life. Melanie Klein, a pioneer in this field, argued that the infant's interactions with primary caregivers are split into "good" and "bad" representations, laying the groundwork for internal conflicts that are unconsciously replayed in later relationships (Rosenfeld, 1983). Klein proposed that these polarized representations form the foundation of the self, influencing how individuals relate to others across their lifespan (Klein, 1932).

Otto Kernberg expanded on Melanie Klein's foundational work, integrating and building upon Edith Jacobson's contributions to the understanding of object relations and affective development (Jacobson, 1964, 1971). While Jacobson focused on how internalized objects contribute to the construction of the self, Kernberg advanced these ideas by introducing the concept of complex triadic structures. These structures consist of an object representation, a self-representation, and an affective tone, which collectively organize the mind's internal world (Kernberg, 1990). For example, a nurturing caregiver may be internalized alongside feelings of love, forming a stable and positive self-representation. Conversely, a rejecting or punitive caregiver might be associated with shame or fear, leading to the development of fragmented or negative self-concepts.

Jacobson (1964) emphasized the centrality of affect in the internalization process, proposing that emotionally charged interactions with early caregivers shape the developing self by becoming embedded in internal object representations. Kernberg (1976) built on the foundation of object relations theory by emphasizing the central role of affective quality in binding self and object representations into dyadic units. These affect-laden dyads evolve through repeated relational interactions, gradually giving rise to more complex psychological structures, including the Superego (Kernberg, 1976, 1984). When early experiences are predominantly negative, internalized dyads may become saturated with aggression and destructive emotions, leading to pathological outcomes such as identity diffusion, emotional dysregulation, and splitting (Kernberg, 1984, 2004). Kernberg (1985) also demonstrated how failures in the integration of these early affective experiences contribute to narcissistic defenses, such as oscillations between grandiosity and devaluation. These disruptions, central to borderline and narcissistic personality organizations, continue to inform contemporary psychodynamic treatment approaches (Kernberg, 2016).These disruptions can manifest in various ways, such as an inability to regulate self-esteem or a tendency to perceive oneself and others in extremes, a phenomenon Kernberg associated with splitting.

Splitting, a defense mechanism extensively theorized by Kernberg, involves maintaining contradictory representations of self and others—such as good and bad—separately to avoid emotional conflict. This defense is particularly prominent in individuals with borderline personality disorder (BPD), where splitting leads to unstable and polarized perceptions of self and others. These individuals often oscillate between idealization and devaluation, struggling to integrate opposing emotional experiences (Kernberg, 1984). The inability to reconcile these fragmented representations poses significant challenges in sustaining emotional stability, self-esteem, and healthy interpersonal relationships.

In psychoanalytic treatment, Kernberg emphasized the importance of integrating these split representations to foster a more cohesive and balanced internal world. The therapeutic goal is to help patients simultaneously hold both positive and negative aspects of themselves and others, thereby enhancing emotional resilience and relational capacity (Yeomans, Clarkin, and Kernberg, 2015). This integration process not only addresses the symptoms of personality disorders but also facilitates deeper psychological growth by reorganizing the internal world around more integrated and adaptive affective experiences.

Kernberg's framework, enriched by Jacobson's focus on the role of affects in building the self, offers a comprehensive understanding of the interplay between early relational experiences, internalized representations, and personality development. By highlighting how affective interactions shape the self and influence relational patterns, his model provides valuable insights into the treatment of personality disorders and other psychological disturbances rooted in early developmental disruptions.

Transference in eating disorders: Anorexia nervosa and bulimia nervosa

In the psychoanalytic perspective, transference dynamics are pivotal in the treatment of patients with EDs, particularly those with AN and BN. These disorders frequently involve distinct transference patterns that provide valuable insights into the patients' internalized representations of self and others. These patterns often manifest through themes of control, attachment, and self-worth, reflecting the deep-seated relational conflicts and emotional struggles underlying their disordered behaviors.

Transference in anorexia nervosa

In patients with AN, transference often appears monotonous, repetitive, and rigid, reflecting limited internalized representations of relationships. This rigidity mirrors a restricted internal world, wherein patients struggle to form complex relational dynamics due to an impaired capacity for mentalization—the ability to comprehend both their own and others' mental states (Fonagy et al., 2002). This limited mentalization capacity presents significant challenges for patients with AN in connecting to their own emotions and understanding others' intentions. As a result, their transference style is often "flat", marked by a distant, detached attitude toward the therapist. This emotional distance serves as a protective barrier, rooted in an internalized need for control and a fear of dependency (Steiner, 1993). This desire for control is not only central in their interpersonal interactions but is also projected onto their relationship with food and their bodies, which become symbols of self-sufficiency and autonomy.

Hilde Bruch, a pioneer in the study of EDs, described a "false self" phenomenon in patients with AN, where they become disconnected from genuine emotions and need to maintain a controlled facade (Bruch, 1973). In therapeutic transference, this "false self" often manifests as a resistance to expressing dependency or vulnerability, as patients view these feelings as threats to their carefully constructed autonomy. Bruch argued that patients suffering from AN employ this resistance as a defense against dependency, perceiving attachment as a risk to their independence and sense of control.

The rigid fixation on control and self-discipline observed in patients with AN often functions as a defense against internal chaos and deep-seated fears of dependency. This rigidity becomes a coping mechanism for emotional instability, reinforcing the individual's reliance on their physical self as a primary object of control. From a psychoanalytic perspective, the body becomes the focus of a symbolic struggle for autonomy, where the restrictive behaviors associated with anorexia mirror an unconscious battle for self-sufficiency and mastery over dependency (Crisp, 1980). In this sense, their relationship with their bodies acts as a substitute for emotional and relational growth, displacing complex feelings onto their physical selves rather than working through them in the therapeutic relationship. This dynamic in therapy underscores the significance of transference as a pathway to understanding deeply embedded conflicts, as it allows the therapist to explore the patient's internalized fears of attachment and loss of control.

In AN, the concept of a "constrained object" captures the restrictive way in which patients relate to the world around them, including themselves, others, and their bodies. For patients with AN, these "objects" become highly constrained, meaning they are limited in depth, complexity, and emotional resonance. This constraint manifests in their interpersonal relationships, emotional life, and how they relate to their own bodies, resulting in a narrow, repetitive, and rigid relational pattern.

These patients tend to treat their bodies as constrained objects, subjecting them to strict control and discipline, reflecting an unconscious attempt to limit vulnerability and dependency by keeping emotions and bodily needs in check. By controlling food intake and weight, they create an illusion of mastery over their physical selves, focusing intensely on this object of control. Crisp (1980) noted that this relentless drive for control over the body symbolizes an underlying struggle for autonomy and self-sufficiency, as patients attempt to free themselves from any perceived dependence on others.

The constrained object in AN also reveals itself in the limited ways patients relate to others. Patients with AN often maintain highly controlled, detached relationships, avoiding emotional dependency and vulnerability. Due to their limited mentalization ability, patients with AN struggle to form nuanced, emotionally fulfilling relationships. Instead, they adopt a more "flat" and rigid approach to others, viewing them as functional entities rather than fully realized individuals with complex internal lives. This constraint allows them to avoid perceived dangers of closeness, intimacy, and emotional interdependence.

Moreover, Hilde Bruch (1973) described how the self can become a constrained object within the psyche of individuals with AN. Patients often experience a "false self", where they become detached from their genuine emotions and needs, adopting a controlled and idealized version of themselves. This false self represents a way of avoiding vulnerability and preserving autonomy. In transference, this manifests as a reluctance to open or depend on the therapist, fearing that revealing their inner self might lead to a loss of control. Consequently, the therapeutic process can feel limited, as patients resist emotional engagement and genuine self-expression.

The concept of the constrained object in AN is closely tied to the dynamics of transference, as it involves the displacement of relational conflicts onto food and body image. In psychoanalytic terms, transference refers to how patients project feelings and relational patterns from past experiences onto new contexts, including the therapeutic relationship. For patients with AN, this displacement onto the body can be seen as a form of transference, where unresolved issues with dependency, control, and intimacy are re-enacted in their relationship with their physical selves rather than through interpersonal connections. The body thus becomes the primary "object" in their internal world, reflecting deep-seated conflicts and offering a controlled outlet for expressing emotional struggles.

In the therapeutic setting, this focus on the body as a constrained object often translates into a rigid and controlled transference style. Patients may resist emotional engagement with the therapist, redirecting their relational energy onto their bodies instead. This dynamic serves as a defense mechanism, protecting them from the perceived unpredictability and vulnerability inherent in human relationships. By treating their body as a concrete, controllable object, they avoid confronting the emotional complexities and dependencies that arise in interpersonal connections, including therapeutic relationships. Consequently, their physical self becomes a substitute for deeper relational engagement, where feelings of dependency and control are acted out rather than explored with the therapist.

Exploring the concept of constrained objects in therapy, therefore, becomes essential for understanding the underlying emotional conflicts driving the ED. Addressing how relational conflicts are displaced onto the body allows therapists to gradually open the patient to more flexible and adaptive transference dynamics. By helping patients recognize the ways in which they limit their relational capacity, therapists can facilitate a shift from a narrow, self-focused transference to a more expansive one, where they feel safer exploring complex feelings within the therapeutic relationship.

This shift in transference opens opportunities for growth, as patients begin to recognize that they can experience intimacy and dependency without losing autonomy or control. Through this process, the body no longer needs to serve as the primary "object" of relational conflict. Instead, the therapeutic relationship itself can become a secure space for patients to work through issues of self-worth, dependency, and vulnerability, helping them develop healthier, more fulfilling ways of relating to themselves and others. This transformation in transference ultimately supports their ability to engage more adaptively with the world, reducing the compulsive focus on body control and allowing for greater emotional resilience.

Transference in bulimia nervosa

In bulimia nervosa (BN), transference often mirrors the complex, turbulent inner world of the patient, marked by instability, dependency, and an intense but ambivalent desire for connection. Psychoanalytically, BN is characterized by a "hunger" for objects—an insatiable need for emotional sustenance, validation, and attachment that parallels the binge-purge cycle. The emotional patterns of BN—oscillating between intense dependency and rejection—are frequently played out in therapy, offering critical insights into the patient's underlying relational dynamics.

Patients with BN often experience a chaotic and fragmented inner world, where intense and conflicting emotions clash, creating a pervasive sense of inner turmoil. This chaotic psychological landscape is closely tied to a lack of emotional containment, with feelings such as anger, shame, and fear lacking stable boundaries and often overwhelming the patient. These individuals may grapple with an underlying sense of emptiness or inadequacy, seeking external validation and attachment to momentarily alleviate these feelings. In transference, this chaotic inner world becomes evident through rapid shifts in their emotional stance toward the therapist, fluctuating from idealization to devaluation and from attachment to anger. This volatility reflects their struggle to find internal stability and to maintain a coherent sense of self (Steiner, 1993).

These patients frequently exhibit unstable and ambivalent relationships, reflecting their internal conflicts with attachment and dependency. According to Kernberg (1984), individuals with unstable object relations tend to alternate between idealizing and devaluing others, reflecting an internalized split between "good" and "bad" self and object representations. Fairburn, Cooper, and Shafran (2003) describe how patients with BN often vacillate between idealizing and devaluing the therapist, reflecting internalized "good" and "bad" object relations (Kernberg, 1990). These oscillating dynamics mirror their relational patterns outside therapy, which are often marked by chaotic attachments. In therapy, this dynamic often results in the idealization of the therapist, followed by disappointment or anger when the therapist cannot meet their emotional needs precisely as desired. This "push-pull" relational pattern mirrors the binge-purge behavior cycle, creating an unstable foundation for relationships where patients vacillate between intense neediness and rejection.

This unstable transference can create significant challenges in therapy, as patients may abruptly detach or lash out if they feel their needs are unmet. This relational pattern reflects a fear of engulfment by the other, alongside a parallel fear of abandonment, making true intimacy both desired and feared. In the therapeutic context, this pattern reveals the deep-seated ambivalence at the core of their disorder, as patients both long for and resist closeness, fearing that dependency may lead to disappointment or betrayal.

The theme of "hunger for objects" is central in BN, reflecting the patient's deep need for connection, love, and validation, often stemming from early unmet attachment needs. This metaphorical hunger mirrors their literal hunger during binge episodes, where food acts as a substitute for the emotional nourishment they lack. Patients with BN frequently demonstrate an insatiable "hunger for the object"—a profound need for validation that drives both their binge-purge cycles and their patterns of relational instability (Jeammet, 1984).

Paul-Claude Racamier (1970) expanded on this theme, describing this intense craving as "narcissistic object hunger". Racamier explained this concept as a powerful, unrelenting need for external sources of validation to fill an internal void. This narcissistic object hunger compels individuals with BN to seek out attachment figures, or "objects", to stabilize their fragile sense of self and bolster their self-worth. Without these external anchors, they often feel an overwhelming emptiness that they attempt to fill with both relationships and compulsive eating behaviors.

In the therapeutic setting, this "hunger for objects" can manifest as an intense dependency on the therapist, where the patient may try to "consume" the therapist's attention, approval, and validation to fill their inner void. The therapist becomes an object of emotional sustenance, a source of stability, and a means of regulating their self-esteem. This dynamic underscores the importance of managing therapeutic boundaries and countertransference, as the patient's profound need for connection may create intense dependency that can complicate the therapeutic process.

This dependency can create a challenging transference dynamic, as patients may oscillate between clinging to the therapist and feeling resentful or disappointed if the therapist does not perfectly fulfill their needs. This dynamic often reflects a childlike need for the therapist to act as a perfect caregiver, coupled with inherent frustration when reality inevitably falls short of this idealized expectation. The "hunger for objects" also manifests as a symbolic need for reassurance and self-worth, making the therapeutic relationship a battleground for the patient's unfulfilled needs and dependency fears.

In the cycle of BN, objects—both people and symbolic sources of attachment—are not only intensely desired but also expelled or rejected once the need for them is momentarily fulfilled. This expulsion mirrors the purging behavior following binge episodes, where the "object" (whether food or emotional attachment) is taken in only to be violently expelled. This behavior can be understood as an attempt to rid oneself of uncomfortable dependency and the vulnerability that comes with closeness. The cyclical nature of binging and purging thus reflects an ambivalence in relationships: while the patient craves closeness, they also reject it to avoid the vulnerability associated with dependency.

In transference, this dynamic of expulsion and rejection can manifest as emotional distancing or sudden anger toward the therapist, particularly when feelings of dependency arise. The need to reject or "expel" the therapist symbolically allows the patient to regain a sense of control over their vulnerability. This cycle often prevents them from forming stable attachments, as they are caught between their hunger for connection and the fear of losing autonomy or being emotionally overwhelmed. Joyce McDougall (1989a) noted that this pattern serves as a "somatic defense", wherein bodily behaviors like purging act as symbolic expressions of psychological conflicts.

Emotional regulation in BN is highly unstable, marked by impulsivity and intense mood fluctuations that mirror the binge-purge cycles. Patients with BN often lack the internal resources to regulate intense emotions, leading them to externalize or act out their feelings through impulsive behaviors. In transference, this instability becomes evident in the patient's shifting emotional responses to the therapist, which can range from deep attachment to sudden anger, reflecting their difficulty in modulating emotions. According to Fonagy et al. (2002), this instability in emotional regulation is tied to impaired mentalization, where patients struggle to understand or process their emotional experiences, leading to sudden outbursts or emotional withdrawal in the therapeutic setting.

In this sense, the binge-purge behavior can be seen as a metaphor for their emotional experience: feelings are taken in with intensity, only to become overwhelming and then expelled. This pattern highlights their difficulty in internalizing and processing emotions, as they lack the means to hold onto and make sense of complex affective states. Therapy can serve as a space to explore and "digest" these emotions without resorting to impulsive behaviors, offering an opportunity to develop healthier ways of managing feelings of dependency, frustration, and self-worth.

Addressing these transference patterns in therapy is crucial, as it allows for the exploration of underlying conflicts that drive the binge-purge cycle and relational instability. By helping the patient become aware of their dependency needs, fear of abandonment, and ambivalence toward intimacy, therapists can work toward building a more stable and secure therapeutic relationship.

The therapist's consistent and non-reactive stance can provide a stable "object" that the patient can rely on, eventually allowing them to internalize healthier relational patterns.

Therapists can encourage patients to explore their "hunger" for emotional connection and validation, helping them recognize that these needs are legitimate and do not have to lead to rejection or expulsion. Over time, the patient may discover how to tolerate the ambivalence between dependency and autonomy, fostering healthier ways of relating to both them and others. This therapeutic journey helps patients replace the symbolic need for binge-purge behavior with more adaptive coping mechanisms, fostering a greater capacity for self-regulation, emotional integration, and relational fulfillment.

Patients with BN often bring intense, chaotic transference dynamics into therapy, marked by acting-out behaviors, emotional upheaval, and risk-taking. This relational turbulence mirrors an unstable internal world where attachment and intimacy are deeply ambivalent experiences. These patients often feel torn between a strong need for connection and an equally powerful fear of dependency, which can lead to an erratic push-and-pull pattern in their relationships (Herzog et al., 1989; Schneider and Irons, 2001). In therapy, these dynamics surface as a desperate need for the therapist's attention, where the therapist becomes a symbolic figure of stability and validation, representing the deep-seated longing for consistent and nurturing connection that the patient may not have experienced in formative relationships.

This need for attachment, however, is complicated by the patient's impulsivity and emotional instability, which can challenge the therapeutic alliance. In particular, the patient's tendency to manage overwhelming emotions through body image and eating behaviors reflects an attempt to express and contain unresolved internal conflicts. Joyce McDougall (1989b) describes such behaviors as creating "theatres of the mind", where the body becomes the stage for acting out psychological distress. For patients with BN, binging, purging, and body fixation are not merely symptoms but are dramatic, symbolic expressions of emotional pain and unresolved conflict. The body, in essence, becomes a vehicle for expressing complex and often contradictory feelings about control, self-worth, and relational boundaries.

McDougall's (1989b) concept of "theatres of the mind" is particularly insightful for understanding the psychodynamic underpinnings of BN. In this framework, physical symptoms serve as performances, a means of externalizing and enacting psychological struggles that the patient cannot consciously articulate. Each episode of binging or purging can be seen as a scene within this internal theatre, representing unspoken fears, unmet needs, or unconscious desires. Through their eating disorder behaviors, patients with BN unconsciously communicate aspects of their emotional world that feel too threatening or overwhelming to confront directly. The therapeutic challenge is to "read" these bodily performances and help the patient begin to symbolize and verbalize the underlying conflicts in ways that promote psychological growth.

In therapy, the impulsivity and neediness in BN patients often lead to boundary-testing behaviors, where the therapist becomes the focus of the patient's intense dependency needs. The therapist's attention and presence are sought as a substitute for the nurturing and stability that the patient longs for but has found difficult to attain. Yet, just as the patient seeks connection, there is also a deep-seated fear of vulnerability, causing them to oscillate between idealizing the therapist and acting out in ways that distance them. This ambivalence complicates the transference and requires the therapist to manage these reactions with both empathy and firm boundaries, providing a stable "holding environment" that allows the patient to safely explore and process their conflicting emotions.

In managing these transference dynamics, the therapist's role is not only to interpret the emotional content behind the patient's symptoms but also to help them gradually replace these bodily enactments with symbolic and verbal expressions of their inner world. This process involves guiding the patient to understand how their behaviors reflect unresolved relational dynamics and helping them develop healthier ways of coping. The therapeutic relationship itself becomes a space where the patient can rehearse new relational patterns, fostering self-awareness and providing the foundation for a more stable and coherent sense of self.

Ultimately, McDougall's "theatres of the mind" framework highlights the depth of the EDs as more than a behavioral pathology; it is a symbolic drama through which patients externalize their internal conflicts. In therapy, by containing and reflecting upon these "performances", the therapist can support the patient in gradually shifting from somatic expressions to psychological insight, enabling them to move toward greater emotional integration and healthier relational patterns (McDougall, 1989b).

Displacement onto food and body image

In both AN and BN, the body serves as a key medium for patients to displace unresolved relational dynamics and internal conflicts. For patients with AN, the body becomes a locus of control, symbolizing an unconscious attempt to manage feelings of dependency, vulnerability, and autonomy by tightly controlling physical needs. In contrast, patients with BN experience cycles of binging and purging that reflect unresolved conflicts around intimacy, attachment, and rejection. These cycles often signify a metaphorical "hunger" for connection, coupled with a deep-seated fear of engulfment and loss of self (Bruch, 1973; Lawrence, 2008). Through their focus on food and body image, patients with BN enact and displace relational needs and conflicts onto their physical selves, turning the body into a battleground for emotional struggles that remain unprocessed.

The dynamics of transference in therapy with BN patients are deeply intertwined with this process of displacement onto the body. Patients often bring their relational patterns into the therapeutic setting, projecting feelings of inadequacy, neediness, or ambivalence toward intimacy onto the therapist. This transference can mirror their relationships outside of therapy, where food and body image act as symbolic stand-ins for emotional needs and conflicts. By engaging with the body as an object of control or nurturance, these patients attempt to resolve unmet attachment needs and feelings of inner emptiness through physical acts rather than interpersonal connection.

Understanding these displacement dynamics is essential in psychoanalytic therapy, as it allows therapists to interpret the transference as a reflection of the patient's underlying relational patterns. For instance, a patient's compulsive focus on food intake or body weight may reveal unconscious feelings of inadequacy or dependency that originated in early attachment relationships. By exploring these projections in therapy, therapists help patients recognize the ways in which their eating behaviors express repressed emotional needs, thereby facilitating greater awareness of the symbolic role the eating disorder plays in their lives. Fonagy et al. (2002) note that through the process of transference interpretation, patients can begin to unravel these unconscious conflicts and identify how their eating behaviors serve as attempts to regulate and express unmet emotional needs.

As the therapeutic work deepens, patients gain insight into the emotional drives fueling their compulsive behaviors, learning to separate relational needs from physical actions. This increased awareness promotes healthier, more adaptive relational dynamics and reduces the reliance on displacement mechanisms. Therapy, therefore, becomes a transformative process, where the compulsive, body-centered aspects of the EDs are gradually replaced with a capacity for more authentic connections and emotional self-regulation.

Countertransference in the treatment of eating disorders: A transformative tool

Countertransference has become an essential concept in psychoanalytic treatment, particularly for patients with EDs. It provides unique insights into the relational dynamics that patients project onto their bodies, behaviors, and interpersonal relationships. When managed effectively, countertransference enables therapists to uncover unconscious conflicts, deepen their understanding of the patient's inner world, and foster meaningful healing.

Historical perspectives on countertransference

The understanding of countertransference has evolved significantly. Originally defined as the analyst's unconscious reaction to the patient's transference, it has expanded into a broader framework for exploring therapeutic relationships. The *"British Psychoanalytic School"*, particularly within the Kleinian framework, emphasized countertransference as deeply tied to processes of projection and introjection (Hinshelwood, 1999). Madeleine and Willy Baranger in Buenos Aires (1969) advanced this perspective with their concept of the "analytic field", framing countertransference as a dynamic intersubjective phenomenon that extends beyond dyadic interactions. This concept has proven invaluable in treating ED patients, who often communicate their struggles through somatic symptoms and relational patterns.

Jacques Lacan critiqued the Kleinian view, suggesting that countertransference is shaped not only by the patient's projections but also by the analyst's unconscious resistances (Lacan, 1951). This dual perspective underscores the importance of distinguishing the analyst's contributions from the patient's material, a balance that is particularly critical when working with ED patients.

Countertransference is inherently tied to the therapist's emotional responses, which serve as reflections of the patient's mental state. Winnicott (1949), in his seminal work *"Hate in the Countertransference"*, emphasized the therapeutic value of tolerating difficult emotions, initially focusing on psychotic and psychopathic patients. These insights are now central to the treatment of EDs, where intense emotions frequently arise.

René Spitz (1956) introduced the concept of a *"diatrophic attitude"* to describe the therapist's role in supporting the regressive and infantile aspects that often emerge during therapy. This term emphasizes the therapeutic stance of nurturing and sustaining the patient through their emotional vulnerabilities, echoing the maternal-infant bond that Spitz identified as crucial for healthy psychological development. However, there appears to be some confusion or misinterpretation of the term, as "atrophic attitude" might also be relevant in describing conditions of emotional and physical decline observed in Spitz's research on maternal deprivation. Spitz's (1945) work on *hospitalism* revealed how the lack of maternal care leads to developmental and emotional deterioration, underlining the critical importance of consistent and attuned caregiving.

Spitz's insights into the maternal-infant relationship inform the therapist's role in providing a "holding function" during treatment. This function mirrors the nurturing role of a primary caregiver, offering patients the emotional safety and support needed for psychological growth and repair. In the context of EDs, this holding function becomes particularly significant, as many patients have experienced early relational environments marked by disruptions in emotional attunement and caregiving. The absence of this foundational connection often leaves ED patients struggling with unresolved dependencies, fragmented self-concepts, and maladaptive coping mechanisms.

By adopting a "diatrophic attitude," the therapist creates a secure and empathetic space where patients can explore their regressive tendencies and unmet emotional needs. This approach fosters the reparation of early relational wounds, enabling patients to develop a stronger sense of self and healthier ways to regulate emotions. Spitz's emphasis on nurturing regressive aspects aligns with the broader psychoanalytic view that the therapeutic relationship can provide a curative emotional experience, one that compensates for earlier developmental deficits and facilitates psychological growth.

Spitz's contributions continue to underscore the essential role of empathy, attunement, and a holding therapeutic environment in treating patients whose early relational experiences have left deep emotional scars. For individuals with EDs, this approach can bridge the gap between past relational failures and the present potential for healing and integration.

Harold Searles (1959) extended the use of countertransference to work with severely disturbed patients, often in cases of schizophrenia, and emphasized the need for frequent sessions and the therapist's capacity to tolerate deep regression. Searles argued that managing intense countertransference responses enables therapists to process the patient's lack of psychic differentiation, supporting a sense of integration within the therapeutic field. He highlighted that tolerating countertransference is not only challenging but also essential for allowing the therapist to contain the patient's projections, fostering a space for healing (Searles, 1959).

Wilfred Bion's container-contained model (1962) has been pivotal in understanding countertransference in the treatment of EDs. Bion posited that therapists act as containers for the patient's unprocessed emotional states, mirroring the nonverbal dynamics of mother-infant interactions. For ED patients, who often communicate their distress through their bodies rather than words, this containment function is particularly critical. The therapist's ability to process and reflect on the patient's projections fosters the potential for emotional integration and growth within the therapeutic relationship.

Building on Bion's framework, Williams (1997) introduced the concept of a "porous psychic membrane" to describe the limitations of the therapeutic apparatus in certain patients. Unlike Bion's model, which emphasizes the successful containment and transformation of emotions, Williams highlights the challenges faced when the psychic membrane is too porous to retain experiences effectively. In therapeutic transference-countertransference dynamics, this porous structure manifests as the patient's inability to recall or build upon material discussed in previous sessions, disrupting the continuity of the therapeutic process.

For patients with EDs, particularly those with severe fragmentation in their psychic structures, this porousness often reflects an inability to internalize or contain their experiences. Sessions can feel disconnected, with the therapist noticing that the patient struggles to integrate insights or recall key emotional events from one session to the next. This dynamic can leave therapists feeling frustrated or helpless, as the therapeutic process seems to lack continuity or cumulative progress.

Williams' concept underscores the therapist's role in working within these fragmented dynamics. Rather than becoming discouraged by the patient's apparent inability to retain or build upon therapeutic material, therapists must adapt their approach to accommodate the patient's limited capacity for psychic containment. This may involve repetition, the gentle reinforcement of key themes, and a focus on grounding the patient in the present session's material.

Otto Kernberg (1965) further refined countertransference theory by identifying two key dimensions. The first, consistent with Freud's view, relates to the analyst's personal neurotic conflicts triggered by the patient's transference. The second is a "totalistic" reaction, where the patient's intense needs and projections draw strong conscious and unconscious responses from the analyst. Kernberg found that these totalistic reactions, which are especially common in patients with personality disorders, serve as diagnostic markers for understanding the patient's regression level and stance toward the therapist. Such responses are crucial for patients with EDs, who often evoke feelings of protectiveness, frustration, and even helplessness in therapists.

Peter Fonagy's (1991) concept of mentalization provided another lens through which to understand countertransference, defining it as the therapist's capacity to grasp both the conscious and unconscious states of others. In EDs treatment, this perspective on countertransference as a mentalization tool helps therapists interpret patients' internal worlds through their own emotional responses, allowing for insights into the patient's underlying conflicts and attachment dynamics.

Adalberto Perrotta (1993) added to this understanding by conceptualizing countertransference as an interpretive tool that helps analysts generate hypotheses about the analytic field, transforming raw emotional material into therapeutic insights.

Glen Gabbard (1995) emphasized the importance of distinguishing between countertransference and projective identification, viewing countertransference as a co-created process shaped by both patient and analyst.

The challenge of narcissistic dynamics

Some patients with AN also presents narcissistic traits or personality disorders. Among the most common countertransference feelings experienced when treating narcissistic personalities are boredom, control, contempt, and admiration (Gabbard, 1998). The feeling of boredom is especially prominent with narcissistic patients, who often disregard the therapist, failing to acknowledge their presence or importance. This dynamic creates a sense of profound exclusion, as if the patient exists entirely alone in their psychological space, rendering the analyst's presence almost irrelevant. Otto Kernberg (1970) referred to this phenomenon as a "satellite existence", describing how the narcissistic patient positions others—including the therapist—as peripheral entities orbiting their central sense of self.

Faced with this exclusion, the therapist may unconsciously withdraw, neglecting the material the patient presents and retreating into their own internal world. Oremland and Windholz (1971) noted that therapists in such situations may find themselves drifting into personal fantasies, inadvertently disengaging from the therapeutic process. This withdrawal reflects a countertransference response to the patient's self-sufficient and dismissive stance, which can evoke feelings of powerlessness, inadequacy, or irrelevance in the therapist (Persano and Ventura, 2006). Recognizing these dynamics is critical, as unchecked countertransference reactions risk reinforcing the patient's sense of isolation and invalidation, perpetuating the very relational patterns the therapy seeks to address.

Countertransference and the intersection of ED and BPD dynamics

Insights from the treatment of borderline personality disorder (BPD) offer valuable perspectives on countertransference in the therapeutic work with ED patients. Both groups share overlapping psychological dynamics, such as fragmented self-concepts, difficulties with emotional regulation, and relational instability (Meissner, 1988). These shared traits mean that countertransference, a vital element in BPD therapy, can provide equally significant insights in ED treatment.

Patients with BPD are often described as highly intuitive and attuned to their therapists' unconscious states. This perceptiveness can bring unresolved aspects of the therapist's psyche to the forefront, creating a dynamic interplay of projections and emotional responses. Similarly, patients with EDs—particularly those with comorbid BPD traits—often display acute sensitivity to the therapist's reactions. They may unconsciously test boundaries or provoke emotional responses as a way of exploring their own unmet needs and fears of rejection.

This heightened sensitivity in EDs and BPD patients frequently complicates the therapeutic process. Their intense projections can evoke a wide range of countertransference responses, including frustration, protectiveness, helplessness, or even a desire to rescue the patient. Frustration may arise when patients engage in self-destructive behaviors, such as extreme restriction, binging, or purging, despite therapeutic efforts to foster insight or change. This mirrors the push-pull dynamics seen in BPD, where patients oscillate between seeking connection and fearing intimacy. Protectiveness may emerge as therapists witness the physical and emotional toll of the patient's behaviors. This reflects the deep caregiving dynamics often provoked by BPD patients, who evoke feelings of both nurturing and exasperation in their relationships.

Persano and Ventura (2006) emphasize the importance of understanding and managing these countertransference reactions to remain grounded in the therapeutic process. For ED patients with BPD traits, therapists must carefully navigate these emotional undercurrents to maintain professional boundaries and foster a supportive environment.

Patients with EDs, like those with BPD, often project their relational conflicts and unconscious fears onto the therapeutic relationship. These projections frequently revolve around core issues such as dependency: Both BPD and ED patients struggle with intense dependency needs, which they may suppress or express ambivalently. For example, a patient with AN may use rigid control over their body to mask a profound fear of dependency, while a patient with BN may oscillate between clinging to and rejecting the therapist. Rejection, the fear of being judged or abandoned is common in both groups, often leading to testing behaviors in therapy. BPD patients may idealize the therapist initially, only to devalue them later, while ED patients may express distrust or defensiveness, particularly if their symptoms feel threatened. Autonomy, the therapeutic relationship, often becomes a microcosm for the patient's struggle between autonomy and connection. This is particularly evident in patients with AN, who may view the therapist as an intruder on their carefully controlled world, or in patients with BN, who may vacillate between craving the therapist's approval and fearing emotional engulfment.

By remaining attuned to these dynamics, therapists can use countertransference to better understand the patient's underlying fears and relational patterns. For instance, a therapist's sense of rejection may mirror the patient's internalized fear of abandonment, providing a pathway for therapeutic exploration.

Managing countertransference in ED and BPD Psychotherapy

Therapists working with ED and BPD patients must strike a delicate balance between empathy and professional boundaries (Persano and Ventura, 2006). Key strategies include:

1 *Self-reflection*: Regular reflection on countertransference responses helps therapists differentiate between their own emotional reactions and the patient's projections. This self-awareness allows for more effective navigation of complex relational dynamics.
2 *Supervision and consultation*: The intense countertransference reactions evoked by these patients underscore the importance of supervision. Discussing these feelings with peers or supervisors helps therapists process their experiences, preventing enactment of unconscious dynamics.
3 *Setting clear boundaries*: Both ED and BPD patients often test the limits of the therapeutic relationship. Establishing and maintaining clear boundaries ensures the therapy remains a safe and structured environment for exploring underlying conflicts.

4   *Focusing on the present moment*: Kernberg (1965) emphasizes the importance of immediate, "here-and-now" interpretations with borderline patients. This approach is equally valuable in ED treatment, where patients often struggle to connect with their emotions or behaviors in real time.

Countertransference in anorexia nervosa

Patients with anorexia nervosa (AN) frequently evoke complementary countertransference, projecting relational dynamics characterized by hyper-control and suppressed emotional needs. For instance, a patient's rigid self-control may provoke feelings of helplessness or frustration in the therapist, mirroring the patient's struggle to maintain autonomy while avoiding dependency.

In these cases, the therapist might feel as though they are embodying the role of a powerless caregiver, reflecting the patient's internalized fear of emotional intrusion. Recognizing these countertransference reactions allows the therapist to approach the patient with empathy and insight, creating a space for the safe exploration of underlying conflicts.

These individuals may evoke feelings of helplessness or irrelevance in the therapist, reflecting their own struggle to suppress dependency and maintain rigid self-control. Therapists may unconsciously align with the role of a powerless caregiver, mirroring the patient's defensive autonomy.

The therapist often experiences a profound sense of helplessness due to the patient's difficulties in developing insight. In such cases, the ability to reflect on what is occurring between the therapist and the patient, and to use these countertransference feelings as a diagnostic inferential tool, becomes critically important. This process enables a deeper understanding of the intimate workings of the patient's psyche within the therapeutic process (Persano, 2006).

It is essential for therapists to reflect on countertransference feelings, particularly those related to adopting a gentle approach during the interpretation process. According to Gianna Williams (2000), therapists may often feel compelled to soften their interventions when working with patients who struggle to tolerate direct interpretations. While this gentleness can foster patient engagement and provide a sense of safety, it does not imply avoiding interpretation altogether. In fact, a patient's request for gentleness may sometimes mask a deeper resistance, serving as an unconscious attempt to deter the therapist from fully engaging in their role. Even when therapists deliberately soften the emotional tone of their interventions, such patients often evoke intensely charged emotions in the therapist's mind. These dynamics underscore the complexity of navigating the therapeutic relationship and the importance of utilizing countertransference feelings as both a diagnostic and therapeutic tool (Persano, 2006).

In my clinical work with restrictive patients with restrictive AN, I have found that managing the intense emotions elicited in countertransference is a delicate and essential process. It requires thoughtful reflection to discern which emotions are genuine reflections of the therapeutic relationship and which might stem from my own subjective experiences. This reflective process allows for interpretations that are offered tentatively and hypothetically rather than as firm or definitive statements, which could feel harsh, intrusive, or even judgmental to patients who are already emotionally vulnerable (Persano, 2006). This approach is particularly effective in creating a safe and tolerable therapeutic environment for individuals with significant psychological fragility.

This approach closely aligns with Gianna Williams's concept of "primary color" interpretations (Williams, 1997), which serves as a metaphor for delivering therapeutic insights in a manner akin to soft, foundational hues rather than stark or overwhelming tones. Just as primary colors provide the essential base for a visual composition without overwhelming the viewer, primary color interpretations aim to gently introduce insights that can be gradually integrated by the patient. These interpretations avoid the "sharpness" of overly vivid or declarative remarks that might feel too intense, threatening, or invasive for the patient.

For patients with restrictive AN, who often struggle with defensiveness and heightened sensitivity, soft interpretations serve multiple purposes. They respect the patient's psychological boundaries by framing insights in a way that feels exploratory rather than prescriptive. For instance, instead of stating, "You're controlling food to suppress your emotions", a soft interpretation might take the form of, "I wonder if focusing on food gives you a sense of control when emotions feel overwhelming". This subtle approach invites collaboration, encouraging the patient to reflect and engage without feeling criticized or coerced.

Soft interpretations, much like soft colors, create an atmosphere of warmth and safety. They allow space for the patient to process difficult emotions and thoughts at their own pace, without the risk of feeling overwhelmed or misunderstood. This is particularly important for patients with restrictive AN, who may already perceive the therapeutic setting as a challenge to their autonomy or as a source of potential judgment.

By integrating Williams's concept of "primary color" interpretations, therapists can build trust and facilitate deeper therapeutic exploration. These interpretations act as gentle invitations rather than demands, fostering a collaborative therapeutic relationship where the patient feels heard, respected, and emotionally secure. Ultimately, this approach helps patients move toward greater self-awareness and resilience, while maintaining the delicate balance needed to support their psychological fragility.

Countertransference in bulimia nervosa

Patients with bulimia nervosa (BN) often evoke complementary counter-transference reactions due to the oscillating and contradictory nature of their relational patterns. During the therapeutic process, the therapist may experience deflected or deferred aspects of the patient's internal object world, as if enacting different facets of the patient's mind. As Racker (1959) noted, in complementary countertransference, the analyst may unconsciously assume the role of the patient's internalized object, offering valuable clinical insight into unconscious dynamics. The binge-purge cycle symbolizes a push-pull dynamic between intense emotional needs and fear of rejection or engulfment. This dynamic frequently manifests in therapy, where the patient's emotional volatility can provoke strong responses.

The emotional turbulence of binge-purge cycles often evokes protec-tiveness or frustration in the therapist. These feelings can reflect the patient's ambivalent longing for intimacy and fear of rejection, high-lighting their internal push-pull dynamic between connection and withdrawal.

Therapists may feel overwhelmed by the patient's impulsivity and emotional intensity, mirroring the patient's inner chaos in concordant countertransference. Therapists may feel compelled to rescue the patient, responding to their unconscious longing for connection. Alternatively, feelings of frustration or rejection may arise, reflecting the patient's inter-nalized fear of abandonment in complementary countertransference.

These countertransference manifestations highlight the defensive pro-cesses of alternating idealization and devaluation, which reveal the struc-tural splitting of the personality, as commonly observed in patients with borderline personality organization.

In these patients, words are not used to assign meaning to psychic phenomena capable of representation but are instead employed to dis-charge primitive emotional states. These archaic emotional states, tied to words used for a cathartic purpose, deeply affect the analyst's mind. The analyst, feeling overwhelmed, may respond with their own primi-tive emotions in a manner resembling a countertransference reaction (Persano, 2006).

The manifestations of countertransference vary significantly between patients with anorexia nervosa (AN) and bulimia nervosa (BN). In patients with AN, their rigid self-sufficiency often evokes feelings of irrelevance or helplessness in the therapist. These reactions mirror the patient's suppression of emotional needs and fear of dependency. In contrast, patients with BN exhibit chaotic and demanding behaviors that can elicit feelings of protectiveness or frustration in the therapist, as they navigate the patient's ambivalent longing for intimacy and simultaneous fear of engulfment.

Managing countertransference in EDs' treatment

Effectively managing countertransference is critical for maintaining an attuned and productive therapeutic relationship. Practical strategies include:

- *Awareness of countertransference*: Therapists must actively monitor their emotional responses to distinguish between their own feelings and the patient's projections. This awareness prevents unconscious enactments that might reinforce the patient's maladaptive patterns.
- *Reflecting on complementary dynamics*: Therapists should explore emotions such as helplessness or protectiveness to uncover the patient's underlying conflicts, such as fear of dependency or unresolved anger.
- *Using countertransference as a diagnostic tool*: Emotional reactions provide valuable insights into the patient's relational world. For example, feelings of frustration might reveal the patient's struggle to express needs without fear of rejection.
- *Balancing boundaries and empathy*: Therapists must maintain a compassionate yet boundaried stance, creating a safe space for the patient to explore their unconscious conflicts.

Navigating countertransference in clinical work with eating disorder patients: Insights from supervision

Countertransference in the treatment of eating disorder (ED) patients presents unique challenges and opportunities, especially when therapists utilize supervision to reflect on their experiences. Supervision provides an essential space for therapists to process the intense emotions that arise during sessions, enabling them to distinguish between their own feelings and the patient's projections. These reflections are critical in navigating the complex relational dynamics often encountered in ED treatment, where transference and countertransference are deeply intertwined.

Supervision becomes a crucial forum for examining therapeutic decisions and emotional responses. For instance, therapists can explore whether their gentle approach stems from a conscious effort to build trust or from unconscious countertransference reactions, such as frustration, protectiveness, or fear of harming the patient. This process allows therapists to discern whether the patient's request for gentleness masks deeper resistance or functions as an unconscious attempt to limit therapeutic interventions.

Refining therapeutic approaches through supervision

In our clinical supervision experience, we have observed how countertransference feelings often mirror the patient's internal conflicts. For example, in working with patients with restrictive AN, therapists may feel helpless or frustrated by the patient's resistance to insight and change. Supervision provides the space to explore these reactions, enabling the therapist to formulate interpretations that address the patient's fear of dependency and vulnerability in a nuanced and constructive manner.

Supervision also facilitates the refinement of therapeutic techniques, such as hypothesized, gentle interpretations. This approach, crucial for patients prone to psychological fragility, aligns with Williams's (1997) concept of "primary color" interpretations, which emphasizes delivering insights in a tolerable, inferred manner rather than through blunt declarations. Supervision discussions highlight the delicate balance between fostering therapeutic engagement and respecting the patient's need for emotional safety, guiding therapists in navigating this complex terrain.

The importance of supervision for junior psychotherapists

For junior therapists, supervision is essential in preventing countertransference enactments during the treatment of severely disturbed patients. Reflecting on clinical material within a structured and supportive framework allows therapists to regain their capacity to think critically about the material. This process aids in understanding the therapeutic dynamics and exploring archaic object relations tied to intense negative emotions that are activated in transference during the analytic process.

Supervision also helps therapists address split-off and expelled material from the patient's psychic apparatus. Such material, often projected into the therapeutic relationship through mechanisms like projective identification, can manifest as overwhelming and disorganized emotional content. By working through these dynamics in supervision, therapists can better process and contain the material within the analytic field, fostering a deeper understanding of the patient's unconscious conflicts and enhancing therapeutic efficacy.

Recognizing concordant and complementary countertransference

Supervision plays a critical role in helping therapists explore their own unconscious contributions to the therapeutic dynamic. Drawing on Heinrich Racker's (1948) concepts of concordant and complementary countertransference, supervisors can guide therapists in recognizing when they are identifying with the patient's feelings (concordant) or unconsciously embodying a significant figure from the patient's past, such as a critical or nurturing caregiver (complementary). By processing these dynamics, therapists can better understand how the patient's relational patterns are projected and reenacted in the therapeutic relationship.

Transforming countertransference into a pathway for healing

Supervision is an indispensable resource for navigating countertransference in the treatment of eating disorders (EDs). It offers therapists a reflective space to explore and process the intense emotional reactions that often arise in therapeutic work with this population. By doing so, supervision helps therapists maintain a compassionate yet appropriately boundaried stance, enabling them to effectively engage with the patient's unconscious conflicts without becoming overwhelmed or entangled. This reflective process is essential for building trust and fostering deeper therapeutic engagement.

Far from being a barrier, countertransference—when supported through supervision—becomes a dynamic and diagnostic tool. Supervision allows therapists to gain insight into the relational dynamics at play, transforming potentially disruptive emotional reactions into valuable sources of understanding about the patient's inner world. By facilitating clarity and confidence, supervision equips therapists to navigate challenging therapeutic encounters with greater skill and empathy.

Ultimately, this process enhances the overall treatment experience, both for the therapist and the patient. Supervision not only strengthens the therapeutic relationship but also supports patients in confronting and integrating their unconscious conflicts. In this way, countertransference becomes a pathway for understanding and resolving the deeper emotional struggles underlying the eating disorder, helping patients move toward healing and psychological growth.

Countertransference challenges: Insights from clinical cases

Supervision is crucial for managing the intense and often chaotic countertransference feelings evoked by patients with bulimia nervosa (BN). These patients tend to oscillate between emotional neediness and withdrawal, creating a challenging and unpredictable therapeutic dynamic. A distinctive feature of communication in patients with BN is their use of cathartic language, which serves not to gain insight but to discharge emotional intensity. This style of interaction can leave therapists feeling overwhelmed, unsure how to interpret or respond effectively to the emotional turbulence presented in sessions.

By providing a structured and reflective space, supervision helps therapists process their reactions and develop strategies to navigate the emotional complexity of the psychotherapeutic process with patients who have bulimia nervosa (BN). It fosters a more grounded therapeutic approach, enabling therapists to remain present, empathetic, and effective, even when faced with the challenges posed by the intense relational dynamics often encountered in this work.

As one therapist described during supervision:

> The patient would flood the session with anger and reproach, leaving me feeling frustrated and ineffective. Supervision helped me understand that her defiance and emotional outbursts reflected her ambivalence about connection and her unconscious fear of rejection.

This example underscores how supervision allows therapists to process their emotions and recognize the defensive processes at play, such as idealization and denigration, which often characterize borderline dynamics in ED patients. These splitting patterns can cause therapists to feel alternately devalued and idealized, leading to emotional imbalance. Supervision becomes a vital tool for maintaining objectivity and addressing these countertransference challenges effectively.

For patients with BN, complementary countertransference may manifest as the therapist feeling like a rescuer, responding to implicit demands for validation and nurturance. While this dynamic may stem from the patient's unconscious desire for connection, it can blur therapeutic boundaries if left unchecked. Supervision offers a space to examine these reactions, ensuring that therapists avoid enacting unconscious relational scripts that might reinforce maladaptive patterns.

A vivid example of this dynamic was shared by a colleague treating a patient with BN:

> Sessions were dynamic until, at a certain point, the patient shifted from self-questioning to criticizing the professionals, one by one. Her anger and reproach filled the sessions, leaving less room for reflection. Her defiant attitude and torrent of words created tension, leaving me angry and frustrated. Only after discussing these feelings in supervision did I feel some relief

This illustrates how supervision can provide therapists with a deeper understanding of their countertransference responses. By reflecting on feelings of frustration or helplessness, therapists can uncover the primitive object relations activated during the analytic process, helping to disentangle their emotions from the patient's projections. This process enables therapists to engage more thoughtfully and effectively with the patient's underlying relational conflicts (Persano, 2006).

The role of supervision in managing countertransference

Supervision is particularly critical for therapists new to the field, as they may struggle to navigate the intensity of countertransference in patients with BN. Without proper support, they risk enacting these emotions, potentially reinforcing the patient's maladaptive relational patterns. For example, cathartic language used by these patients may feel over-whelming to therapists, leaving them emotionally flooded. Supervision offers a framework to process these feelings and regain perspective.

Discussing countertransference in supervision also highlights how patients with BN often use emotional discharge as a defense against exploring deeper meanings. These defenses, rooted in splitting and projective identification, require the therapist to maintain a balanced and reflective stance. As Persano (2006) notes, supervision enables therapists to understand these dynamics while preventing emotional acting-out in sessions.

Working with patients with BN demands careful navigation of coun-tertransference dynamics, which often mirror the patients' internal con-flicts and relational patterns. Supervision serves as an indispensable resource for processing the complex emotions that arise, fostering a deeper understanding of the patient's unconscious defenses. By addressing these challenges within a supportive framework, therapists can maintain their therapeutic effectiveness, transforming countertransference into a valuable tool for healing and integration.

Managing exhaustion in therapy with severely disorganized patients

Another colleague shared her experiences with a severely disorganized patient, describing the profound feelings of powerlessness, anger, and exhaustion that arose in therapy. She observed:

> The patient seemed 'dead inside', and my attempts to connect with her were met with silence or 'I don't know'. She was unable to orga-nize herself or ask for help. Only after psychiatric hospitalization did she gain structure in her life, finally achieving a sense of order she could not establish on her own
>
> (Persano, 2006).

This exhaustion and confusion reflect the "totalistic countertransference" that Kernberg (1993; 2016) and Gabbard (1995) discuss, where severe per-sonality disorganization triggers strong emotions in the therapist. For such patients, establishing limits within outpatient treatment is often necessary, as their demands can overwhelm the therapist's capacity for containment. In some cases, psychiatric or clinical-nutritional hospitalization becomes essential—not as a countertransference reaction but as a genuine contain-ment measure to help the therapist reflect on the treatment without being overwhelmed by the patient's chaotic behaviors (Persano, 2006).

The therapist's fear for the patient's life

A particular challenge in working with severe eating disorders is the therapist's fear for the patient's life, given the risks associated with malnutrition, cardiac issues, and self-harm. Treating high-risk patients requires a coordinated interdisciplinary team, with each member maintaining open communication about the patient's well-being. This teamwork allows the analyst to focus on psychoanalytic work without feeling they are constantly in an emergency, which could lead to counter-transferential acting-out and even rescue fantasies that risk enmeshment with the patient's dynamics (Persano, 2006).

Navigating concealment and deception in eating disorder treatment

Another challenge is the frequent concealment and deception observed in these patients, often tied to an inability to verbalize their symptoms and a defensive need to preserve a symptom-based identity. The patient's unconscious maneuvers may lead to confrontations with family members in adolescent cases, as parents share information the patient has withheld. This dynamic can draw the therapist into conflict, especially if parents request consultations to disclose hidden behaviors. In such cases, countertransference awareness is critical, as these patients seek autonomy but unconsciously desire parental substitutes in their therapists. Recognizing these dynamics is crucial to avoid enacting unconscious fantasies and to understand the patient's ambivalence about autonomy.

Countertransference: A pathway to healing in eating disorder treatment

Countertransference is not merely a challenge but a transformative tool in the psychoanalytic treatment of eating disorders (EDs). Patients with EDs often project their internal conflicts onto the therapeutic relationship, externalizing their struggles through symptoms and relational patterns. By tolerating and reflecting on their emotional responses, therapists gain critical insights into the unconscious dynamics driving these behaviors, fostering trust, collaboration, and the integration of healthier relational patterns. As Glen Gabbard (1995) emphasized, countertransference becomes a co-created process shaped by both the patient and the therapist, offering a pathway to navigate the intense emotional landscapes of ED patients with greater understanding and empathy.

Countertransference serves as a dynamic and diagnostic tool, enabling therapists to uncover unconscious relational patterns that fuel the patient's symptoms. By recognizing and reflecting on their countertransference responses, therapists can transform these reactions into meaningful therapeutic insights. For example, patients with AN may evoke feelings of helplessness or frustration in the therapist, mirroring their internal struggle to suppress dependency and maintain rigid self-control. Conversely, patients with BN often elicit protectiveness or frustration, reflecting their oscillation between emotional neediness and withdrawal. Understanding these dynamics allows therapists to address the core conflicts around dependency, autonomy, and self-worth that underpin the patient's behaviors.

Effectively managing countertransference involves viewing it as a series of inferences rather than reactionary responses. Combining bottom-up strategies—inferring from the patient's presented material—and top-down approaches rooted in countertransference theory allows therapists to tailor interventions to each patient's unique dynamics. For ED patients, this method broadens the therapeutic scope, offering valuable insights into their psychic organization while addressing the relational conflicts that maintain their symptoms.

Through collaborative exploration, countertransference fosters deeper emotional integration and healing. Therapists can use their emotional responses as a diagnostic and therapeutic resource, illuminating the patient's unconscious fears and unmet needs. This process not only disrupts the destructive cycles of EDs but also facilitates the development of healthier relational patterns and a more cohesive sense of self. By remaining attuned to their countertransference reactions, therapists transform potential pitfalls into opportunities for growth, making countertransference an indispensable cornerstone of psychoanalytic treatment and a pathway to lasting emotional healing.

Bibliography

Baranger, M. and Baranger, W. (1969). La situación analítica como campo dinámico. In *Problemas del Campo Psicoanalítico*, Buenos Aires: Ed. Kargieman, (chapter 7, 1993 edition).

Bion, W. R. (1962). *Learning from Experience*. London: Heinemann.

Breuer, J. and Freud, S. (1893a). Studies on hysteria: Case histories, Case 2: Frau Emmy von N. *The Standard Edition of the Complete Psychological Works of Sigmund Freud, (2)*. London: The Hogarth Press, 48–105 (1991 edition).

Breuer, J. and Freud, S. (1893b). Studies on hysteria: Case histories, Case 4: Katharina. *The Standard Edition of the Complete Psychological Works of Sigmund Freud, (2)*. London: The Hogarth Press, 125–134 (1991 edition).

Bruch, H. (1973). *Eating Disorders: Obesity, Anorexia Nervosa and the Person Within*. New York: Basic Books.

Crisp, A. H. (1980). *Anorexia Nervosa: Let Me Be*. Academic Press.

Fairburn, C. G., Cooper, Z., and Shafran, R. (2003). Cognitive behavior therapy for eating disorders: A "transdiagnostic" theory and treatment. *Behaviour Research and Therapy*, 41(5): 509–528.

Fonagy, P. (1991). Thinking about thinking: Some clinical and theoretical considerations in the treatment of a borderline patient. *International Journal of Psychoanalysis*, 72(4): 639–656.

Fonagy, P., Gergely, G., Jurist, E. L., and Target, M. (2002). *Affect Regulation, Mentalization and the Development of the Self*. New York: Other Press.

Freud, S. (1912). The Dynamics of transference. *The Standard Edition of the Complete Psychological Works of Sigmund Freud, (18)*. London: The Hogarth Press, 3–64 (1991 edition).

Gabbard, G. O. (1995). Countertransference: The emerging common ground. *International Journal of Psychoanalysis*, 76(3): 475–486.

Gabbard, G. O. (1998). Transference and countertransference in the treatment of narcissistic patients. In E. Ronningstam (ed.) *Disorders of Narcissism. Diagnostic, Clinical and Empirical Implications*. Washington DC: American Psychiatric Press, 125–145.

Gabbard, G. O. (2001). *Love and Hate in the Analytic Setting*. London: Karnac Books.

Heimann, P. (1950). On counter-transference. *International Journal of Psychoanalysis*, 31: 81–84.

Herzog, D. B., Keller, M. B., Sacks, N. R., Yeh, C. J., and Lavori, P. W. (1989). Psychiatric comorbidity in treatment-seeking anorexics and bulimics. *Journal of the American Academy of Child & Adolescent Psychiatry*, 28(6): 829–835.

Hinshelwood, R. D. (1999). Countertransference. *International Journal of Psychoanalysis*, 80(4): 797–818.

Jacobson, E. (1964). *The Self and the Object World*. New York: International Universities Press.

Jacobson, E. (1971). *Depression: Comparative Studies of Normal, Neurotic, and Psychotic Conditions*. Madison, CT: International Universities Press.

Jeammet, P. (1984). L'anorexie mentale. *Encyclo. Med. Chir. Psychiatrie Vol. 3*, 37350: A10 et A15; 2. París: Elsevier.

Kernberg, O. F. (1965). Notes on countertransference. *Journal of the American Psychoanalytic Association*, 13(1): 38–56.

Kernberg, O. F. (1970). Factors in the psychoanalytic treatment of narcissistic personalities. *Journal of the American Psychoanalytic Association*, 18(1): 51–85.

Kernberg, O. F. (1976). *Object Relations Theory and Clinical Psychoanalysis*. New York: Jason Aronson.

Kernberg, O. F. (1984). *Severe Personality Disorders: Psychotherapeutic Strategies*. New Haven, CT: Yale University Press.

Kernberg, O. F. (1985). Object relations theory and the psychoanalytic treatment of narcissistic personalities. In A. J. Cooper (ed.), *Narcissism and the Interpersonal Self*. Madison, CT: International Universities Press, 65–89.

Kernberg, O. F. (1990). New perspectives in psychoanalytic affect theory. In R. Plutchik and H. Kellerman (eds.) *Emotion, Psychopathology, and Psychotherapy*. New York: Academic Press, 115–131.

Kernberg, O. F. (1993). The psychotherapeutic management of psychotic transferences in borderline patients. *Journal of Clinical Psychoanalysis*, 2(1): 23–36.

Kernberg, O. F. (2004). *Aggression in Personality Disorders and Perversions*. New Haven, CT: Yale University Press.

Kernberg, O. F. (2016). The treatment of patients with borderline personality organization. *Bulletin of the Menninger Clinic*, 80(4): 307–328.

Klein, M. (1932). Melanie Klein: Subject relations. In L. Gomez *An Introduction to Object Relations*. New York: New York University Press, 29–53.

Lacan, J. (1951). Intervención sobre la Transferencia. In *Escritos1*. Buenos Aires: Siglo XXI Editores, 204–215.

Lawrence, M. (2008). *The Anorexic Mind*. London: Routledge.

McDougall, J. (1989a). *Théâtres du Corps*. Paris: Éd. Gallimard.

McDougall, J. (1989b). *Theatres of the Mind: Illusion and Truth on the Psychoanalytic Stage*. New York: Free Association Books.

Meissner, W. W. (1988). Countertransference. In *Treatment of Patients in the Borderline Spectrum*. New Jersey: Jason Aronson, 209–249 (chapter 7).

Oremland, J. and Windholz, E. (1971). Some specific transference, countertransference and supervisory problems in the analysis of a narcissistic personality. *International Journal of Psychoanalysis*, 52(3): 267–274.

Perrotta, A. (1993). *Contratransferencia y Regresión: Un Modelo Científicono Tradicional Aplicado a la Clínica Psicoanalítica*. Buenos Aires: Editorial de la Fundación, Ediciones Machi.

Persano, H. L. (2006). Contratransferência em pacientes com transtornos alimentares. In J. Zaslavsky and M. J. Pires dos Santos (eds.) *Contratransferência: Teoria e Prática Clínica*. Porto Alegre: Artmed, 150–166 (chapter 10).

Persano, H. L. and Ventura, A. D. (2006). Contratransferência em pacientes com transtornos da personalidade borderline e narcisista. In J. Zaslavsky and M. J. Pires dos Santos (eds.) *Contratransferência: Teoria e Prática Clínica*. Porto Alegre: Artmed, 103–124 (chapter 7).

Racamier, P. C. (1970). *Le Psychanalyste Sans Divan*. Paris: Ed. Payot.

Racker, H. (1948). A contribution to the problem of counter-transference. *International Journal of Psychoanalysis*, 34: 313–324.

Racker, H. (1959). *Transference and Countertransference*. London: Karnac Books, (1968 edition).

Rosenfeld, H. (1983). Primitive object relations and mechanisms. *International Journal of Psychoanalysis*, 64(3): 261–267.

Schneider, J. A. and Irons, R. R. (2001). Eating disorders and sexuality. *Psychiatric Clinics of North America*, 24(2): 291–303.

Searles, H. (1959). Integration and differentiation in schizophrenia. In *Collected Papers on Schizophrenia and Related Subjects*. New York: International Universities Press, 304–316 (chapter 10) (19th Printing 1988).

Spitz, R. A. (1945). Hospitalism: An inquiry into the genesis of psychiatric conditions in early childhood. *Psychoanalytic Study of the Child*, 1: 53–74.

Spitz, R. (1956). Countertransference: Comments on its varying role in analytic situation. *Journal of American Psychoanalyst Association*, 4(2): 256–265.

Stefana, A., Hinshelwood, R. D., and Borensztejn, C. L. (2021). Racker and Heimann on countertransference: Similarities and differences. *The Psychoanalytic Quarterly*, 90(1): 105–137.

Steiner, J. (1993). *Psychic Retreats: Pathological Organizations in Psychotic, Neurotic, and Borderline Patients*. London: Routledge.

Stern, A. (1938). Psychoanalytic investigation of and therapy in the border line group of neuroses. *The Psychoanalytic Quarterly*, 7(4): 467–489.

Williams, G. (1997). Reflections on some dynamics of eating disorders: "No entry" defences and foreign bodies. *International Journal of Psychoanalysis*, 78(5): 927–941.

Williams, G. (2000). *Internal Landscapes and Foreign Bodies: Eating Disorders and other Pathologies*. London: Duckworth, Tavistock Clinic Series.

Winnicott, D. W. (1949). Hate in the counter-transference. *International Journal of Psychoanalysis*, 30: 69–74.

Yeomans, F. E., Clarkin, J. F., and Kernberg, O. F. (2015). *Transference-Focused Psychotherapy for Borderline Personality Disorder: A Clinical Guide*. Washington DC and London: American Psychiatric Publishing.

8 Dream analysis and imagery in eating disorder treatment

Utilizing dreams and imagery as tools for understanding eating disorders

Freud's early theoretical framework on dreams

In Freud's early theoretical framework on dreams, he posits that sleep occurs when no excitations are intense enough to stimulate the psyche's core (Ψ), creating an ideal state of inertia or rest and relieving the reservoir of psychic energy ($Q\eta$). Freud suggests that, in adults, the Ego serves as this reservoir of energy, and its discharge facilitates sleep, establishing the foundation for primary psychic processes (Freud, 1895). These primary processes become prominent as external perceptions are suspended and motor activity and willpower are paralyzed, allowing the psyche to shift from reality-bound functions to more primitive, internally driven processes (Persano, 2019).

Freud emphasizes the fundamentally hallucinatory nature of dream representations, describing them as states where "...one closes their eyes and hallucinates, opens them and thinks with words" (Freud, 1895). He proposes that the suppression of consciousness and motor activity during sleep allows for a backward flow of psychic energy from the Φ system to the Ψ system, endowing internal representations with perceptual qualities that blur the boundary between thought and sensory experience (Persano, 2019).

Furthermore, Freud notes that, during wakefulness, the Ego inhibits these hallucinatory processes by preventing perceptions from transferring backward from the Φ system. This inhibition is essential; without it, distinctions between perceptions and memory representations would collapse, resulting in a hallucinatory state. By maintaining this function, the Ego introduces the "objective reality marker"—a key aspect of consciousness that differentiates internal from external experiences. Freud draws a subtle yet important distinction between clarity and vividness in representations: a memory may appear clear if it is sufficiently invested but does not reach the vividness of perceptual reality. This distinction depends on the psychic value the individual assigns, allowing one to differentiate between a clear memory and a vivid hallucination (Freud, 1895).

DOI: 10.4324/9781032724997-8

These concepts shed light on the unique psychological challenges faced by patients with EDs, particularly those struggling with distorted body image. In these individuals, disruptions in the primary process—the unconscious mechanisms responsible for symbolic thought and dreaming—may impair their ability to differentiate between objective reality and imagined perceptions. This disruption blurs the boundaries between their inner world and external reality, intensifying their distorted views of their bodies and fuelling the psychological conflicts underlying their symptoms.

Many of these patients experience intense, vivid dreams revolving around daily concerns about food and body image. Given that eating disorder patients often struggle with developing an enriched representational world, the Ego's function of distinguishing between sensory perceptions and memory representations may be weakened. As a result, their dreams become more vivid and their ability to distinguish between the real and imagined body is further impaired. For these patients, perceptions of their body become closer to memories, blurring the line between inner and outer worlds. In Freudian terms, the "objective reality marker" is weakened, leaving the individual less able to differentiate accurately between the inner and external realms.

In *"The Interpretation of Dreams"* Freud introduces the enduring psychoanalytic concept of dreams as wish fulfillments, which became a cornerstone in understanding the unconscious. Published at the turn of the 20th century, this work marked a significant shift in approaches to investigating the mind (Freud, 1900[1899]). Freud moved from "bottom-up" approaches that focused on neural mechanisms to "top-down" methods that sought to explore the depths of the mind by examining its products, such as dreams. This approach allowed Freud to connect the mind's complex symbolic processes with foundational psychoanalytic concepts, expanding his theoretical landscape. Through this work, Freud introduced his topographic model of the mind and expanded on the concept of regression—wherein the mind reverts to more primitive or infantile modes of expression, especially evident in the dreaming process (Persano, 2019).

Freud's study of dreams emphasized the significance of symbolism as a critical mechanism for understanding both dreams and symptoms, particularly through processes like condensation and figurability. Rangell (1987) highlighted that Freud regarded symbolism as one of the most extraordinary contributions of *"The Interpretation of Dreams"*, suggesting that it could even substitute for free association in unlocking unconscious material. Freud theorized that symbolic representations within dreams serve as a disguised pathway for repressed or unfulfilled wishes to emerge, enabling the dreamer to encounter otherwise unacceptable impulses or desires without the constraints of conscious awareness (Persano, 2019).

These foundational ideas in Freud's dream theory provide a lens for understanding mechanisms in EDs, where internal conflicts often manifest as distorted bodily perceptions and behaviors. Just as dreams use symbolic language to communicate hidden desires and fears, the body in EDs can become a symbolic canvas upon which patients project unconscious struggles. The hallucinatory aspect of dreams and the Ego's regulation of clarity versus vividness echo the ways in which individuals with EDs struggle to separate internalized ideals or fears from physical experiences, resulting in compulsive or distorted behavior patterns. This connection suggests that primary processes and unconscious representations manifest not only in dreams but also in the deeply ingrained self-perceptions seen in EDs.

Using Freud's model of dreams in eating disorders

In the context of EDs, food and body image often take on symbolic meanings that are archaic and concrete, mirroring the primitive symbolism found in dreams. For example, food in dreams may represent nurturance, comfort, or even guilt—themes that can also appear concretely in the lives of individuals with EDs, where food becomes loaded with unconscious meaning and symbolism. Severe eating disorder patients, particularly those with anorexia nervosa (AN) or bulimia nervosa (BN), often relate to food in ways that go beyond mere sustenance; food may embody control, self-worth, or punishment, transforming daily acts of eating or restriction into symbolic expressions of their inner psychic world.

Furthermore, the dream process offers insights into the symbolic nature of bodily experiences in EDs. Just as the dream work process condenses and disguises latent wishes through symbols, individuals with EDs may condense complex emotional and psychological conflicts into symbolic acts of restriction, binging, or purging. This somatic symbolization bypasses verbal representation, allowing individuals to express unconscious content through their bodies in a way reminiscent of Freud's concept of compromise formation in dreams. Here, the body becomes the site where unconscious conflicts play out, much like the dream functions as a canvas for repressed wishes.

In this light, the study of dreams provides a valuable framework for understanding the symbolic underpinnings of EDs. By recognizing the parallels between dream symbolism and bodily symbolism in EDs, psychoanalytic treatment can help patients uncover the hidden meanings underlying their eating behaviors, offering a pathway toward integrating these unconscious conflicts into more adaptive modes of expression. Thus, Freud's dream theory not only sheds light on the workings of the unconscious but also offers a roadmap for exploring and addressing the symbolic layers within EDs.

Both Freud and Bion saw dreaming as a unique form of thinking that operates in a different mode than conscious thought. For them, dreams represent thoughts without words, processed through the primary process. Bion considered "dream thoughts" to belong to the same category as myths and symbols, carrying meaning without the use of linguistic structures (Bion, 1967). This nonverbal, imagistic form of expression allows for complex psychic material to emerge in a way that is not accessible through ordinary language, revealing aspects of the unconscious mind in symbolized, sensory images (Persano, 2019).

Elizabeth Auchincloss complements Freud's views by defining a dream as a mental experience occurring during sleep that encompasses images, thoughts, and feelings remembered upon waking. For patients with EDs, the symbolic content of dreams can provide a profound window into their internal conflicts, often reflecting struggles with self-worth, control, and identity. These symbolic processes parallel the symbolic nature of their symptoms, where food, body image, and behaviors serve as metaphors for deeper psychological struggles. Integrating these perspectives in psychoanalytic treatment allows for a deeper exploration of how unconscious material is expressed both in dreams and in the lived experiences of patients (Auchincloss, 2015).

Psychoanalytic mind: Symbolization

Fred Busch, drawing on Loewald's ideas, adds another layer to this understanding by observing that some patients, especially at the beginning of analysis, use words more as a language of action rather than as representations of genuine mental states. For instance, while recounting a dream or describing an event, these patients may convey an overwhelming emotional intensity that the analyst can feel but that lacks symbolic depth or conscious meaning (Busch, 2014). This differs from the free association process, where words are meant to communicate inner states. Busch suggests that this "language of action" is a preliminary manifestation of the unconscious, a stage where raw affect is expressed before it can transform into symbolic language as analysis deepens. Over time, through the analytic process, this language of action may evolve into words that genuinely represent symbolic meaning (Persano, 2019).

As Busch explains, "Transformations of words as actions into symbolic, representational thinking is part of helping the analysand to develop a psychoanalytic mind, as the capacity to play with thoughts is dependent on their being representable" (Busch, 2014). In this process, the analyst's task is to help patients move from acting out feelings or conflicts to articulating them in words, allowing for more abstract and symbolic thinking to emerge.

In understanding EDs, this framework is particularly relevant. Individuals with these conditions often act out their inner conflicts through their bodies, using compulsive behaviors as a substitute for symbolic expression. Initially, these actions—such as restriction, binging, or purging—may lack symbolic content, functioning instead as a language of action. However, as in the dream process, these behaviors hold the potential to transform within a therapeutic context, where they can begin to represent underlying psychic conflicts in a meaningful way. The transition from action-driven communication to symbolic thinking, like the evolution of language in dream work, allows patients to externalize and work through complex emotions in ways that words alone could not initially achieve.

Freud's concept of "day residues" also provides insight into how waking life impacts the content of dreams. When an individual is consciously thinking about a topic or event during the day, this content often carries over into sleep and can serve as raw material for dream formation. In psychoanalytic terms, these are referred to as day residues, elements of daily experience that fuel the imagery and scenarios of dreams. Additionally, events or situations that leave an emotional impact—even if not consciously processed—can also form part of day residues as unconscious mnemonic traces, lending emotional weight and depth to the dream's symbolic content (Persano, 2019).

In patients with EDs, day residues may often consist of distressing or charged experiences related to body image, food, and self-worth. These traces, embedded in dreams, can then be processed through the primary process, which reworks them into symbolic representations. For instance, food-related imagery in dreams may take on exaggerated or surreal forms, symbolizing not just nourishment but also deeper emotional conflicts—such as longing, shame, or guilt.

The symbolization process that unfolds in dreams provides a model for understanding how these patients might begin to engage with their experiences in a more representational way. In dreams, their compulsive actions and obsessive thoughts about food and body image may transform into visual symbols that communicate internal struggles. Over time, this symbolic approach to understanding dreams can parallel a similar shift in therapeutic work, where patients gradually move from acting out inner conflicts to expressing them in ways that reveal underlying meaning and promote healing.

This symbolization process aligns with Freud's concept of compromise formation, where the unconscious seeks to express repressed material in a disguised but meaningful way. In both dreams and eating disorder behaviors, symbols emerge through a blend of conscious and unconscious elements, condensed and often bizarre, that communicate inner conflicts without direct language. Just as dreams offer a symbolic arena for repressed wishes and fears, the body can become a similar canvas for those with eating disorders. Food, body image, and physical behaviors are imbued with symbolic meanings, providing an outlet for expressing conflicts around control, self-worth, and dependency in a form the individual may find more tolerable.

The relationship between dreams and EDS has been explored, with particular attention given to the prevalence of food-related themes in the dreams of individuals with EDs. Studies, such as those by Schredl and

Montasser (1999), found an increased occurrence of food-related content in the dreams of individuals with AN. This finding has been interpreted as a reflection of the intense preoccupation with food and eating that dominates the waking lives of individuals in this group. Dream analysis thus offers a unique lens through which to understand the pervasive influence of food-related concerns in the psychological landscape of individuals with AN.

In the therapeutic setting, recognizing the symbolic dimension of eating disorder behaviors allows for a richer understanding of the patient's inner life. As patients work through the meanings embedded in their dreams and actions, the analyst can guide them toward integrating these insights, transforming raw actions into symbol-laden representations. This approach not only deepens the analytic work but also helps patients develop a more adaptive and flexible relationship with their inner conflicts, enabling the mind to play with thoughts and meanings rather than compulsively enacting them.

Dreams from neuroscientific and neuro-psychoanalysis viewpoint

From a neuro-psychoanalytic perspective, Mark Solms describes how visual images flow in dreams, outlining three key brain areas involved. The first, linked to the retina, is the primary visual cortex at the back of the occipital lobes, serving as the entry region. Moving forward, there is a zone focused on processing information, especially for moving and colorful images. Further forward lies a third area where more abstract visual processing occurs, linked to functions such as arithmetic, writing, constructive operations, and spatial attention (Solms and Turnbull, 2002). Interestingly, during sleep—and particularly dreaming—this flow appears to reverse; zone three becomes the entry point, with dream images breaking down into discrete elements by the time they reach zone one, which functions as a "projection screen" where dreams are "seen". This finding seems to confirm certain psychoanalytic theories, including the concept of regressive flow in dreams, primary process thinking, and the regression of complex waking thoughts into symbolic dream images.

Neuroscience research also indicates that dreams play a significant role in consolidating memory processes during sleep. Long-term memories are especially consolidated during REM sleep, though NREM sleep also contributes, demonstrating a complementary relationship between the two. Events from waking life are integrated during sleep, particularly through dreaming, with other life events in a continuous nightly process that becomes part of autobiographical memory.

Sleep enables the linking of new units of personally meaningful information, while irrelevant information is excluded from memory integration; only emotionally significant content is incorporated into existing memory circuits. This process occurs in two stages: initially, during

NREM sleep, when circuits related to recent learning—such as a new motor skill or language—are still active. Later, these memory traces are reactivated during REM sleep, where they are linked with older memories stored in long-term memory circuits.

In the early minutes of sleep, NREM dreams are associated with networks involved in semantic knowledge processing, where images are linked to previously stored memories. This stage of dreaming is thought to engage cognitive processes that organize and consolidate learned information. In contrast, REM dreams are characterized by emotionally charged perceptual images that are integrated with past experiences. During REM sleep, new experiences are fused with older memories, often in ways that appear bizarre or illogical—a phenomenon Freud likened to dreams being a "form of psychosis" (Cartwright, 2010). This distinction highlights how different stages of sleep contribute uniquely to the processing of emotions, memories, and experiences in the dreaming mind.

According to Kandel, REM dreams tend to be longer, primarily visual, and closely tied to emotions, often appearing disconnected from daily life events. This corresponds to Freud's concept of latent dream content, where underlying, often unconscious emotions and desires surface in symbolic form (Kandel et al., 2013). In contrast, NREM dreams are shorter, contain fewer visual elements, have less emotional intensity, and are more abstract, resembling what Freud considered manifest content—directly reflecting daily experiences without deep emotional undercurrents (Kandel et al., 2013).

Kandel and colleagues also identified the most frequently activated emotions in dreams as, in descending order: anxiety, surprise, joy, sadness, and shame, with the majority linked to unpleasant or negative states. Additionally, emotions experienced in dreams trigger neurotransmitter cascades, activating complex circuits from the brainstem to the cortex and producing neurohormonal releases (Damasio, 2000; Solms and Turnbull, 2002; Cartwright, 2010). This neurohormonal activity may relate to the heightened levels of ghrelin observed in individuals experiencing starvation, which can increase worries about food throughout the day and potentially manifest as food-related dreams (Personal communication, *Nutritionist* Paula Rodríguez, November 2024).

The 1940s "Minnesota Semi-Starvation Experiment" documented the extensive effects of prolonged semi-starvation, including irritability, insomnia, metabolic disturbances, depression, and notable changes in dream content. Conducted during World War II to explore the impact of severe caloric restriction, the study revealed that participants not only suffered physical symptoms but also intense psychological effects, such as an obsessive preoccupation with food and vivid, food-centered dreams. These findings enhance our understanding of how hunger profoundly shapes both emotional and dream life, illustrating how starvation-induced neurohormonal changes can influence dream content, linking physical deprivation to vivid and symbolic expressions in dreams.

These findings suggest that, in psychoanalytic treatments, it may be valuable to refocus on the emotional world expressed through dreams and how these emotions are communicated when patients recount their dreams in sessions. For patients with EDs, where food, body image, and self-worth are so intricately tied to emotional experiences, dreams can become a symbolic landscape where unresolved conflicts and anxieties are processed. By engaging with the emotional content in these dreams, psychoanalytic work can help patients explore and address unconscious fears, desires, and symbolic representations tied to their daily struggles with food and body image, offering a pathway toward deeper understanding and transformation.

Symbolic representations of the self, body, and food in dreams

Self and symbolization in dreams of eating disorder patients

Severe eating disorder (ED) patients often face significant challenges with mentalization and symbolization—crucial processes that enable individuals to interpret and make sense of internal experiences. For patients with chronic restrictive AN, the physiological and psychological effects of intense starvation frequently led to severe sleep disturbances. Their dreams are often dominated by food imagery, reflecting the persistent preoccupation with hunger and nourishment in their waking lives. Conversely, individuals with BN tend to experience dreams filled with themes of violence and anxiety, mirroring the emotional turmoil and loss of control that define their daily struggles.

Wilma Bucci (1997) introduces the concept of sub-symbolic processing, a style of information processing rooted in sensory and emotional experiences rather than language-based symbols. For patients with EDs, this often translates into dreams that are directly connected to visceral, bodily sensations and raw affective states, rather than being organized into coherent, abstract representations or symbolic narratives. These sub-symbolic dreams provide a glimpse into the pre-verbal and deeply embodied emotional states of ED patients, revealing the intensity of their internal conflicts and unmet needs.

By understanding the connection between sub-symbolic processing and the dream content of ED patients, clinicians can gain valuable insights into the nonverbal and often unarticulated emotional struggles that underpin their disorders. This perspective emphasizes the importance of addressing both the physiological and psychological dimensions of EDs in therapy, fostering a more integrated approach to treatment and recovery.

Patients with EDs often experience dreams that are fragmented and lack coherent narratives, reflecting a concrete, sensory-driven mode of processing rather than the associative, symbolic thinking typically seen in dream narratives. This phenomenon is closely related to their use of "concretized metaphors", a concept explored by Robinson and Skårderud. In this context, metaphors are not abstract or figurative but are instead experienced as direct, physical sensations, blurring the line between physical and emotional experiences (Skårderud, 2007; Robinson, Skårderud, and Sommerfeldt, 2017).

For instance, a patient might describe feeling "weighed down" not just as an emotional burden but as a literal sensation of heaviness. This concretization indicates a difficulty in mentalizing—the ability to understand and interpret one's own and others' mental states—which is often impaired in individuals with EDs. Skårderud notes that this impairment can lead to a diminished capacity for reflective functioning, where emotional experiences are not symbolized but are instead acted out or somatized (Robinson, Skårderud, and Sommerfeldt, 2019).

This mode of experiencing can extend to their dream life, where the lack of symbolic processing results in dreams that are more literal and less interpretive. Such dreams may not provide the psychological insight typically gained from symbolic dream analysis, as the content remains tied to concrete experiences and sensations. Understanding this concretized mode of processing is crucial for therapists working with ED patients, as it highlights the need to develop the patient's capacity for mentalization and symbolic thinking, thereby facilitating a more integrated and reflective self-experience.

This blurs the line between physical and emotional experience. For example, a feeling of being "weighed down" might not just represent an emotional burden but is felt as a literal sensation of heaviness. These concrete metaphors bypass the psychological flexibility of symbolic representation, becoming instead rigid, immediate realities. This limits the patient's ability to gain psychological distance and reflect on their experiences from a broader perspective.

Despite this challenge with symbolic thinking, certain recurring themes in ED patients' dreams do reveal significant underlying issues with self-representation. Common dream themes include violence—whether directed at or enacted by the dreamer—helplessness, entrapment, engulfment, guilt, and a sense of being scrutinized or judged (Brink, Allan, and Boldt, 1995).

Hilde Bruch (1978) observed that feelings of ineffectiveness, self-hate, and loss of autonomy are central to AN and frequently appear in dream content. Younger patients suffering from anorexia nervosa, as Magagna (2000) reported, often have dreams tied to themes of autonomy loss and emotional suppression (Lask and Bryant-Waugh, 2000). Bruch (1985) also noted a pairing between feelings of being judged and a fixation on food, which manifests in dreams where the dreamer feels guilty or observed, as if accused of wrongdoing. Some patients report a sense of relief upon waking from dreams in which they ate forbidden foods, reassuring themselves that the event was not real and did not impact their bodies.

For patients with AN, fear of eating and weight gain extends far beyond mere aversion to food. Eating becomes a metaphor for an emotional state of being "filled" or overwhelmed; the fear of "too much" encompasses not just food but also difficult thoughts and emotions. This fear of excess creates a longing for emptiness, which can drive restrictive or purging behaviors. Other patients feel a direct link between the sensation of physical heaviness and negative emotions, reinforcing a sense of burden and an urgent need to control both physical and emotional experiences (Skårderud, 2007).

Mara Selvini Palazzoli (1974) observed that dreams of patients with anorexia nervosa (AN) often contain themes of constant surveillance or an inability to nourish themselves. These dream themes appear to bypass the patients' well-established defense mechanisms, revealing underlying feelings of vulnerability and helplessness that contrast sharply with their outward facade of control (Selvini Palazzoli, 1974). Such dreams offer a window into the emotional struggles of AN patients, highlighting their internal conflicts between autonomy and the pressure to conform to external expectations.

For many patients suffering from AN, particularly those from highly controlling families, the pervasive feeling of being scrutinized or directed by others is a recurring source of distress. Stern (1986) described this phenomenon as "malignant control", where parental expectations dominate and suppress the child's individual needs and desires, creating a repressive and emotionally stifling dynamic. This dynamic often manifests in the patients' dreams as scenes of surveillance, judgment, or external control, symbolizing the oppressive familial influences that they have internalized.

Brink, Allan, and Boldt, (1995) further emphasized how these themes of invasive oversight reflect the broader emotional environment of patients with AN. The constant sense of being watched or judged in their dreams mirrors the real-life experiences of being subjected to rigid family structures and high expectations. These dream scenarios not only symbolize the patients' internalized sense of oppression but also provide a valuable therapeutic avenue for exploring the emotional roots of their disorder. Recognizing these underlying dynamics can guide more empathetic and effective therapeutic interventions, helping patients reconcile their need for autonomy with the internalized pressures they carry.

For many individuals with AN, the pursuit of emptiness is fueled by a deep-seated fear that their inner void, originating in feelings of worthlessness, can never truly be filled. This inability to self-nurture, paired with an obsession with food, underscores food's dual role in dreams as both a symbol of unachievable self-worth and a reminder of denied self-care. Dreams in patients with AN often lack relational depth, showing the dreamer as isolated, sometimes with family figures present but few male figures, reflecting a rejection of relational roles and underscoring themes of control and self-isolation (Schredl and Montasser, 1999).

Narcissistic themes also emerge in the self-representations of ED patients, particularly those with AN. The patient's grandiosity, exhibitionism, and desire for external validation reveal a narcissistic vulnerability, with dreams often expressing a heightened sense of surveillance and judgment in those who suffer from AN (Bruch, 1985; Goodsit, 1985; Weizsäcker, 1964). This pervasive sense of being watched in dreams symbolizes the relentless pursuit of approval and the profound fear of exposure.

For BN patients, dream content tends to reflect intense negative emotions, with few positive themes, mirroring the depressive mood and low self-esteem common in BN. Dreams of chaos, aggression, and loss of control reflect the emotional dynamics inherent in binge-purge cycles. The absence of positive affect aligns with their heightened self-criticism and perceived inability to regulate impulses, often manifesting as self-loathing and emotional turbulence in their dreams (Schredl and Montasser, 1999).

In summary, dreams in ED patients offer a unique insight into their inner struggles. For patients with AN, dreams reflect themes of isolation, control, and rejection of nurturing, symbolizing self-worth struggles and the reliance on physical emptiness to manage overwhelming emotions. For patients with BN, dreams of chaos and negativity echo the psychological turmoil surrounding binge-purge cycles, capturing conflicts around control, self-image, and emotional regulation. These dream themes highlight the depth of unconscious processes that shape the emotional lives and self-perceptions of individuals with EDs, reinforcing the necessity of therapeutic interventions that address both symbolic understanding and emotional processing.

Dreams, body, and symbolization in eating disorder patients

In patients with EDs, dreams are often intricately entwined with physical sensations and deep emotional states. Many patients report a visceral link between physical experiences—such as body weight or sensations of heaviness—and negative emotions. For instance, a sensation of lightness may bring not only physical relief but also a profound emotional release, reflecting a sense of inner ease (Skårderud, 2007).

Among those patients with AN, dream themes frequently involve feelings of stomach heaviness or discomfort, closely tied to anxieties surrounding food and eating. Upon waking, patients often experience a lingering sensation of fullness or distress, which quickly dissipates once they realize they have not actually eaten, bringing significant relief. MacLeod (1981) describes the anorexic's struggle to assess her physical needs, noting an impaired ability to gauge hunger or fullness. This drive toward emptiness reflects a deeper fear of emotional "filling"—of being overwhelmed by emotions connected to a perceived inner unworthiness that dates to childhood. This unprocessed fear creates a fragile sense of self, one that depends on constant external validation to feel secure (Goodsit, 1985).

For patients with AN, fear of eating and weight gain extends beyond mere food aversion. Eating symbolizes an emotional flood, a sense of "too much" that applies not only to physical intake but also to difficult emotions and overwhelming thoughts. In dreams, this fear often manifests as intense bodily sensations of weight gain, evoking panic that feels very real. These dreams highlight how weight concerns go beyond the physical, touching on core anxieties about managing emotional boundaries and self-control (Schredl and Montasser, 1999).

The effects of starvation can also bring a strange predictability for patients with restrictive AN, who may find comfort in the familiarity of their emaciated state. Touching their own skeletal body or hardened muscles can provide a feeling of stability and control. In dreams, however, encountering a body perceived as "fat" can provoke intense disgust, fear, and anxiety, whereas dreams of weight loss bring feelings of relief. For these patients, losing body weight becomes synonymous with shedding something negative, reinforcing the connection between physical control and emotional well-being (Skårderud, 2007).

In AN, compound body metaphors arise, where various physical sensations merge into a symbolic whole. Control might be represented by an empty stomach, a firm or thin body, and a feeling of purity. These complex metaphors create a direct link between physical sensations and emotional states, where bodily experiences serve as concrete expressions of psychological struggles. However, while the body can function as a medium for symbolic expression, it lacks the capacity for self-reflection. This underscores the need for a "metalanguage"—a way to articulate and interpret these embodied expressions within a reflective psychological framework.

AN can be shown as a response to deep-seated vulnerability and a sense of exposure—an "openness" that is both physical and emotional. This perceived exposure leads to a symbolic "closing" of the body, expressed through food refusal and the physical act of keeping the mouth closed. This perspective explains why AN is difficult to understand from the outside and why patients often resist therapy: they are confined within a literal, rigid symbolic system in which complex emotions are expressed through restrictive, physical acts.

For BN, the complexity of emotional experience is condensed into the act of eating, forming what can be described as a metaphorical "economics of supply". Before a binge, patients report feeling a painful emptiness—an aching void accompanied by a restless, almost desperate hunger. This hunger is not just physical but a humiliating need that demands to be satisfied. Food initially serves as a "magic drug" to soothe this void. However, once ingested, it quickly transforms into a source of shame, a perceived poison that must be expelled before it can become "ugly fat" (Hamburg, 1989). Thus, excess is linked with impurity, imperfection, and shame, reinforcing a view that desiring anything is inherently wrong. In this "anal world", the goal becomes complete purging of this perceived badness. After purging, patients are left exhausted and empty, but the cycle resumes.

BN also engages a "genital world" of excitement, where hunger takes on a sexualized quality. The anticipation of a binge induces a frenzied excitement, temporarily filling the void and masking loneliness. However, this stimulation is fleeting, leaving only dissatisfaction and renewed emptiness (Hamburg, 1989).

Dreams in patients with BN often reflect the symbolic patterns and emotional dynamics that characterize the bulimic cycle. As described by Hamburg the bulimic cycle alternates between an "oral world", where food symbolizes comfort but becomes toxic, and an "anal world", where purging serves as an attempt to rid the self of perceived "badness". This process is deeply tied to the symbolic and affective content of dreams, where unresolved conflicts around hunger, fullness, and cleansing frequently manifest (Hamburg, 1989).

In patients suffering from bulimic conditions, dreams may metaphorically represent their internal dynamics through vivid imagery of consuming or expelling substances, reflecting their psychological struggle with control and self-perception. For instance, dreams involving chaotic eating scenarios or uncontrollable consumption can mirror the desperation felt before a binge, while imagery of rejection or loss might symbolize the purging phase, where the patient attempts to eliminate perceived contamination.

The description of inner space in BN as a cloacal cavity—hollow, aching, and unfillable—finds parallels in the symbolic content of their dreams. These dreams may include imagery of voids, caves, or endless corridors, symbolizing an internal emptiness that demands to be filled but remains perpetually unsatisfied. Such dreams reveal the patient's unconscious struggle with feelings of inadequacy and unworthiness, mirroring their waking experience of cyclical hunger and purging.

The "genital world" of excitement described in the bulimic cycle also finds expression in dreams that transition from moments of exhilaration or indulgence to irritation or disgust. This mirrors the fleeting satisfaction followed by shame and discomfort that characterize the bulimic experience. Dreams of rapid changes in emotional or physical states—such as indulging in forbidden pleasures and then facing catastrophic consequences—highlight the internal conflict and oscillation between desire and rejection (Hamburg, 1989).

Thus, the cyclical dynamics of BN, as described by Hamburg, resonate deeply with the content and structure of bulimic dreams. These dreams provide insight into the patient's unconscious struggles, where food and bodily processes serve as metaphors for unresolved emotional conflicts and distorted self-perception. By exploring these dream symbols in therapy, therapists can help patients uncover and process the underlying fears, desires, and self-representations that fuel the bulimic cycle (Hamburg, 1989).

In sum, the dreams and bodily sensations of both AN and BN patients offer insights into the symbolic language of these disorders. For patients with AN, themes of isolation, control, and avoidance of nurturing reflect their struggles with self-worth, dependence on physical emptiness, and rigid self-control. Dreams of patients with bulimic conditions, characterized by chaotic intensity and pervasive negativity, mirror the psychological cycles of binging and purging, capturing the profound conflicts around control, body image, and self-worth. Through these dream patterns, we can see how each disorder's symbolic expressions underscore the potent role of unconscious processes in shaping the emotional life and self-perception of individuals with EDs.

Dreams, food, and symbolization in eating disorder patients

For individuals with EDs, food is a powerful, often distressing symbol. In dreams, food becomes a battleground for issues like self-worth, control, and unprocessed emotional needs. For patients with AN and BN, food in dreams embodies the deep-seated conflicts they experience in daily life— longing, rejection, fear, and struggle. These symbolic representations not only reflect the distress of waking life but also reveal a profound disconnection between their physical and emotional selves.

The emotional landscape of food dreams

Food frequently appears in ED patients' dreams, but it rarely brings comfort or satisfaction. Instead, these dreams evoke strong negative emotions like guilt, anxiety, and tension. For patients suffering from BN, food often takes on a monstrous or overwhelming quality, representing excess that is both desirable and terrifying. These dreams feature enormous portions, distorted shapes, and other symbols of loss of control, reinforcing the sense of food as a forbidden, overpowering force in their lives. For patients suffering from AN, the focus in dreams is less on the food itself and more on rejecting it. These dreams serve as symbols of self-denial and control, where restraint provides a sense of power over desires and needs. As one patient expressed, "Food appears as aggression, something forbidden or unavailable", mirroring the strict self-imposed restrictions of AN.

These dreams leave patients with intense emotional responses, including feelings of guilt and panic upon dreaming of consuming forbidden foods. When they wake, realizing the event was not real, they often feel relief. This cycle of anxiety and relief highlights the constant tension surrounding food that defines their waking lives as well.

Symbolic distortion: Food as monstrous and overpowering

In the dreams of individuals with eating disorders (EDs), food frequently takes on surreal and grotesque dimensions, appearing exaggerated or even monstrous. This distorted imagery mirrors research on size perception distortions in ED patients, who often perceive food portions as disproportionately large. Studies by Gutnisky, Persano, and Campos (2019) and Gutnisky and Campos (2024) demonstrate that ED patients experience more significant size distortion with food than with their own bodies.

These findings suggest that food occupies a uniquely overwhelming and intrusive space in the minds of ED patients, surpassing even the intensity of their distorted self-image. The exaggerated representation of food in both waking perceptions and dreams highlights its symbolic significance, reflecting the profound emotional conflicts and anxieties associated with nourishment, control, and identity. This connection underscores the central role that food plays in the psychological landscape of individuals with EDs, offering important insights for therapeutic intervention.

In dreams, the outsized portrayal of food symbolizes the terrifying loss of control that patients associate with consumption, indulgence, and nourishment itself. This imagery underscores the profound inner conflicts that food represents for individuals with EDs, amplifying feelings of helplessness, fear, and emotional paralysis. The surreal quality of these dreams reflects not only the patients' anxieties about food but also their struggle to reconcile the act of nourishment with their need for control and self-discipline.

These insights allow for the hypothesis that self-distortion in object representations—such as the exaggerated perception of food—may be as pronounced, if not more so, than body distortion in ED patients. This perspective highlights how food, as both a physical object and a psychological symbol, becomes a focal point of anxiety, representing not just sustenance but the complex emotional battles tied to identity, control, and self-perception. Understanding these dynamics provides valuable avenues for therapeutic exploration, addressing both the symbolic and tangible aspects of food in the context of EDs.

Self-nurturing deficits and feelings of unworthiness

Dreams about food among ED patients go beyond simple hunger or cravings—they highlight profound self-nurturing deficits and feelings of unworthiness. Brink, Allan, and Boldt (1995) described food dreams as unconscious reflections of a patient's inability to feel deserving of care or nourishment. For many patients with AN, food restriction becomes a core part of identity, where restraint is seen as a measure of self-control, discipline, and purity. These patients often view restrictive eating as an act of self-worth, masking deeper emotional needs for self-compassion and acceptance.

In patients with AN, food is often a fixation symbolized in dreams by avoidance and rigid control. While they may be unconsciously aware of the emotional significance behind these behaviors, their conscious focus is on calories, weight, and self-restraint, leaving unprocessed emotional needs unaddressed.

Purity and control: The role of food in anorexia nervosa

For patients with AN, the concept of "purity" is deeply tied to their relationship with food. Pure food is often defined as low-calorie, low-fat, and artfully arranged. Food is meant to be sparse, separated, and unblended, creating a sense of order and certainty. This purity represents a longing for simplicity and control in life, allowing these patients to distill their experience to its most manageable form, free from the "contamination" of indulgence or emotional expression.

In this framework, food is not just sustenance but a reward, a luxury that must be earned. Many patients feel that they must work hard to "deserve" food, reflecting an ingrained belief that even basic comforts must be earned. This sense of undeserving extends beyond food, encompassing a broader perception of self-worth that equates worthiness with self-denial and achievement.

Food as emotional balm in bulimia nervosa

For patients with BN, food symbolizes emotional relief rather than reward. Many of these patients describe food as a comforting escape, temporarily soothing their inner turmoil. In dreams, food often appears as an endless resource—a bottomless supply intended to numb feelings of tension and inadequacy. Hamburg (1989) aptly described food in these cases as a "giant filling place", representing an attempt to fill the "empty tension of desire".

However, this reliance on food as comfort creates inner conflict for BN patients, whose bodies often become sources of shame. Food in dreams embodies both comfort and shame, reflecting the duality of their waking struggles. BN patients' obsession with food mirrors their desire for affirmation, making them feel vulnerable, appreciated not for who they are but for what they can provide.

The battleground of food dreams

Food in dreams offers a profound symbolic arena for ED patients, where it becomes far more than mere sustenance. Food dreams capture the complex ways patients both fear and seek comfort in food, illustrating a web of conflicting emotions around self-worth, control, and unmet emotional needs. The recurrent themes of these dreams highlight the intricate connections between ED symptoms and the patient's psyche, revealing the necessity of addressing not just eating behaviors but also the underlying emotional wounds.

For ED patients, food dreams underline a painful irony: those most in need of self-care and nurturing often feel most alienated from these basic needs. True recovery requires a reconnection with the self that transcends food as a measure of worth or purity. By transforming the meaning of food in their lives—from a symbol of control to a source of genuine self-nourishment—patients can begin to find inner peace. Through this reimagined relationship, dreams of food may evolve from scenes of conflict to expressions of healing and self-acceptance.

Eating disorders, childhood trauma, sexual abuse, and dreams

For patients with histories of childhood trauma, particularly sexual abuse, dreams take on a uniquely charged and symbolic role, often carrying layers of fear, anxiety, and unprocessed emotional pain. Such patients frequently experience dreams dominated by catastrophic imagery—monstrous figures, natural disasters, or even their own death. These dreams, reflecting unresolved trauma, often mirror the fragmented sense of self and distorted body image characteristic of EDs.

The role of trauma in EDs symptoms and dream content

Research and clinical observations underscore the significant correlation between histories of abuse and the severity of ED symptoms. Childhood trauma profoundly disrupts the natural development of trust, safety, and bodily autonomy, leaving lasting imprints on how patients perceive their self-worth and bodily boundaries. Survivors of sexual abuse, for example, frequently report an overwhelming sense of shame and a disconnection from their physical selves—experiences that are often vividly mirrored in their dreams.

In the Day Hospital Unit for Eating Disorders, the dream workshop has become a critical tool for uncovering the complex psychological struggles faced by patients. Many participants not only contend with severe eating disorder symptoms but also experience a range of co-occurring conditions, including depression, self-harm behaviors, and suicidal ideation. The dream workshop provides a unique and non-threatening avenue for these individuals to explore their inner worlds, often revealing emotional conflicts and traumatic experiences that are difficult to express directly (Personal communication, *Psychologist* Ariana Muñoz, November 2024).

The content of their dreams frequently features scenarios imbued with feelings of entrapment, violation, or annihilation. These intense and disturbing dream narratives serve as symbolic representations of the patients' psychological wounds. For instance, recurring images of being trapped or pursued often mirror their struggles with control and helplessness, core themes in EDs. Dreams of violation or destruction can reflect feelings of vulnerability, shame, and the internalized impacts of relational trauma, such as neglect or abuse. These symbolic dreamscapes offer a profound glimpse into their inner emotional and psychic worlds, often bypassing the defenses they rely on in waking life to shield themselves from these painful realities.

The workshop also reveals the intersection of trauma and ED symptoms, where the dreams act as a bridge to understanding the roots of disordered behaviors. Dreams of annihilation or consumption, for example, may symbolize the patients' perception of their bodies as battlegrounds where the forces of self-worth, control, and external pressures collide. These dreams provide valuable material for therapeutic work, as they highlight the deeply entrenched emotional struggles that fuel their eating disorders.

Sharing and analyzing dreams in a supportive group setting fosters a profound sense of connection and validation among patients. Many participants report feeling less isolated upon realizing that others share similar dream experiences, reinforcing the understanding that their struggles are not uniquely personal, but part of a broader context linked to their disorder. This collective exploration helps patients feel seen and understood, reducing the shame and alienation that often accompanies EDs.

For therapists, the dream workshop provides invaluable insights into patients' unconscious fears, desires, and conflicts. These symbolic narratives offer a window into the deeper emotional and psychological struggles that may not easily surface in conventional dialogue. By uncovering these hidden dynamics, the workshop enriches the therapeutic process, creating opportunities for deeper exploration and more targeted interventions. This collaborative approach not only enhances individual treatment but also strengthens the sense of community and shared healing within the group.

Ultimately, the dream workshop serves as more than a diagnostic tool; it becomes a therapeutic space where patients can confront their inner turmoil in a creative and symbolic manner. By decoding the rich, often fragmented language of dreams, therapists and patients alike gain a clearer understanding of the emotional scars underlying EDs, paving the way for healing and psychological growth.

Food dreams: A mirror of trauma and suffering

In patients with EDs, food dreams can become a metaphorical battlefield where past trauma and current struggles intersect. These dreams frequently represent themes of unworthiness, guilt, and suffering. For instance, for individuals with BN, food dreams may involve uncontrollable binges or grotesque imagery of food as contamination, symbolizing their inner conflict between hunger for emotional fulfillment and the fear of losing control. Similarly, for patients with AN, food dreams often depict scenarios of forced feeding or punishment, illustrating the internalized belief that nourishment equates to failure or weakness.

Catastrophic and monstrous dream imagery

The catastrophic events and monstrous figures commonly reported in these dreams symbolize not only the external dangers these patients have faced but also their internalized fears and unresolved conflicts. Monstrous dream figures may represent the abuser, a punitive Super-ego, or the patient's own distorted self-image, experienced as grotesque or unworthy. Catastrophic dreams—of falling, drowning, or being devoured—often reflect the patient's unconscious fears of engulfment or annihilation, echoing their struggles with dependency, control, and vulnerability.

Dreams and the body: A reflection of trauma

For patients with histories of sexual abuse, the body often becomes a site of shame and alienation, a perception that is reflected and amplified in their dreams. These patients frequently describe dreams where their bodies are violated, dismembered, or transformed into monstrous forms, symbolizing the fractured sense of bodily autonomy and self-worth rooted in their trauma. Food dreams for these patients often revolve around themes of contamination, punishment, or insatiable hunger, highlighting their conflicted relationship with nourishment and survival.

Clinical implications: Working with dream content

Understanding the dream content of ED patients with traumatic histories offers a vital avenue for therapeutic intervention. Dreams serve as a window into the patient's unconscious, providing insight into their fears, desires, and unresolved conflicts. By exploring the symbolic meaning of these dreams, therapists can help patients process their trauma, challenge internalized beliefs of unworthiness, and rebuild a more compassionate relationship with their bodies.

Integration of dream work in EDs treatment

Incorporating dream analysis into the treatment of ED patients with trauma histories requires sensitivity and skill. Therapists must navigate the intense emotions these dreams evoke while fostering a safe space for exploration. Interpreting food dreams can help patients uncover how their past experiences shape their present struggles, allowing them to reclaim a sense of agency and connection to their bodies. This process not only addresses the symptoms of the EDs but also supports broader healing from the psychological wounds of trauma

Bibliography

Auchincloss, E. (2015). The world of dreams. In *The Psychoanalytic Model of the Mind*. Arlington. VA: American Psychiatric Publishing, 93–103.

Bion, W. R. (1967). *Second Thoughts: Selected Papers on Psychoanalysis*. Oxford: Butterworth-Heinemann.

Brink, S. M., Allan, J. A., and Boldt, W. (1995). Symbolic representation of psychological states in the dreams of women with eating disorders. *Canadian Journal of Counselling and Psychotherapy*, 29(4): 332–344.

Bruch, H. (1978). *The Golden Cage: The Enigma of Anorexia Nervosa*. Cambridge, MA: Harvard University Press.

Bruch, H. (1985). Four decades of eating disorders. In D. M. Gamer and P. E. Garfinkel (eds.) *Handbook of Psychotherapy for Anorexia Nervosa and Bulimia*. New York: Guilford Press, 7–18.

Bucci, W. (1997). *Psychoanalysis and Cognitive Science: A Multiple Code Theory*. New York: Guilford Press.

Busch, F. (2014). *Creating a Psychoanalytic Mind: A Psychoanalytic Method and Theory*. London and New York: Routledge.

Cartwright, R. D. (2010). *The Twenty-four Hour Mind: The Role of Sleep and Dreaming in Our Emotional Lives*. New York: Oxford University Press.

Damasio, A. (2000): *The Feeling of What Happens: Body and Emotion in the Making of Consciousness*. London: Vintage.

Freud, S. (1895). Project for Scientific Psychology. In *The Standard Edition of the Complete Psychological Works of Sigmund Freud, (1)*. London: The Hogarth Press, 283–397 (1991 edition).

Freud, S. (1900[1899]). The interpretation of Dreams. In *The Standard Edition of the Complete Psychological Works of Sigmund Freud, (4) (5)*. London: The Hogarth Press, (1991 edition).

Goodsit, A. (1985). Self-psychology and the treatment of anorexia nervosa. In D. M. Gamer and P. E. Garfinkel (eds.) *Handbook of Psychotherapy for Anorexia Nervosa and Bulimia*. New York: Guilford Press, 513–572.

Gutnisky, D. A., Persano, H. L., and Campos, D. (2019). *Food Size Distortion in Eating Disorders: Development of a Simple Photographic Test*. International Congress of Psychiatry, June 2019. London: Royal College of Psychiatrists, UK. doi:10.13140/RG.2.2.29509.60645.

Gutnisky, D. A. and Campos, D. (2024). *Meal Portion Distortion in Eating Disorders* Conference: Poster Displayed at the Faculty of Eating Disorders Spring Conference 2024. London: Royal College of Psychiatrists, UK. doi:10.13140/RG.2.2.26060.83849.

Hamburg, P. (1989). Bulimia: The construction of a symptom. *Journal of the American Academy of Psychoanalysis*, 17(1): 131–140.

Kandell, E. R., Schwartz, J. H., Jesell, T. M., Siegelbaum, S. A., and Hudspeth, A. J. (2013). Sleep and Dreaming. In *Principles of Neural Sciences, Fifth Edition*. New York: Mc Graw Hill, 1140–1158 (chapter 51).

Lask, B., and Bryant-Waugh, R. (2000). *Anorexia Nervosa and Related Eating Disorders in Childhood and Adolescence* (2nd edition). Hove, UK: Psychology Press.

Magagna, J. (2000). Dreams, the internal world and eating disorders. In M. Williams (ed.) *Winnicott and the Future of Psychoanalysis*. London: Karnac Books, 157–172.

MacCleod, S. (1981). *The Art of Starvation*. London: Virago.

Persano, H. L. (2019). Los sueños revisitados a la luz de algunas teorías psicoanalíticas y extra-psicoanalíticas actuales. In F. M. Gómez (ed.) *Percepción y Sueño: Perspectivas actuales*. Buenos Aires: APA Editorial, 409–453.

Rangell, L. (1987). Historical perspectives and current status of the interpretation of dreams in clinical work. In A. Rothstein (ed.) *The Interpretations of Dreams in Clinical Work*. Madison, CT: International Universities Press, 3–24 (chapter 1).

Robinson, P., Skårderud, F., and Sommerfeldt, B. (2017). *Hunger: Mentalization-based Treatments for Eating Disorders*. Cham: Springer.

Robinson, P., Skårderud, F., and Sommerfeldt, B. (2019). Eating disorders as clinical examples of impaired mentalizing: Theory and descriptions. In *Hunger: Mentalization-based Treatments for Eating Disorders*. Cham: Springer, 15–34.

Skårderud, F. (2007). Eating one's words, Part I: 'Concretised metaphors' and reflective function in anorexia nervosa—An interview study. *European Eating Disorders Review*, 15(3): 163–174.

Schredl, M. and Montasser, A. (1999). Dreaming and eating disorders. *Sleep and Hypnosis*, 1(4): 225–231.

Selvini Palazzoli, M. (1974). *Self-Starvation*. New York: Jason Aronson, (1978 edition).

Solms, M. and Turnbull, O. (2002). Dreams and hallucinations. In *The Brain and the Inner World: An Introduction to the Neuroscience of Subjective Experience*. London and New York: Routledge.

Stern, S. (1986). The dynamics of clinical management in the treatment of anorexia nervosa and bulimia: An organizing theory. *International Journal of Eating Disorders*, 5(2): 233–254.

Weizsacker, V. V. (1964). Dreams in so-called endogenic magersucht (anorexia). In M. R. Kaufmann and M. Heiman (eds. and trans.) *Evolution of Psychosomatic Concepts: Anorexia Nervosa: A Paradigm*. London: Hogarth Press, 181–197.

9 Treatment approaches in psychoanalytic therapy

Psychodynamic psychotherapy of eating disorders

Introduction

This chapter explores psychoanalytic approaches to the treatment of eating disorders, divided into four key topics: the psychoanalytic understanding of EDs, working with resistance, identifying defensive mechanisms in clinical practice, and the application of transference-focused psychotherapy (TFP) and mentalization-based therapy (MBT).

Introduction to the psychoanalytic comprehension of EDs for psychotherapeutic processes challenges and complexities in ED treatment

The psychodynamic psychotherapeutic treatment of eating disorders (EDs) poses significant challenges for therapists, given the complexity and multifaceted nature of these conditions. Effective treatment requires an interdisciplinary approach, as no single professional can address the wide-ranging needs of this population in isolation. Collaboration with a multidisciplinary team—including a nutritionist, general practitioner, and, frequently, a psychiatrist—is essential for providing comprehensive care.

The high prevalence of psychiatric comorbidities among patients with eating disorders (EDs) often calls for the integration of psychopharmacological treatments. These interventions play a crucial role in supporting the psychotherapeutic process and managing co-occurring conditions that can complicate clinical presentation. While Chapter 11 will explore interdisciplinary collaboration and pharmacological strategies in detail, this chapter emphasizes the importance of seamlessly incorporating these elements into a cohesive and comprehensive treatment framework within individual psychotherapy.

Such integration is essential for achieving optimal therapeutic outcomes, as it ensures that all dimensions of the patient's mental and physical health are addressed. By weaving psychopharmacology and psychotherapy into a unified approach, clinicians can better support patients in

DOI: 10.4324/9781032724997-9

navigating the complex interplay of symptoms and underlying emotional struggles, ultimately fostering more effective and sustainable recovery.

Navigating the clinical and emotional terrain

ED patients present a range of complications that demand careful management to ensure the continuity of treatment and prevent early abandonment. These include malnutrition, self-harming behaviors, suicide attempts, emotional dysregulation, and behaviors such as the indiscriminate use of laxatives, diuretics, vomiting, and binge-eating episodes. Emotional outbursts and frequent acting out further underscore the complexity of maintaining therapeutic engagement.

To address these challenges, therapists must adopt technical parameters that provide a stable framework for treatment, ensuring that patients remain within the therapeutic process despite their intense emotional and behavioral fluctuations.

Psychoanalytic characteristics of ED patients

From a psychodynamic perspective, ED patients often present profound disturbances within their psychic apparatus. These include:

- *Dominance of archaic mental functioning*: As André Green (1999) notes, ED patients often operate at a level where archaic mental states dominate, reflecting primitive modes of thought and interaction.
- *Deficits in symbolization and mentalization*: Patients frequently struggle with processes of symbolization and mentalization, often stemming from early attachment disruptions. Studies indicate a prevalence of insecure or disorganized attachment patterns in this population (Bateman and Fonagy, 2019); (Robinson, Skårderud, and Sommerfeldt, 2019); (Zeeck et al., 2021); (Tasca, 2010).
- *Action-oriented communication*: Rather than expressing themselves through thought and language, these patients often communicate through actions, such as self-harming behaviors, binging, or purging (Kernberg, 2018).
- *Splitting and lack of integration*: Following Kernberg's (2012) conceptualizations, ED patients exhibit splitting of mental representations, reflecting difficulties in integrating conflicting aspects of their identity and experiences.
- *Primitive defensive mechanisms*: These patients rely heavily on primitive defenses, including denial, projection, and omnipotence, to cope with emotional pain and internal conflicts (Kernberg, 1984).
- *Distortions of reality and body image*: Reality testing is often impaired (Frosch, 1983), and body image distortion becomes a central feature of

their psychopathology, reflecting difficulties in achieving an integrated sense of self.

- *Object craving and emotional dependency*: Jeammet (1992, 1994) high-lights the role of object craving and relational voracity in EDs, reflecting a compensatory response to emotional emptiness and unstable object constancy.
- *Tyranny of the Ideal of the Ego*: Patients are often dominated by an unattainable Ideal of the Ego that imposes impossible standards, contributing to their sense of failure and self-criticism (Persano, 2005).
- *Difficulties in autonomy and separation*: ED patients frequently struggle with achieving emotional autonomy and effective separation from primary objects (Robinson, Skårderud, and Sommerfeldt, 2019); (Bateman and Fonagy, 2004, 2019); (Kernberg, 2004); (Petrucelli, 2015).

Therapeutic implications

Understanding the unique psychoanalytic dimensions of ED patients is critical for tailoring effective psychodynamic interventions. Therapists must adopt an approach that acknowledges the primitive nature of their psychic functioning, providing containment while fostering the development of more mature defenses, symbolic capacities, and relational stability.

The interdisciplinary team plays a pivotal role in addressing the multi-faceted needs of these patients, while the therapist's ability to tolerate and interpret the archaic transference manifestations is central to facilitating psychic integration and long-term recovery. Psychoanalytic insights offer a roadmap for navigating the profound challenges of ED treatment, ensuring that interventions address not only the symptoms but also the deep-rooted emotional and relational disturbances that underlie these disorders.

Choosing the psychotherapist

The selection of the therapist is a critical aspect of the treatment process for patients with EDs and warrants careful consideration. The passive, silent stance traditionally associated with psychoanalysis is generally counterproductive for this patient population, as they are unlikely to tolerate it. Given the centrality of aggression—both internal and in their relationships with significant others—it is crucial that the therapeutic relationship serves as a secure space for the expression and exploration of emotions and feelings. As Winnicott (1949) aptly stated, the patient must be allowed to be "aggressive, but not destructible".

Attributes of an effective psychotherapist

Patients with EDs often present a marked deficit in symbolic capacity, which manifests as impaired mentalization and reflective functioning

(Bateman and Fonagy, 2004, 2019; Robinson, Skårderud, and Sommerfeldt, 2019). Therefore, one of the primary attributes to consider when selecting a therapist is a strong capacity for mentalization. The therapeutic process itself may temporarily compromise the therapist's ability to mentalize, particularly in the face of the patient's intense emotional states and defenses (Robinson, Skårderud, and Sommerfeldt, 2019). For this reason, ongoing supervision and reflective practice are essential components of the therapist's work.

The psychotherapist must also possess a high tolerance for frustration. The complexities and crises that inevitably arise during the treatment of severe cases demand resilience and the ability to remain composed under pressure. This includes tolerating criticism from peers or colleagues that may emerge during challenging phases of treatment. Empathy, warmth, and firmness are equally important traits, as is a genuine belief in the patient's capacity to improve and the therapist's ability to facilitate that improvement (Gunderson, 2000).

Technical training and supervision

A therapist treating ED patients must be well-trained in psychotherapeutic techniques appropriate to this population and committed to ongoing professional development. Regular supervision is critical for addressing difficulties that may arise during treatment and for maintaining the therapist's reflective capacity (Ventura, 2014). Supervision also provides a forum for processing countertransference and refining interventions to better align with the patient's needs.

The crucial role of patience in eating disorder treatment

Patience is an indispensable quality for therapists working with patients suffering from EDs. The therapeutic process is often characterized by slow, incremental progress, particularly in the early stages, which can feel stagnant and discouraging. As though traversing a labyrinth without a clear exit, therapists must navigate the complexities of their patients' defenses, fears, and resistance to change. This slow pace can test even the most seasoned professionals, but it is precisely this patience that forms the cornerstone of successful treatment.

Maintaining curiosity and hope

As Izydorczyk (2022), Bruch (1978), and Selvini Palazolli (1974) emphasize, maintaining curiosity, interest, and hope is not merely a recommendation but a therapeutic imperative. Without these qualities, the therapist risks becoming disengaged or disheartened, which can disrupt the delicate process of building trust and fostering growth. Curiosity keeps the therapist attuned to the subtle nuances of the patient's internal world, while hope provides a counterbalance to the despair that often permeates the patient's experience.

Patients with EDs frequently exhibit intense ambivalence about treatment. They may simultaneously desire change and resist it, clinging to the perceived safety of their symptoms. This paradox places significant demands on the therapist's ability to tolerate uncertainty and avoid imposing their own agenda on the patient. Instead, the therapist must patiently hold the space for the patient to explore their motivations, fears, and conflicts, allowing change to emerge organically over time.

"Knowing how to wait"

The idea that therapists must "know how to wait" is rooted in the understanding that genuine engagement with the therapeutic process cannot be forced. For patients with EDs, who often operate from a defensive posture rooted in fear and mistrust, premature efforts to push for change can reinforce resistance and deepen the patient's sense of alienation. As Bruch (1978) notes, therapists must adopt a stance of steady availability, signaling to the patient that they are present, consistent, and unconditionally invested in the process.

This patience extends beyond the immediate therapeutic encounter to encompass the broader trajectory of treatment. Changes in EDs often occur in fits and starts, with periods of progress interspersed with setbacks. The therapist's ability to maintain a long-term perspective, even in the face of apparent regression, provides the patient with a sense of stability and safety.

Organization of treatment

The treatment of patients with EDs presents a series of profound therapeutic challenges that necessitate careful organization and a thoughtful psychotherapeutic approach. These challenges are rooted in the complex dynamics of the patient's internal world, their relationships, and their interaction with the therapeutic setting (Yeomans, Clarkin, and Kernberg, 2002, 2015).

The evolution of the therapeutic relationship

Over time, as trust builds and defenses begin to soften, the therapeutic relationship evolves into a powerful vessel for change. It becomes a space where the patient feels seen, heard, and understood—perhaps for the first time. This relational experience is transformative, allowing the patient to internalize new ways of relating to themselves and others. Progress may initially manifest in small ways, such as a willingness to share more openly or a reduction in self-critical thoughts. However, these subtle shifts often herald deeper, more enduring changes.

As the patient begins to engage more fully with the therapeutic process, the therapist's patience is rewarded with moments of profound connection and insight. These moments, though sometimes fleeting, provide a glimpse of the potential for growth and healing. They reaffirm the value of the therapist's steadfast presence and their commitment to holding space for the patient's journey (Yeomans, Clarkin, and Kernberg, 2002, 2015).

Patience as a therapeutic tool

Patience is not merely a passive quality but an active component of the therapeutic process. It requires the therapist to regulate their own emotional responses, manage frustration, and maintain a sense of hope even when progress is slow. It also involves creating an environment where the patient feels free to explore their vulnerabilities without fear of judgment or pressure.

Through this deliberate practice of patience, the therapist models a way of being that the patient can begin to internalize. Over time, the patient may develop greater self-compassion and an increased capacity to tolerate their own emotional experiences, paving the way for meaningful and sustained recovery.

Patience in the treatment of EDs is more than a professional virtue; it is a therapeutic necessity. By "knowing how to wait", therapists provide the conditions for genuine engagement and transformation. As the therapeutic relationship deepens, the slow, steady work of change takes root, allowing patients to move beyond the confines of their symptoms and toward a fuller, more authentic engagement with life. In this way, patience becomes not only a tool for the therapist but also a gift to the patient—a testament to the enduring power of human connection and the possibilities of healing.

The therapeutic relationship in the treatment of EDs is a complex and demanding endeavor. The selection of a therapist equipped with the skills, resilience, and empathy to navigate this process is critical. Through a combination of technical expertise, reflective capacity, and unwavering patience, the therapist becomes not only a facilitator of change but also a stable and reliable presence in the patient's journey toward recovery.

Structural diagnostic interviews: Evaluating personality organization

Preliminary diagnostic interviews are essential for understanding the patient's level of personality organization and tailoring the treatment accordingly (Kernberg, 1984; McWilliams and Shedler, 2017). These interviews assess several key dimensions, including:

- *Identity integration or identity diffusion*: The degree to which the patient possesses a coherent sense of self.

- *Prevalent defense mechanisms*: From mature defenses like repression in neurotic organizations to primitive defenses like splitting in borderline personality organizations and withdrawal on massive projection in psychotic organizations.
- *Reality testing*: The ability to differentiate internal experiences from external reality.
- *Dominant anxieties and object relationships*: Including separation and abandonment fears, and the quality and stability of interpersonal relationships.
- *Impulse control and aggression regulation*: Including tendencies toward self-harm or externalized aggression.
- *Integration of moral values*: Reflecting the functionality and cohesiveness of the superego.

These assessments guide the organization of treatment, offering insights into the patient's prognosis, potential adherence, and the types of crises that may arise during therapy (Kernberg et al., 1989; Clarkin et al., 1999; Ventura, 2014).

For research purposes, Kernberg's team designed a self-report instrument (the Interview for Personality Organization, IPO) and a semi-structured interview version (STIPO). We have used the IPO for a long time during the diagnostic process, often in combination with the DIB-R (Zanarini et al., 1989). We found that many patients suffering from EDs diagnosis, especially those suffering from BN, present a borderline personality disorder and borderline personality organization (Persano et al., 2011, 2016)

The role of trauma and attachment

Many ED patients have histories of developmental trauma, including physical, emotional, or sexual abuse, neglect, or abandonment. Such experiences often lead to insecure or disorganized attachment patterns, resulting in impairments in mentalization and reflective functioning (Bateman and Fonagy, 2019); (Zeeck et al., 2021). This manifests as deficits in symbolization and impoverished mental representations, along with object cravings—a hallmark feature in bulimic conditions, as described by Jeammet (1994). These dynamics frequently lead to overwhelming demands on the therapist in BN or withdrawal and isolation in AN.

Levels of personality organization and therapeutic implications

Understanding personality organization levels provides a foundation for selecting appropriate therapeutic techniques:

- *Normal and neurotic personality organization*: Both are marked by an integrated identity, stable object relations, and reliance on mature defense mechanisms. However, neurotic personality organization tends to exhibit greater rigidity in defenses and heightened Superego functioning, often leading to more pronounced internal conflict and self-critical tendencies.

- *Borderline personality organization*: Defined by identity diffusion and the use of primitive defense mechanisms such as splitting, idealization, and devaluation. While reality testing remains intact, borderline organization is dominated by separation and abandonment anxieties. Aggressive drives frequently overshadow libidinal ones, contributing to unstable relationships and heightened emotional reactivity.

- *Psychotic personality organization*: This organization is characterized by delusions involving identity, reliance on primitive defenses, and impaired reality testing. These impairments often present as delusions or hallucinations that persist despite confrontation or clarification. The absence of an integrated sense of self further exacerbates difficulties in interpersonal functioning and adaptive behavior, making it challenging for individuals to navigate relationships and daily life effectively.

In our clinical experience, EDs are most associated with borderline personality organization (BPO). Consequently, psychotherapeutic approaches must incorporate strategies designed for patients with personality disorders. EDs are frequently categorized as self-disorders (Petrucelli, 2015; Robinson, Skårderud, and Sommerfeldt, 2019).

Implementing protective parameters in treatment

Before initiating therapy, the diagnostic interviews and contract discussions serve to establish parameters that safeguard the treatment's progression. These parameters protect both the therapeutic alliance and the patient's ability to engage with the process, ensuring that treatment remains focused and effective despite the significant challenges inherent in treating personality disorders and EDs. By doing so, therapists create a structured yet flexible environment in which patients can begin the journey toward recovery.

The importance of the therapeutic contract

The therapeutic contract is a foundational element in the treatment of personality disorders, including EDs. As outlined by Clarkin, Yeomans, and Kernberg (1999), the contract establishes the minimal conditions necessary for treatment to proceed effectively. It functions as a formal agreement defining the boundaries, expectations, and responsibilities of both therapist and patient. This structured framework not only supports adherence but also mitigates the risk of early dropout—a frequent challenge in the initial stages of therapy.

Safeguarding treatment through clear agreements

The contract serves multiple purposes, providing clarity and accountability while fostering a therapeutic alliance essential for the success of treatment. During the preliminary diagnostic interviews, the therapist informs the patient that therapy has not yet commenced until these interviews are completed, and both parties have agreed upon the rules and framework for the process. This approach aligns with the principles proposed by Clarkin, Yeomans, and Kernberg (1999), emphasizing the importance of a collaborative and transparent foundation for therapy.

The agreement must explicitly address key parameters, including:

- *Attendance and commitment*: Emphasizing the necessity of regular participation in therapy.
- *Treatment scope*: Clearly defining how the therapeutic process will proceed, including expectations for sessions and goals.
- *Crisis management*: Outlining how to address critical situations such as weight loss, purgative measures, self-harm, and suicide attempts.
- *Responsibilities*: Ensuring both patient and therapist understand their roles within the treatment framework.

Customizing the contract to individual needs

Typically, the process of establishing a contract takes two sessions. In the first session, general rules are discussed, such as the need for consistent attendance and the overall therapeutic approach. The second session focuses on individualizing the contract to address specific parameters relevant to the patient's needs. This may include conditions for managing high-risk behaviors or clarifying how external interventions, such as hospitalization, will be handled if necessary (Yeomans, Selzer, and Clarkin, 1992; Kernberg et al., 1989).

Addressing complexities in ED treatment

Eating disorder patients often present unique challenges that require careful incorporation into the therapeutic contract. These may include behaviors such as extreme weight loss, purging, or other self-harming actions. By setting clear boundaries and expectations around these behaviors, the contract ensures that treatment can continue safely and effectively. Parameters should also include the need for multidisciplinary collaboration with nutritionists, psychiatrists, and general practitioners, particularly when medical risks are present (Persano, 2022).

Fostering the therapeutic alliance

The process of developing the therapeutic contract inherently strengthens the therapeutic alliance. By engaging the patient in a transparent dialogue about expectations and responsibilities, the therapist demonstrates respect for the patient's autonomy while ensuring that the treatment structure is robust enough to handle crises. This collaboration helps build trust and reduces resistance, creating a stable foundation for the therapeutic journey.

In summary, the therapeutic contract is not merely an administrative step but a dynamic tool that integrates clinical, relational, and practical elements into the treatment of personality disorders and EDs. Its careful implementation ensures that both patient and therapist are aligned in their goals and approach, paving the way for meaningful and sustained progress.

According with Adrian Ventura´s expertise in conducting psychotherapeutic processes, he explains initial phase of the treatment with patients suffering from ED in this way:

> This treatment is intended to help you solve the problems that brought you here. If we are going to work together, it is important that you commit to it. It is very important that you attend the sessions regularly, since you cannot help or work with someone who is not present.
>
> It is also very important that you feel free to express your thoughts and feelings, even if they are related to the relationship we are going to establish. In principle, you should come to talk about the problems that brought you to the consultation, about those things that worry you the most and that you want to solve.
>
> If during a session you think that there is no topic that worries you, then you should communicate anything that comes to your mind, without censoring it.
>
> It is also important that if you dream and remember what you dreamed, you bring it as material for analysis, since dreams are important to discover the unconscious motives that condition conscious behavior.
>
> If there is an important reason that threatens the continuity of the treatment, this is the first thing we should address in the sessions.
>
> For my part, I promise to be available at the agreed times and days and I will let you know in advance if one day I am not available, unless something urgent happens (a rare situation), for example, if one day I wake up sick with a fever and I am unable to attend to you. At the same time, I promise to listen to you carefully and help you so that you can understand more deeply what the unknown reasons for your difficulties are.

Finally, I would like to clarify that my commitment is limited to the times of the sessions that we will arrange and that I will not be available outside of these times. What do you think about this?

The importance of patient collaboration and establishing special rules in treatment.

Engaging from the patient's perspective is a critical aspect of initiating effective treatment. It is common for patients with EDs to underestimate the importance of consistent attendance at sessions. Absences, which often manifest as a form of resistance, present significant obstacles during the early stages of treatment and are a frequent cause of therapeutic failure or premature termination.

Evaluating patient commitment and past experiences

Observing the patient's compliance during preliminary evaluation interviews can provide valuable insight into their readiness for therapy. It is also essential to gather detailed information about previous treatments. Key areas to explore include:

- The advantages and disadvantages of past therapeutic approaches.
- Reasons for treatment abandonment.
- Specific challenges or difficulties that emerged during prior interventions.

Whenever possible, obtaining the patient's permission to communicate with their previous therapist can offer additional context and help identify patterns likely to reappear in the current treatment. Awareness of these recurring issues allows therapists to anticipate potential obstacles and plan strategies to address them effectively.

Working with resistance in eating disorders

Paranoid dynamics and initial resistance

Patients with EDs frequently exhibit significant resistance at the beginning of treatment. This resistance often takes the form of paranoid attitudes toward the therapist, regardless of whether the patient has entered treatment voluntarily or has been urged to seek help by concerned family members. As Jeammet (1992) observes, patients with AN may perceive the therapist as an intrusive figure representing those who want to "fatten them", reinforcing their defensive stance. Conversely, patients with BN may view the therapist as someone intent on depriving them of the sensory pleasure and relief their symptoms provide. These perceptions create a dynamic of distrust and suspicion, often leading to initial withdrawal and posing challenges to establishing rapport and therapeutic engagement.

Resistance and the emotional significance of weight

The centrality of weight in EDs makes it an emotionally charged topic and a potential source of resistance. Addressing weight directly in psychotherapy can inadvertently reinforce defensive structures, such as splitting or denial, and may provoke further mistrust. For this reason, it is essential to delegate weight management to a nutrition professional, ensuring that psychotherapy remains focused on the patient's psychological and emotional experiences rather than on their physical symptoms.

Discussions about weight should only enter the therapeutic space when initiated by the patient, allowing it to become a topic for analysis rather than confrontation. This strategy preserves psychotherapeutic space as one of reflection and exploration.

However, in situations where the patient's weight reaches life-threatening levels, therapists must address the issue with sensitivity and precision. Collaborating closely with the nutritionist, the therapist can frame the discussion in terms of the patient's omnipotent beliefs and the risks to their life. For example, extreme weight loss can be explored as a manifestation of unconscious suicidal ideation or as a desire to assert control in the face of overwhelming emotional distress. This approach aligns with the reality principle, gently confronting the patient's defenses while opening a pathway for deeper exploration of their internal world.

Resistance and the reality principle

Resistance often manifests in ED patients as a rejection of the reality principle, replaced by omnipotent fantasies of control over their body and environment. For example, patients suffering from AN may believe they are immune to the physical consequences of starvation, while patients with BN may minimize the health risks associated with purging behaviors. Introducing reality-based interventions, such as the potential need for hospitalization in life-threatening situations, must be handled delicately.

By linking these behaviors to the patient's unconscious conflicts, the therapist can foster insight into the underlying dynamics driving their symptoms. For example, framing extreme weight loss as an expression of self-destructive tendencies allows the patient to begin bridging the gap between their inner world and external reality. This approach does not merely impose external authority but helps patients recognize the connections between their symptoms, unconscious conflicts, and relational patterns.

Resistance and defensive processes

Resistance in eating disorder (ED) patients is deeply interwoven with their reliance on primitive defense mechanisms such as splitting, denial, and projective identification. These defenses serve an unconscious purpose: protecting the individual from overwhelming emotional states and internal conflicts. However, they simultaneously hinder therapeutic progress by distorting the patient's perception of both the therapist and the treatment process.

For example, the defense of splitting often leads the patient to categorize the therapist as either an "all-bad" figure—perceived as coercive, judgmental, or controlling—or an "all-good" figure who is idealized and burdened with the unrealistic expectation of resolving all the patient's struggles. This oscillation undermines the development of a stable and balanced therapeutic alliance, perpetuating resistance.

Understanding and managing resistance in ED patients

Recognizing defensive patterns

Resistance often manifests as overt or covert behaviors that serve to maintain psychic equilibrium but obstruct the therapeutic process. For instance:

Withdrawal and hostility in patients with AN are frequently defenses against perceived intrusion or threats to autonomy. The patient's rigid refusal to eat or gain weight reflects their need to assert control and avoid emotional vulnerability.

Apparent compliance in patients with BN may disguise deeper feelings of resentment, fear of dependency, or a need to maintain control through superficial agreement.

Exploring the role of resistance

Resistance should not be viewed merely as an obstacle but as a meaningful expression of the patient's internal struggles and defenses. For example:

- Withdrawal might indicate a profound fear of intimacy or a history of relational trauma where closeness led to harm.
- Hostility may be a projection of self-directed aggression onto the therapist, reflecting the patient's internal battle with shame, guilt, or self-criticism.

By interpreting resistance in this way, therapists can uncover its underlying meaning and address the patient's deeper conflicts.

Strategies for managing resistance

1   *Acknowledging the defensive function*

- It is crucial to validate the protective role that resistance plays for the patient. For example, acknowledging that the patient's reluctance to discuss certain topics stems from a need to feel safe can create a space for openness.

- Recognizing and naming the defense without judgment helps the patient begin to differentiate between past relational dynamics and the therapeutic relationship.

2 *Maintaining neutrality*

- Therapists must remain attuned to their countertransference reactions, such as frustration or a desire to overcompensate. Neutrality and emotional regulation allow the therapist to avoid enacting the split perceptions of being "all-bad" or "all-good."
- For instance, when a patient accuses the therapist of being controlling, the therapist can explore this perception collaboratively rather than reacting defensively.

3 *Gradual confrontation*

- Resistance should be confronted gently and incrementally. For example:
  "It seems like discussing your eating behaviors makes you feel uncomfortable, and I wonder if it feels like I'm trying to take control away from you".
- This approach validates the patient's experience while inviting reflection on the relational dynamics at play.

4 *Fostering reflective functioning*

- Encouraging the patient to reflect on their emotional states and relational patterns helps them transition from action (e.g., splitting or withdrawal) to thought. This shift is a critical step in reducing resistance and fostering engagement.
- For instance, helping a patient with BN recognize how their apparent compliance masks fears of abandonment can deepen their understanding of their relational and emotional needs.

5 *Strengthening the therapeutic alliance*

- Building trust is fundamental in managing resistance. By consistently maintaining a nonjudgmental and supportive stance, therapists can demonstrate that the therapeutic relationship is a safe space for exploration and growth.
- This is particularly important for patients who have experienced attachment disruptions, as they may test the therapist's reliability through acts of resistance.

Resistance as a pathway to growth

Resistance in ED patients reflects the intricate interplay of primitive defense mechanisms—splitting, denial, projective identification, and related behaviors—and deeply rooted fears of vulnerability, dependency, and loss of control. These defenses, while initially adaptive in shielding the patient from emotional overwhelm, can impede therapeutic progress by distorting perceptions of the therapist and the treatment process. However, rather than viewing resistance as a barrier, therapists can reframe it as an opportunity for meaningful engagement and insight.

By understanding the defensive function of resistance, the therapeutic process can transform these behaviors into a pathway for psychic integration and emotional growth. Through validation, neutrality, and gradual confrontation of defenses, resistance becomes a bridge to deeper self-awareness, helping patients to address the unconscious conflicts that underpin their maladaptive patterns.

Resistance and the therapeutic relationship

Successfully addressing resistance requires the creation of a therapeutic relationship that is both stable and flexible. The therapist must establish clear boundaries and a structured framework while remaining deeply attuned to the patient's emotional and relational needs.

This balance transforms the therapeutic space into a secure environment where resistance can be explored rather than enacted.

Building trust is a gradual process, especially for patients whose early attachment experiences have left them distrustful of dependency or hypersensitive to perceived rejection. For these patients, resistance often reflects their inner fears and struggles. By engaging with resistance rather than avoiding or opposing it, therapists can foster a deeper understanding of the patient's inner world.

Transforming resistance into insight

Resistance can manifest in various forms, from withdrawal and hostility to apparent compliance masking deeper fears. Each form provides valuable material for therapeutic exploration:

- Withdrawal might signal fears of intrusion or a need for autonomy.
- Hostility could reflect projections of self-directed aggression or unresolved relational trauma.
- Compliance may mask ambivalence, resentment, or fears of dependency.

The therapist's role is to meet these behaviors with curiosity, empathy, and firmness, creating a space where the patient feels safe enough to confront their defenses and the underlying conflicts they protect.

From resistance to psychic integration

As resistance is gradually worked through, the therapeutic relationship evolves into a vessel for integration and growth. Patients begin to transition from action-oriented defenses (e.g., splitting, acting out, withdrawal) to reflective engagement, developing the capacity to mentalize their own emotions and those of others. This shift fosters:

- Greater emotional regulation.
- Improved relational stability.
- A cohesive sense of self.

Overcoming resistance is not a linear process but a dynamic one, requiring the therapist's patience, neutrality, and unwavering presence. The therapeutic alliance becomes the foundation for navigating these challenges, transforming resistance from an obstacle into a cornerstone of meaningful change.

By embracing resistance as a vital element of the therapeutic journey, both patient and therapist can engage in a collaborative process of healing and transformation, paving the way for enduring psychic and emotional well-being.

Countertransference and resistance in eating disorders

The interplay of countertransference and resistance

Working with resistance in EDs inevitably evokes countertransference reactions in therapists, given the intensity of the relational dynamics involved. Patients with EDs often project their internal conflicts onto the therapist, triggering emotional responses that can either hinder or enhance the therapeutic process. Recognizing and managing countertransference effectively is critical to maintaining therapeutic boundaries and using these reactions as tools for deeper understanding and intervention.

For example, a patient with AN exhibiting a rigid refusal to gain weight may provoke feelings of frustration or helplessness in the therapist, while a patient with BN with repeated relapses into purging behaviors can elicit exasperation or discouragement. These responses, although challenging, offer valuable insights into the patient's unconscious dynamics and relational patterns. As Corcos and Jeammet (2001) emphasize, countertransference can serve as a window into the patient's internal world, reflecting the primitive defenses and unresolved conflicts that underlie their symptoms.

Countertransference as a diagnostic and interpretative tool

Using countertransference constructively involves acknowledging it as a reflection of the patient's unconscious projections and integrating it into the interpretative process. For instance, if a therapist feels criticized or rejected by a patient, this dynamic can be explored to illuminate how the patient navigates attachment, conflict, and dependency in other relationships. These insights are particularly relevant in EDs, where patterns of splitting, projection, and idealization are frequently observed (Persano and Ventura, 2006; Persano, 2006).

The activation of primitive object relations in the therapeutic relationship often exacerbates countertransference reactions. Patients with EDs may relate to the therapist as a "bad object", embodying their fears of intrusion or abandonment, or as an "all-good object", idealized as a source of salvation. These polarized dynamics must be carefully navigated to avoid enactment and to facilitate the integration of split representations.

Navigating countertransference in anorexia nervosa and bulimia nervosa

Patients with AN often evoke countertransference characterized by helplessness, frustration, or even a sense of inadequacy. Their rigid defenses and withdrawal from engagement can make the therapist feel excluded or powerless. These reactions mirror the patient's internal struggle with autonomy and control, highlighting their fear of dependency and loss of identity (Persano, 2006).

Conversely, patients with BN frequently overwhelm the therapist with their relational voracity and insatiable demands for attention. These behaviors can elicit feelings of depletion or resentment, reflecting the patient's struggle with boundary-setting and emotional regulation. Recognizing these dynamics helps the therapist address the patient's underlying fear of abandonment and need for validation (Persano, 2006).

The prevalence of the death drive and aggressive dynamics

As Corcos and Jeammet (2001) note, the prevalence of the death drive is particularly evident in ED patients. This manifests in self-directed aggression, such as self-harm, suicide attempts, or severe malnutrition, and in interpersonal aggression, characterized by conflictual relationships and emotional volatility. These dynamics inevitably surface in the transference and must be carefully managed to prevent disruptions in the therapeutic alliance.

Countertransference reactions, such as anxiety, anger, or despair, often mirror the patient's unprocessed feelings and unresolved conflicts. For instance, feelings of dread in the therapist may reflect the patient's unconscious fear of annihilation or failure. Recognizing these projections allows the therapist to empathize with the patient's experience while maintaining a grounded and reflective stance.

Managing countertransference and resistance: A structured approach

Effectively addressing countertransference and resistance requires a structured therapeutic framework that prioritizes containment, collaboration, and interpretation (Persano and Ventura, 2006); (Persano, 2006). This involves:

- *Self-awareness and supervision*: Therapists must remain attuned to their emotional responses and seek supervision or peer consultation to process and contextualize countertransference reactions. This practice helps prevent enactment and maintains the therapist's capacity for reflection.
- *Establishing boundaries*: Clear therapeutic boundaries are essential to managing the intense relational dynamics of ED treatment. For example, the therapist may need to clarify their role in the patient's care, avoiding over-involvement while remaining consistently available and empathetic.
- *Linking behaviors to internal conflicts*: Countertransference can be used to explore the connections between the patient's external behaviors (e.g., purging, restricting) and their internal conflicts. For instance, a therapist feeling drained by a patient with BN demands might interpret these behaviors as attempts to regulate feelings of emptiness or abandonment.
- *Addressing splitting and projection*: Therapists must work to integrate the polarized representations of self and others that underlie the patient's defensive patterns. This involves interpreting the dynamics of splitting and projection within the therapeutic relationship and helping the patient develop a more cohesive sense of identity.

Countertransference and the therapeutic alliance

Managing countertransference effectively strengthens the therapeutic alliance, transforming resistance into an opportunity for growth and insight. By maintaining a stance of neutrality and empathy, the therapist can help the patient navigate their fears of dependency, vulnerability, and loss of control. This process fosters trust and collaboration, creating a safe space for the patient to explore their defenses and underlying conflicts.

Countertransference as a pathway to understanding

Countertransference in ED treatment is both a challenge and an invaluable tool. It reflects the intensity of the patient's relational dynamics and offers a pathway for understanding their unconscious processes. By navigating countertransference with awareness and skill, therapists can transform resistance into a vehicle for therapeutic engagement and psychic integration. This approach not only supports the patient's recovery but also enriches the therapist's capacity for empathy, insight, and professional growth (Persano and Ventura, 2006).

Transforming resistance into insight

Resistance in EDs is not merely an obstacle to treatment but a window into the patient's unconscious conflicts and relational dynamics. By understanding and addressing resistance through the lens of psychoanalytic principles, therapists can foster a therapeutic process that respects the patient's defenses while encouraging growth and insight. This approach transforms resistance from a barrier into a meaningful avenue for exploration, helping patients move toward greater self-awareness and emotional integration.

Avoiding resistance in the initial phase of treatment

In the psychodynamic treatment of EDs, resistance often emerges as a significant obstacle, especially during the initial phase of therapy. This resistance can take various forms, such as reluctance to engage in the therapeutic process, emotional withdrawal, denial of the severity of the disorder, or overt defiance of treatment goals. These behaviors reflect the deeply entrenched nature of the disorder, as well as the patient's fear of relinquishing the control that the ED provides. Resistance is not merely an oppositional stance; it often represents the patient's struggle with vulnerability, trust, and ambivalence about change.

Addressing resistance early in the therapeutic relationship is critical for ensuring long-term success. The therapist must approach resistance with empathy and curiosity, understanding it as a defense mechanism rather than a personal affront or failure of treatment. Openly exploring the underlying fears and conflicts driving resistance can help patients feel validated and understood, fostering a stronger therapeutic alliance.

A key strategy to mitigate resistance involves establishing clear, structured guidelines from the outset. These guidelines should address critical aspects such as maintaining minimum weight requirements, consistent attendance, and adherence to agreed-upon goals. Such structure provides a sense of safety and predictability, reducing the patient's anxiety about the therapeutic process. At the same time, it creates accountability, ensuring that both therapist and patient remain committed to the treatment plan.

Another essential component is the therapist's ability to balance firmness with flexibility. While structured guidelines are important, they must be implemented in a way that respects the patient's autonomy and fosters collaboration rather than control. For instance, engaging the patient in discussions about treatment goals and strategies can help them feel more involved and less coerced, reducing resistance over time.

Finally, addressing resistance involves recognizing and working through the transference and countertransference dynamics that may arise in therapy. Patients with EDs often project their struggles with control, trust, and self-worth onto the therapeutic relationship. Therapists must remain attuned to these dynamics, using them as opportunities to deepen insight and facilitate change. By approaching resistance as a gateway to understanding the patient's inner world, rather than as a barrier to progress, therapists can transform it into a powerful tool for growth and healing.

Establishing a minimum weight: A collaborative framework

For patients with EDs, particularly those who suffer from AN, establishing a minimum weight threshold is a critical component of treatment, ensuring both the safety of the patient and the continuity of therapeutic work. This threshold serves as a tangible boundary, clearly communicated and agreed upon at the outset of treatment, helping to create structure and accountability while fostering a collaborative therapeutic relationship.

Determining and maintaining the minimum weight requires close collaboration with a nutrition specialist, who plays an integral role in the multidisciplinary care team. The nutritionist assesses the patient's overall health status, analyzes weight trends, and considers individual factors such as body composition, medical history, and energy needs. Based on this comprehensive evaluation, the nutritionist works with the therapist and medical team to set a realistic and safe weight threshold.

Throughout treatment, the nutritionist monitors the patient's progress, ensuring that any weight fluctuations are addressed promptly. If the patient approaches or drops below the established minimum weight, the nutritionist informs the therapist and broader treatment team, signaling the need for an urgent intervention. This communication is crucial for addressing potential risks and adjusting the treatment plan as necessary.

Setting a minimum weight threshold as part of a collaborative framework has psychological as well as physical benefits. Involving the patient in the process helps to create a sense of shared responsibility, emphasizing that the guidelines are not punitive but rather a vital part of their care and recovery. Framing these boundaries as a cooperative effort reduces resistance, as the patient feels respected and included in the decision-making process, rather than feeling controlled or coerced.

This collaborative approach is also essential for maintaining the therapeutic alliance. By fostering open communication and mutual understanding, the therapist helps the patient recognize the importance of adhering to the weight guidelines for their health and the continuation of treatment. This balance of structure and empathy strengthens trust and reinforces the patient's commitment to recovery.

Despite its importance, establishing and maintaining a minimum weight can present challenges. Patients with AN often have a heightened fear of weight gain and may resist even the idea of setting a weight target. Therapists must approach this process with sensitivity, validating the patient's fears while emphasizing the necessity of the guidelines for their well-being. Creating a supportive environment where the patient feels safe to express their concerns can mitigate these challenges and promote a more positive engagement with the process.

Additionally, therapists must remain attuned to the emotional and relational dynamics surrounding weight discussions. These conversations can trigger feelings of shame, fear, or defiance in the patient, requiring the therapist to use skills such as active listening and reflective responses to address these emotions constructively.

Establishing a minimum weight threshold is not merely about physical health; it is also a symbolic step toward recovery. By creating a framework that integrates physical, psychological, and relational considerations, the treatment team provides the patient with a sense of safety and stability. This foundation allows the patient to focus on deeper therapeutic work, addressing the underlying emotional and psychological factors driving their ED.

Ultimately, the collaborative establishment and enforcement of a minimum weight threshold is an essential element of a holistic treatment approach. It aligns the efforts of the patient, therapist, and multidisciplinary team, ensuring that all aspects of the patient's health and recovery are addressed with care, structure, and compassion.

Framing special rules to avoid resistance

To avoid early resistance, it is essential to establish a therapeutic contract that includes special rules for managing potential crises or behaviors that could undermine treatment. These rules might include parameters for how to address self-harming behaviors, the use of purgative measures, or even suicidal ideation—frequent issues in this patient population.

The patient must be aware from the outset that violating these rules, such as dropping below the minimum weight threshold or failing to attend sessions, will necessitate a reassessment of the treatment plan, possibly involving hospitalization. However, it is crucial to frame these rules as protective measures rather than punitive, emphasizing that they exist to ensure the patient's safety and progress.

Presenting these rules in a clear, compassionate, and collaborative way reduces the likelihood that the patient will view them as oppressive or threatening, thereby decreasing resistance. This framework helps the patient understand that the treatment team is not only supportive but also committed to their well-being, creating a sense of partnership rather than conflict.

Addressing attendance and avoiding early dropout

Attendance issues, particularly frequent absences or lateness are common forms of resistance in the early stages of ED treatment. It is essential for the therapist to establish a firm yet empathetic stance on the importance of regular attendance. As with the weight guidelines, the patient must understand that attending sessions regularly is not just a matter of compliance but a crucial part of their recovery process.

To minimize the risk of early dropout, therapists can engage the patient in a dialogue about past treatment experiences, particularly addressing any failures or difficulties that might have led to disengagement. Exploring the reasons for previous treatment abandonment helps the therapist anticipate similar challenges in the current treatment and create strategies to mitigate them.

Proactive strategies to anticipate challenges

Proactively addressing challenges that may arise during the initial phase of treatment is essential for minimizing resistance. By anticipating common issues, such as the patient's reluctance to engage in weight-related discussions or their tendency to avoid difficult emotions, the therapist can create a safe, structured framework for exploration and reflection.

Additionally, by framing rules around weight thresholds and attendance as non-negotiable, but framed within a compassionate and collaborative treatment process, the therapist emphasizes the importance of patient accountability. This strategy enhances the patient's sense of agency and involvement in their care, thus reducing resistance.

Ensuring continuity of care

Maintaining continuity in ED treatment is a major concern, particularly given the high dropout rates in psychodynamic therapy for this population. By setting clear guidelines, including the need for regular attendance and weight management, therapists ensure that the patient understands the structure and expectations of the therapeutic process.

At the same time, flexibility in how the patient's needs are addressed is key. Although rules are important for creating a sense of safety, the therapeutic relationship should remain adaptive and responsive to the patient's emerging needs and difficulties. In this way, the framework becomes a stabilizing force that supports the patient through their initial ambivalence and resistance.

The initial phase of treatment for EDs is often fraught with resistance, but through clear, compassionate, and structured guidelines—especially regarding minimum weight and attendance—therapists can build a solid foundation for ongoing therapeutic work. By collaborating with the patient, the multidisciplinary team, and carefully managing expectations, therapists can foster patient engagement, minimize resistance, and ensure continuity of care. This structured yet flexible approach helps create the conditions necessary for long-term recovery and therapeutic success.

Finally, integrating patient feedback, monitoring compliance, and establishing clear guidelines are essential for fostering a therapeutic alliance and navigating the complexities of ED treatment with greater resilience and success.

Ventura's example of according a minimum weight with the patient:

> I'd like you to know that you must agree on a minimum weight with the nutritionistand that you must stay above that weight throughout the treatment.
>
> The weight you agree on is a weight that will guarantee that we won't have to worry about suspending our work because of your need to be hospitalized.
>
> I'm not interested in how much you weigh if you stay a little above that agreed minimum weight. We'll only address the issue of weight if the treatment or your life is in danger. Do you think you can commit to this?

The possibility of discussing treatment rules should always remain open for two important reasons:

- *Avoiding false consent*: Allowing open dialogue ensures that the patient does not simply agree to the rules superficially while secretly intending to disregard them. This prevents a disconnect between the patient's verbal agreement and their actual behavior, fostering genuine commitment.
- *Addressing resistance*: Discussions about the rules provide an early opportunity to explore the patient's resistance. Resistance is a natural part of the therapeutic process and addressing it from the outset lays the groundwork for deeper work in the initial phase of treatment. It allows the therapist to understand the patient's objections, fears, or ambivalence, turning these into productive areas of focus for the therapeutic journey.

This approach fosters trust, collaboration, and a sense of shared responsibility between the patient and therapist, creating a solid foundation for successful treatment.

At the outset of treatment, patients with AN often approach the therapeutic relationship with feelings of suspicion and distrust. They may perceive the therapist as a persecutory figure intent on making them gain weight, which reinforces their defensive stance. To address this, it is crucial to clearly communicate from the beginning that weight will not be a focus of the sessions unless the patient brings it up as a topic for discussion. The only exception to this rule arises if the patient approaches the minimum agreed-upon weight threshold determined by the nutritionist, thereby endangering their health and necessitating hospitalization. Clarifying this boundary can help reduce the patient's anxiety and build trust.

For patients with BN, the initial focus should be on reducing and ideally stopping purgative behaviors, particularly frequent vomiting. Persistent purging not only obstructs therapeutic progress but also poses severe risks to the patient's health due to hydro-electrolytic imbalances, which can be life-threatening. Vomiting often follows a binge episode and provides a perceptual satisfaction akin to the pleasure derived from addictive substances (Jeammet, 1992, 1994). Addressing this cycle early in treatment is critical for ensuring the patient's safety and supporting their ability to engage in therapy.

In both AN and BN, it is essential to establish clear agreements regarding how crises will be managed, including hospitalization for physical complications, self-harm, suicide attempts, or other high-risk behaviors. From the outset, it should be made explicit that hospitalization, when required, must be accepted as a non-negotiable aspect of care. Furthermore, any decision to discharge against medical advice would result in the discontinuation of the therapeutic process, as it would undermine the treatment framework and patient safety.

Setting these parameters early in the therapeutic relationship creates a foundation of transparency and mutual understanding, allowing both patient and therapist to navigate the complexities of eating disorder treatment with clear guidelines and shared expectations.

Establishing rules for managing suicide risk and self-harm

In the case of suicide attempts, it is essential to establish clear and non-negotiable rules. The patient must agree not to act on suicidal thoughts and, if the urge to self-harm becomes overwhelming, they are required to seek immediate help by going to an emergency room.

They must also commit to accepting the decision of the emergency team, whether it involves hospitalization or another intervention. Furthermore, the patient must return to treatment at the scheduled time and provide a report from the emergency room. This report serves as a basis for analyzing the triggers and underlying causes of their self-harming ideation, helping to frame these behaviors within the therapeutic process.

For self-harm, which is typically superficial and not immediately life-threatening, the therapist must first evaluate how much these actions disrupt the course of psychotherapy. Self-harm often serves as a behavioral equivalent of psychological pain, with physical pain acting as a coping mechanism to alleviate emotional distress. The primary goal is to address and diminish self-harming behaviors in the short term by helping patients identify and manage the underlying emotional triggers, such as feelings of emptiness, futility, or abandonment.

The role of defense mechanisms: Identifying common defense mechanisms and their function in maintaining maladaptive eating patterns

The role of defense mechanisms in eating disorders: Maintaining maladaptive patterns

Defense mechanisms are pivotal in understanding the persistence of maladaptive behaviors in individuals with EDs. These unconscious strategies protect the individual from overwhelming emotional pain or conflict but often perpetuate the disorder by maintaining rigid patterns of thought and behavior. Identifying and addressing these mechanisms within the therapeutic process is essential for promoting meaningful change.

Hierarchy of defense mechanisms in ED patients

As outlined by Perry, Kardos, and Pagano (1993) and Persano (2019), among other authors, the defense mechanisms employed by individuals vary significantly depending on their level of personality organization. Patients with more integrated psychic structures primarily rely on mature and neurotic defenses, while those with more primitive or fragmented organizations depend on immature or psychotic defenses.

J. Christopher Perry's (1991) hierarchy of defense mechanisms categorizes defenses based on their adaptiveness and complexity. Persano (2019) suggests that Perry's levels 6 and 5, which include neurotic defenses, should often be considered together, as they frequently overlap in clinical presentations. In addition, Berta Varela (2016) highlights the importance of recognizing a level 0 in Perry's hierarchy, corresponding to psychotic defenses, which include primitive mechanisms such as delusional projection and fragmentation.

For children and adolescents, Paulina Kernberg (Kernberg, Weiner, and Bardenstein, 2000) stresses the need to identify, dedifferentiation, constriction, de-animation, dispersal, dismantling, autistic encapsulation, fusion, freezing, hypochondriasis, and reversal of the affect as defenses at the psychotic (fourth) level, as these can indicate severe developmental challenges and impaired mental organization.

The focus in clinical practice is not solely on identifying individual defense mechanisms but rather on understanding the overall pattern of defensive functioning (*overall defensive functioning ODF*). These patterns provide insight into the individual's level of mental organization and the interplay between their defenses and underlying personality structure. Tracking shifts in these patterns over the course of psychotherapy is critical for evaluating meaningful psychic changes and the progression of the therapeutic process.

By examining these levels within the therapeutic process, clinicians can better understand how defense mechanisms both reflect and influence a patient's psychological resilience, adaptability, and overall mental health. Observing shifts from primitive to more mature defenses during treatment serves as a marker of therapeutic progress and deeper psychic integration.

High-adaptive (Mature) defenses (Level 7): These mechanisms promote optimal adaptation to stress and are associated with healthy functioning. Function: Enable adaptation to reality while maintaining emotional balance. Prevalence: Rare in severe ED cases, where more primitive defenses dominate: *Affiliation, altruism, anticipation, self-assertion, humor, self-observation, sublimation, suppression, fantasy.*

Obsessional Defenses (Level 6): These involve mechanisms for individuals to manage internal conflicts through excessive control. Function: Mitigate anxiety by distorting or isolating emotions. Prevalence: Found in patients with less severe EDs or higher functioning: *Reaction formation, displacement, isolation, intellectualization, undoing.*

Other neurotic defenses (Level 5): This category includes defenses such as repression and displacement, which are common in neurotic conditions and involve managing anxiety by keeping distressing thoughts out of conscious awareness. Function: Mitigate anxiety by repressing or dissociating representations from emotions. Prevalence: Found in patients with less severe EDs or higher functioning, principally in hysteric conditions: *Repression, dissociation, projection of impulses, neurotic denial.*

Minor image-distorting (Narcissistic) defenses (Level 4): These mechanisms, like devaluation and idealization, involve slight distortions in the perception of self or others to maintain self-esteem. Function protects against unbearable emotions but often leads to minor distorted perceptions of self and others. Prevalence: Common in individuals with narcissistic personality disorders and frequently co-occurring with EDs: *Self-devaluation/ Devaluation of others, idealization of self/others, omnipotence.*

Disavowal defenses (Level 3): This level includes mechanisms such as denial and projection, where individuals refuse to accept reality or attribute their own unacceptable thoughts to others. Function protects against unbearable emotions but often leads to dismissing perceptions of self and others. Prevalence: Common in individuals which avoid reality in severe personality disorders frequently co-occurring with EDs, when they deny reality of body image: *Denial, rationalization, primitive non-delusional projection, autistic fantasy.*

Major image-distorting (Borderline) defenses (Level 2): These involve significant distortions in self or others' perception, such as splitting, leading to unstable relationships and self-image. Function: Protect against unbearable emotions but often lead to distorted perceptions of self and others. Prevalence: Common in individuals with borderline personality organization, frequently co-occurring with EDs, especially in those who suffer from BN: *Splitting of self/Splitting of object representations, projective identification.*

Action defenses(Level 1): The most primitive level where internal conflicts are expressed through actions rather than mental processes. Function: To expel from the psychic apparatus thoughts or feelings to the external world or to their own body. Prevalence: High in borderline personality organizations and EDs specifically BN: *Acting out, passive aggression, hypochondriasis.*

Psychotic defenses (Level 0): Function: Severely distort reality to defend against psychic fragmentation. Prevalence: Rare but may appear transiently under extreme stress in patients with severe EDs: *Rejection of reality, delusional projection, distortion, withdrawal.*

Joaquín Gratch (2016) developed his master's thesis in psychoanalysis under the direction of Humberto Persano, focusing on the role of defensive mechanisms in EDs. His research highlights the complex and heterogeneous nature of defensive styles in this population. Despite this variability, most studies, including Gratch's work, indicate a predominant reliance on immature defensive styles. These include maladaptive defenses (Style 1) and/or image-distorting defenses (Style 2), as classified by Michael Bond through the "Defensive Style Questionnaire (DSQ)" (Bond, 1995).

Among the defensive mechanisms frequently identified, splitting emerges as the most prominent. Additionally, mechanisms such as denial, dissociation, projection, projective identification, idealization, and devaluation are remarkably prevalent, underscoring the psychological complexity inherent in EDs. Gratch's research contributes to a deeper understanding of these patterns, offering valuable insights into the psychoanalytic interpretation of defensive processes in individuals with eating disorders.

Primitive defense mechanisms in EDs: Their role and manifestations

Splitting:

- *Definition*: Dividing experiences, relationships, and self-perceptions into "all good" or "all bad."
- *Manifestation in EDs*:

- Patients may idealize certain behaviors (e.g., restriction) while devaluing others (e.g., emotional expression or relational closeness).
- Relationships with therapists or caregivers may oscillate between admiration and hostility, complicating treatment.

- *Therapeutic implication*:

  - Highlighting and integrating these polarized perceptions is essential for fostering a more cohesive sense of self and relational stability.

Idealization and devaluation:

- *Definition*:

  - *Idealization*: Overvaluing certain aspects of self, others, or behaviors.
  - *Devaluation*: Viewing oneself or others as entirely flawed or worthless.

- *Manifestation in EDs*:

  - Patients may idealize thinness or control over food while devaluing perceived vulnerability or dependence.
  - Therapists may be alternately idealized as saviors or devalued as failures when progress stalls.

- *Therapeutic implication*:

  - Gently confronting these extremes helps patients recognize their defensive function and build more nuanced views of self and others.

Omnipotence and denial:

- *Definition*:

  - *Omnipotence:* Believing one has absolute control or immunity from consequences.
  - *Denial*: Refusing to acknowledge reality.

- *Manifestation in EDs*:

  - Patients with AN may believe they can control their bodies indefinitely without harm.
  - Patients with BN may deny the severity of physical or emotional consequences associated with purging.

- *Therapeutic implication*:
    - Linking these defenses to underlying fears (e.g., vulnerability, loss of control) allows the patient to begin confronting reality.

Acting out:

- *Definition*: Expressing unresolved conflicts through impulsive actions rather than reflective thought.
- *Manifestation in EDs*:
    - Self-harm, binging, purging, or substance misuse often serve as outlets for unarticulated emotional pain.

- *Therapeutic implication*:
    - Addressing acting-out behaviors through clear boundaries (e.g., therapeutic contracts) and providing alternative coping strategies (e.g., relational support) fosters reflective engagement.

Withdrawal and autistic fantasy:

- *Definition*:
    - *Withdrawal*: Retreating from reality as a protective measure.
    - *Autistic Fantasy*: Escaping into a self-created, idealized mental world.

- *Manifestation in EDs*:
    - Patients with AN may withdraw physically and emotionally, retreating into rigid self-control.
    - Both withdrawal and fantasy may reinforce isolation and the avoidance of relational or emotional engagement.

- *Therapeutic implication*:
    - Encouraging small, manageable steps toward relational connection helps break the cycle of isolation and avoidance.

Acting out in EDs: A reflection of underlying conflicts

During early phases of treatment and during regression during therapeutic process acting out is used as a pattern from coping in an archaic way with painful situations (Persano, 2022) and it is used for several unconscious functions:

- Relieving internal tension.
- Regulating overwhelming emotions.
- Seeking masochistic gratification.
- Establishing connections, particularly in social contexts (e.g., online groups that normalize disordered behaviors).

Self-harm as a primitive acting-out defense

Self-harm represents another acting-out behavior rooted in primitive defense mechanisms and is particularly prevalent in individuals with low representational capacity. As Persano (2022) emphasizes, self-harm often replaces the verbal articulation of psychological pain, serving as a non-verbal means to communicate distress. In these patients, the capacity to process and express emotions symbolically is underdeveloped, leading to behaviors that externalize internal conflicts.

This defense mechanism offers a temporary sense of control or relief, allowing patients to momentarily regulate overwhelming emotional states or escape feelings of inner chaos. However, while it may provide immediate gratification or a reprieve from psychic pain, self-harm perpetuates the cycle of emotional dysregulation and avoidance. Rather than addressing the root causes of their distress, patients become entrenched in maladaptive behaviors that reinforce their reliance on acting out.

Unconscious functions of self-harm

Self-harm serves multiple unconscious functions that sustain its use as a defense mechanism:

- *Relief from internal tension*: The physical act of self-harm diverts attention from unbearable psychological pain.
- *Masochistic gratification*: It may unconsciously fulfill a need for punishment or serve as a substitute for libidinal expression.
- *Regulation of emotional states*: By externalizing pain, patients achieve a sense of control over unmanageable emotions.
- *Connection and identity formation*:Particularly in social contexts, such as online communities, self-harm can create a shared identity or offer validation through others who engage in similar behaviors (Persano, 2022).

Implications for treatment

Self-harm, as a primitive defense mechanism, reflects the patient's inability to mentalize or symbolically process their experiences. Effective psychotherapeutic interventions must address this deficit by fostering the patient's capacity for symbolic thought and reflective functioning. This involves:

- *Naming and validating emotional states*: Helping patients articulate and label their feelings reduces their reliance on self-harm as a means of communication.
- *Exploring underlying conflicts*: Therapists must gently guide patients toward understanding the unconscious motivations and relational dynamics underpinning their self-harming behavior.
- *Establishing alternative coping strategies*: Collaboratively identifying healthier ways to regulate emotions, such as reaching out to trusted individuals or engaging in grounding techniques, provides patients with tools to replace self-harm.

Transitioning from action to reflection

Self-harm exemplifies the broader challenge in treating individuals with EDs, where action replaces reflection. The therapeutic process aims to transform these behaviors into opportunities for insight, enabling patients to:

- Transition from acting out to verbalizing emotions.
- Develop a capacity for mentalization and reflective engagement.
- Achieve greater emotional regulation and relational stability.

By addressing self-harm within the context of primitive defense mechanisms, therapists can help patients move beyond destructive behaviors, fostering the growth of a more cohesive and adaptive psychic structure. As Persano (2022) observes, the gradual shift from action to reflection is central to the therapeutic journey, allowing patients to move from avoidance to meaningful engagement with their inner world.

Substance Misuse could be also a primitive acting out defense

- Alcohol, cocaine and marijuana, often used by ED patients, reflect avoidant defenses, bypassing psychological pain with external solutions.
- Substance misuse disrupts reflective functioning, underscoring the need for therapeutic contracts prohibiting substance use before sessions.

Overall therapeutic strategies: Moving from action to reflection

Therapeutic contract is the initial intervention for blocking acting out behaviors and to invite a focus in introspections. It functions in creating clear boundaries around behaviors like weight thresholds, purging, and self-harm to create a framework for managing acting-out behaviors. As well it makes a collaboration in setting these rules fosters patient accountability and reduces resistance.

During the therapeutical process the interpretation of acting out breaches of the therapeutic contract provide opportunities for exploring unconscious conflicts. For example:

- A missed session might reflect fear of intimacy or failure.
- Self-harm after a difficult session may indicate unprocessed anger or despair.

The therapeutic process gradually helps patients move from primitive defenses toward more adaptive mechanisms, by integration of self and object representation while reconciling fragmented aspects of identity and relationships, as well, as through mentalization process the patients can develop the capacity to reflect on emotional states rather than acting them out. If sublimation high level defense mechanism arises, the individual suffering from EDs can redirect destructive impulses into creative or productive outlets.

Conclusion: Toward reflective engagement

The persistent use of primitive defense mechanisms—splitting, acting out, idealization, omnipotence, and withdrawal—maintains the maladaptive patterns central to EDs. By addressing these defenses through a structured therapeutic approach, therapists can help patients transition from action to reflection. This shift not only fosters emotional regulation and relational stability but also promotes the development of a cohesive and integrated sense of self. Through consistent interpretation and containment, the therapeutic process lays the foundation for meaningful psychic and emotional transformation.

Incorporating Transference-Focused Psychotherapy (TFP) and mentalization techniques for eating disorders: Transference-Focused Psychotherapy in EDs

Transference-Focused Psychotherapy (TFP) provides a structured and psychoanalytic framework particularly suited to treating individuals with EDs, where intense relational dynamics and primitive defense mechanisms dominate the therapeutic process. TFP, grounded in the object relations model, addresses the split representations of self and others while fostering identity integration (Kernberg et al., 1989; Clarkin, Yeomans, and Kernberg, 1999, 2006). This approach integrates well with mentalization techniques to strengthen reflective functioning, an area often underdeveloped in ED patients.

Phases of TFP treatment for eating disorders

Transference-Focused Psychotherapy (TFP) for EDs provides a structured, phased approach to address the complex interplay of primitive defenses, relational dynamics, and identity disturbances typical of ED patients.

The three distinct phases—Initial, Middle, and Final—guide the therapeutic process toward integration and emotional growth.

1. Initial phase: Confronting resistance and stabilizing the therapeutic alliance

The initial phase focuses on managing intense resistance, often expressed through primitive defense mechanisms like splitting, denial, and acting out. These behaviors reflect the patient's attempt to maintain psychic equilibrium amidst overwhelming emotional states.

Common manifestations of resistance include:

- Suicidal ideation or threats.
- Self-harm behaviors.
- Significant weight loss in anorexia nervosa (AN).
- Frequent purging in bulimia nervosa (BN).
- Absences from therapy sessions.
- Concealment or distortion of information.
- Acting out within and outside the therapeutic relationship.

Prioritizing intervention

Managing behaviors that pose immediate risks to safety, or the therapeutic process is the primary focus in this phase. Suicidal ideation, self-harm, and severe weight loss take precedence, requiring reality-based interventions that address immediate risks while preserving the therapeutic frame.

Building the therapeutic alliance

The therapist works to establish a stable and secure therapeutic relationship, despite the intensity of resistance. This involves validating the patient's feelings, addressing destructive behaviors, and maintaining consistent boundaries. As Kernberg et al. (1989) emphasize, the therapist must adopt a neutral yet active stance, avoiding collusion with maladaptive patterns while fostering trust.

Key techniques:

- *Clarification*: Exploring ambiguities in the patient's speech or actions. Examples:

- "You mentioned skipping meals and feeling fine; could you explain more about that feeling?"
- "You just told me that every time you argue with your mother you eat and vomit. Could you explain to me what feelings you experience at those times and why they are transferred to food?"

Another important point is that we must work from a shared reality. We must interpret any distortion or deviation from reality until we come to an agreement. Example:

- You were telling me that you are fat, but we also agreed that you are still wearing the same small sizes as when you started treatment. So, we agreed that you see yourself in a way that is not real, that, although you see yourself as fat and I accept that is your perception, this perception is wrong?

Confrontation: Highlighting contradictions in the patient's behavior or thought processes. Examples:

- "You said therapy is important to you, yet you've missed two sessions. How do you make sense of this?"
- When the session started you were very angry with me and told me that coming to treatment was a waste of time, that nothing was going to change and now ten minutes later you tell me that one of the most important things that is happening to you is the bond with me. Could you explain that to me?
- A few minutes ago, we were talking about your desire to die and yet I notice that every time you tell me that you think about killing yourself, I see that you smile. Could you explain to me how, when faced with something as painful as the possibility of killing yourself, you sketch a smile?
- There is something I don't understand. You keep saying how important the treatment is for you, but nevertheless, you have been absent for two of the last five sessions and you arrived ten minutes late today. How do you explain this?

Containment: Establishing a predictable therapeutic structure to help the patient regulate their emotions.

The therapist's role

The therapist must tolerate frustration, accept ambiguity, and understand the patient's projections as opportunities to uncover relational patterns.

Resistance is viewed not as a barrier but as a starting point for exploration and understanding.

2. Middle phase: Addressing split representations and facilitating reflection

Once resistance diminishes and the therapeutic alliance stabilizes, the middle phase focuses on addressing split representations, exploring body image distortions, and fostering reflective functioning.

Core objectives:

- *Integration of split internalized representations*: Helping the patient move from polarized perceptions of self and others to a more integrated understanding.
- *Exploration of body image distortions*: Addressing how fragmented identity and relational dynamics contribute to distorted body perceptions.
- *Fostering reflective functioning*: Encouraging the patient's ability to reflect on their emotional experiences and relational interactions.

Techniques for integration:

- *Interpretation in the here and now*: Linking relational dynamics and emotional states to the therapeutic context.
  - Example: "You're angry with me for discussing your purging behaviors, yet you've also said you want to stop. Could we explore this contradiction together?"
- *Connecting actions to feelings*: Identifying the emotional triggers behind ED behaviors like bingeing or restricting.
  - Example: "When you described feeling abandoned after your argument with your friend, you mentioned skipping meals. Could these be connected?"

Managing body image distortion

As the patient becomes more receptive to interpretations, the therapist can address distorted self-perceptions with greater precision. This work helps patients challenge rigid body image beliefs, laying the groundwork for identity integration.

As Izydorczyk (2022) highlights, this phase is pivotal for addressing the relational and emotional underpinnings of body image disturbances.

3. Final phase: Identity integration and emotional growth

In the final phase, patients exhibit increased mentalization, identity cohesion, and relational stability, marking a shift from reliance on primitive defenses to adaptive emotional processing.

Core objectives:

- *Mentalization*: Enhancing the patient's capacity to understand their own and others' mental states.
- *Cohesion of identity*: Reconciling fragmented aspects of self into a more stable and integrated identity.
- *Relational stability*: Developing healthier, more reciprocal relationships.

Addressing dependency and separation-individuation

Themes of dependency and autonomy become central as the patient explores their relationship with their ED identity and moves toward a more authentic sense of self.

Example of interpretation in this issue:

- "It seems like letting go of your eating disorder feels like losing a part of yourself. Could we explore what that part represents for you?"

Separation-individuation and the false self

The therapist helps patients navigate the relinquishment of the anorexic or bulimic identity, which has functioned as a defensive substitute for an integrated and true self (Farrell, 2000; Mahler, 1968; Mahler, Pine, and Bergman, 1975).

- Example Interpretation: "It sounds like letting go of your eating disorder feels like losing a familiar part of yourself. What might it mean to imagine yourself without it?"

Dealing with depressive symptoms

As defenses are relinquished, underlying depressive symptoms may surface, including feelings of guilt, mourning, and loss. These emotions are processed through a supportive and interpretative approach, helping the patient navigate the complexities of their emotional experiences (Blatt, 1974).

In the final phase, patients often experience depressive symptoms, reflecting the loss of the "false self" associated with their ED. These symptoms, characterized by anaclitic depression and feelings of guilt and mourning, are addressed through supportive and interpretative work (Blatt, 1974).

Processing guilt and mourning

Patients often feel guilt or shame for the impact of their illness on others or mourn the loss of the protective role their symptoms played. This work is critical for resolving depressive states and fostering emotional growth.

- Example: "You've mentioned feeling guilty about how your parents have worried about you. Could we explore what that guilt means to you and how it affects your feelings about recovery?"

Dealing with trauma in the final phase of TFP for ED patients

Addressing traumatic experiences in ED patients is a pivotal component of the final phase of TFP. Many patients reveal histories of childhood sexual abuse, physical abuse, or neglect, but these deeply painful issues should only be explored after a strong therapeutic alliance has been established. A secure, predictable framework is essential to support the patient through the challenging process of revisiting and processing these traumas.

Timing and approach to trauma work

In-depth trauma work must occur after the patient has achieved emotional stability and developed trust in the therapist. Koenisberg et al., (2000) emphasize that the therapist should anticipate powerful transference dynamics, including:

- *Alternating roles in transference*: The therapist may be perceived as a perpetrator, victim, or seducer, reflecting the patient's internalized relational conflicts.
- *Unconscious guilt and shame*: Feelings of guilt over perceived complicity or moments of enjoyment during abuse often complicate the patient's emotional processing, manifesting themselves as shame or self-punishment.

For example, one patient alternated between viewing her therapist as a sadistic authority figure and a supportive ally, highlighting her struggle to reconcile her experiences of both love and hatred toward her abusive father. These transference paradigms required careful exploration to facilitate emotional integration.

Trauma and behavioral manifestations

Traumatic experiences frequently resurface in ED patients through behaviors like binging, purging, or avoidance of intimacy. Clinical case example demonstrates how trauma can shape behaviors:

- *Case example*: A patient who had been raped multiple times during adolescence, experienced binging and vomiting episodes triggered by the presence of her abuser. Initially, she could not connect these behaviors to her trauma. Through transference work, she processed her anger toward her mother's lack of protection and her guilt over feelings of desire and fear. This enabled her to break free from patterns of avoidance and form healthier relationships.

Goals of trauma work

- *Processing guilt and anger*: Patients explore and resolve feelings of betrayal, anger, and guilt toward perpetrators and enablers.
- *Reclaiming agency*: Trauma work empowers patients to redefine their narrative, moving from victimization to autonomy.
- *Relational healing*: Patients address how trauma has impacted their ability to form stable, reciprocal relationships.

Therapeutic techniques in EDs patient's trauma

- *Analytical neutrality*: Maintaining neutrality allows the therapist to help patients explore their conflicting feelings without judgment or reinforcement of maladaptive defenses.
- *Gradual confrontation of transference*: Through interpretations, the therapist helps the patient recognize and integrate fragmented aspects of their experiences.
- *Supportive framework*: Agreeing on the patient's readiness and willingness to address trauma ensures a collaborative approach and minimizes reexperiencing traumatization.

Outcomes of trauma work

As patients process trauma in the final phase of TFP, they often experience:

- *Improved mentalization*: Enhanced capacity to reflect on their internal states and relational dynamics.
- *Resolution of splitting*: Ability to reconcile good and bad aspects of self and others, reducing reliance on primitive defenses.
- *Greater relational stability*: Improved relationships, characterized by mutuality and emotional reciprocity.

Conclusion on dealing with trauma through TFP in EDs patients

Trauma work in TFP offers ED patients a profound opportunity for healing and integration. By addressing the lasting impact of trauma within a safe and structured therapeutic framework, patients can reconcile their past experiences, achieve a cohesive sense of self, and build healthier relationships. As Yeomans and Diamond (2010) highlight, this transformative process fosters reflection, emotional growth, and the modulation of affect, marking a pivotal step toward recovery.

Another important aspect of TFP in EDs patients

Maintaining analytical neutrality and abstinence

The therapist's stance is crucial in the final phase, balancing neutrality with active engagement:

- *Analytical Neutrality*: The therapist refrains from taking sides or imposing judgments, allowing the patient to explore their conflicts freely.
- *Rule of Abstinence*: The therapist avoids providing gratification beyond what the therapeutic process itself offers, ensuring that the work remains focused on internal growth rather than external validation.

Navigating breaks in neutrality

Occasional breaks in neutrality may occur, particularly when safety or immediate needs are at stake. These moments are later analyzed to understand the dynamics that led to such actions and their implications for the therapeutic process (Yeomans, Clarkin, and Kernberg, 2002, 2015).

- Example: "Two weeks ago, I spoke with your parents about your concerns. Now that the situation has passed, let's explore why you felt unable to address them yourself and what it means for our work together."

Addressing transference and relational patterns

The final phase provides an opportunity to resolve transference dynamics, both positive and negative. Patients may revisit themes of dependency, anger, and abandonment, which are explored and reworked within the therapeutic relationship.

- Example: "You've mentioned feeling abandoned when I challenged your troubles with eating behaviors. Could we explore how this mirrors other relationships in your life?"

As transference evolves, patients develop a more cohesive sense of self and greater relational stability, marking the culmination of the therapeutic journey.

The interpretative process in the final phase of treatment for eating disorders

The interpretative process in psychodynamic therapy for eating disorders (EDs) represents a gradual unfolding, moving from addressing surface defenses to exploring deeper unconscious conflicts. By the final phase of treatment, the interpretative work achieves greater depth, focusing on integration, identity, and emotional growth. This phase marks a critical period of reflection and transformation, where the therapist helps the patient navigate unresolved intrapsychic conflicts while maintaining a stable therapeutic frame.

Interpretation: From surface to depth

Interpretation involves making unconscious material conscious, helping the patient recognize the underlying dynamics of their behaviors and emotions. In ED treatment, this process follows a structured path:

- *Early Phases*: Interpretations focus on defenses and immediate behaviors. For example, addressing behaviors like acting out, purging, or self-harm as defenses against overwhelming emotions or relational fears.
- *Final Phase*: The focus shifts to interpreting deeper drives and conflicts, including issues of identity, dependency, and separation-individuation.

As Persano (1999) observes, the immediacy of patients' internal worlds during earlier phases often makes it challenging to historicize interpersonal relationships. However, by the final phase, with actions stabilized and transference patterns clarified, patients are better equipped to engage in reflective work.

Key features of interpretation in the final phase

1 *Here and now focus*: Interpretations continue to prioritize the immediate therapeutic relationship. This allows patients to explore how their relational patterns and defenses manifest in real-time within the therapy setting.

    - Example: "You mentioned feeling criticized when I asked about your purging behaviors. Could we explore how this reaction might relate to experiences outside therapy?"

2 *Integration of split representations:*As Kernberg et al., (1989) highlight, a key goal is integrating polarized perceptions of self and others, moving beyond "all-good" and "all-bad" representations.

    - Example: "You describe your mother as both overly critical and deeply caring. How do these aspects coexist in your experience of her?"

3 *Body image distortion*: By this stage, patients are more capable of addressing distorted body perceptions. This work is critical for resolving the fragmented identity often reflected in their body image struggles (Izydorczyk, 2022).

- Example: "You've said you see yourself as 'fat', yet you recognize that your clothes still fit the same. Could we explore why this perception feels so persistent?"

4 *Addressing secondary gains*: Secondary benefits from illness, such as parental attention or avoiding responsibilities, are explored and dismantled to prevent perpetuation of symptoms.

- Example: "It seems like your troubles with eating disorder have sometimes brought you closer to your parents' concern. Could we think about other ways to maintain that connection?"

Integration and transformation

The interpretative process in the final phase of ED treatment represents the pinnacle of therapeutic work, addressing the deepest layers of identity, relational patterns, and emotional conflicts. By guiding patients through the integration of fragmented representations, the relinquishment of defensive identities, and the resolution of depressive symptoms, the therapist facilitates profound psychic transformation. The final phase not only resolves symptoms but also fosters a sense of wholeness and authenticity, empowering patients to move beyond their eating disorder into a fuller, more integrated life.

Progressing toward psychic integration and emotional growth

Each phase of TFP builds progressively, guiding patients from states of resistance and fragmentation toward integration and emotional growth. By targeting primitive defense mechanisms such as splitting, denial, and acting out, TFP offers a structured framework for transforming destructive patterns into opportunities for self-awareness and relational healing. This phased approach not only addresses immediate risks but also establishes a foundation for long-term recovery and identity cohesion. Furthermore, as Kernberg (2018) highlights, this process facilitates the resolution of aggression and the re-emergence of healthy eroticism, integral to achieving psychological balance.

To summarize, the basic concepts of TFP treatment include:

- Stability of the therapeutic setting and treatment limits.
- Active attitude of the therapist (especially predominance of verbal interventions, not necessarily interpretive).

- Tolerance of the patient's hostility without engaging in retaliatory behavior or emotional withdrawal (since anger is the most characteristic and predominant affect, its presence is a diagnostic indicator and, at the same time, the greatest difficulty for treatment).
- Treating self-harming behaviors from becoming unsatisfactory for the patient (ego-dystonia).
- Promote the ability to anticipate the real consequences of one's own actions.
- Focus on the connection between actions and feelings.
- Promote the ability to recognize one's own internal world, as well as differentiate the therapist's emotional internal world.
- Imposing limits by blocking acting-out behaviors, behaviors that threaten the safety of the patient, the therapist, or the psychotherapy itself.
- Focus interventions on clarifications and interpretations in the here and now.
- Monitoring countertransference feelings.

Mentalization-based treatment for eating behavior disorders: A coherent approach

Mentalization-Based Therapy (MBT) presents an innovative and effective approach to addressing the complex challenges of treating EDs. These disorders are often characterized by deficits in mental representation, reflective functioning, and emotional regulation. Originally developed for borderline personality disorder (BPD), MBT focuses on improving the capacity for mentalization—the ability to understand and interpret one's own mental states and those of others. For ED patients, who frequently struggle with self-awareness and relational dynamics, enhancing mentalization is a crucial therapeutic goal.

MBT has been specifically adapted to address eating behavior disorders, integrating individual therapy with group psychotherapy—an aspect explored in depth in chapter 11. Individual sessions, conducted weekly, aim to enhance mentalization, which is often impaired or underdeveloped in these patients. This approach also focuses on improving emotional recognition and expression, fostering better emotional regulation, and repairing fragmented and deteriorated object relations (Robinson and Skårderud, 2019; Skårderud and Fonagy, 2012).

The therapist's role

A critical element of MBT is the careful selection of the therapist, whose mentalization skills are essential. The therapist's capacity to mentalize is often tested during the therapeutic process, necessitating resilience and adaptability. The therapist must adopt a stance characterized by curiosity and a "not-knowing" attitude, free from preconceived notions. This openness allows the therapist to explore the patient's inner world with a sense of discovery, uncovering hidden motives and fostering deeper understanding. Warmth and active engagement are also key, as many patients with EDs have felt unaccepted or misunderstood in prior treatments. Moreover, families often struggle to understand the patient's condition, and their well-meaning but misguided attempts to help can inadvertently lead to further isolation or conflict, exacerbating the patient's difficulties (Robinson, Skårderud, and Sommerfeldt, 2019).

Core therapeutic processes

Encouraging patients to articulate their mental experiences is central to MBT. This involves collaboratively exploring their mental states and examining the interpersonal processes that connect their internal world to their mental representations. Before treatment begins, the therapist gathers comprehensive information to construct an understanding of the patient's issues. This includes evaluating the role of mentalization deficits, current and past attachment patterns, and relational vulnerabilities (Robinson and Skårderud, 2019).

Therapists employ standard MBT techniques, emphasizing supportive and empathetic attitudes. Praising patients when they successfully apply mentalization to achieve positive outcomes fosters change and strengthens their reflective capacity.

Clarification in mentalization-based treatment (MBT)

Clarification is a cornerstone technique in MBT, designed to help patients with EDs develop a deeper understanding of their emotions, behaviors, and interpersonal patterns. For patients who struggle with symbolic thought and emotional regulation, clarification facilitates the development of reflective capacity, allowing them to make sense of their internal experiences and their connections to external behaviors.

Key features of clarification in MBT

- *Elucidating behavior-emotion links*: Patients with EDs often struggle to recognize how their actions are connected to underlying emotions or mental states. Clarification involves exploring these links to make unconscious or ambiguous processes more explicit. For instance, a patient might binge eat when feeling overwhelmed but not realize that the behavior is an attempt to soothe emotional distress. Clarification helps them articulate this link.
- *Highlighting behavioral sequences*: Therapists work with patients to break down events into a sequence of thoughts, feelings, and actions. This step-by-step analysis allows patients to see how their mental

states evolve and lead to specific behaviors. For example, understanding how feelings of rejection might lead to restrictive eating behaviors can provide insight into their patterns.

- *Exploring misinterpretations and biases*: Patients with EDs often misinterpret interpersonal cues or internalize distorted beliefs about themselves and others. Clarification helps identify these cognitive distortions, such as the belief that others' criticisms reflect their intrinsic inadequacy and encourages patients to evaluate their accuracy.
- *Encouraging narrative coherence*: By clarifying the connections between past experiences and current behaviors, therapists help patients construct a more coherent narrative of their life experiences. This promotes a better understanding of how early attachment patterns or relational dynamics influence present-day challenges.
- *Facilitating emotional awareness*: Patients with EDs often have difficulty identifying or naming emotions, a phenomenon known as alexithymia. Clarification helps expand their emotional vocabulary and awareness, enabling them to identify, label, and express feelings more effectively.
- *Addressing avoidance and defensiveness*: Eating disorder symptoms often serve as defenses against painful emotions. Clarification gently explores the functions of these defenses, encouraging patients to reflect on what they might be avoiding and why. This helps reduce reliance on maladaptive coping mechanisms, such as restricting or binging.

Therapeutic application of clarification

- *Collaboration and curiosity*: The therapist adopts a collaborative stance, working with the patient as a partner in discovery. Rather than imposing interpretations, the therapist uses open-ended questions to guide the patient toward their own insights, fostering a sense of agency.
- *Empathy and validation*: Clarification is conducted with empathy, ensuring the patient feels understood and supported. Validating the patient's experiences while gently probing deeper promotes trust and openness.
- *Here-and-now focus*: Clarification often draws on current interactions and events within the therapeutic relationship. Exploring misunderstandings or emotional reactions during sessions provides a concrete and immediate context for mentalization.
- *Iterative process*: Clarification is not a one-time intervention but an ongoing process. It involves revisiting and refining insights as the patient's mentalization skills improve and new patterns emerge.

Benefits of clarification in MBT for eating disorders

- *Increased reflective functioning*: Patients develop the capacity to think about their own and others' mental states, leading to improved emotional regulation and relational functioning.

- *Reduction of symptomatology*: By addressing the emotional underpinnings of eating disorder behaviors, clarification helps diminish their frequency and intensity over time.
- *Enhanced interpersonal relationships*: As patients gain a clearer understanding of their emotional and relational patterns, they are better equipped to navigate relationships and reduce conflict.

In summary, clarification in MBT plays a pivotal role in bridging the gap between a patient's internal experiences and external behaviors. By fostering self-awareness and reflective thinking, it empowers patients with eating disorders to make meaningful changes in their emotional and relational lives.

The therapeutic relationship

Close attention to the dynamics of the therapeutic relationship, particularly transference and countertransference, is essential in MBT. The here-and-now interactions between patient and therapist provide a valuable space for identifying mentalization failures and exploring their consequences. These relational dynamics serve as a microcosm of the patient's broader relational patterns, offering insights that can be used to strengthen their ability to mentalize.

In general, MBT may enhance treatment strategies by adapting interventions to the mental capacities of a patient with an ED, help to maintain a secure and trusting therapeutic relationship and reduce relapse rates through reducing psychological difficulties that maintain the disorder (improve affect regulation and a sense of self, reduce interpersonal difficulties). Furthermore, MBT might help therapists to keep a focus on their own capacity to mentalize, which in the treatment of patients with an ED is repeatedly endangered by intense affects and dysfunctional interpersonal reactions (Skårderud and Fonagy, 2012; Zeeck et al., 2021)

As Robinson, Skårderud, and Sommerfeldt (2019) emphasize, a therapist's initial stance should be one of curiosity and openness: "An attitude of curiosity, a certain ignorance, and a desire to understand the patient's experience" creates a foundation of trust and engagement. This is particularly important for ED patients, as their struggles with introspection and emotional articulation often necessitate a therapeutic approach that prioritizes simplicity and clarity. Izydorczyk (2022) and Petrucelli (2015) further recommend using straightforward language and avoiding metaphors, which may confuse patients with limited representational capacities.

Representation deficits and their impact on ED patients

Deficits in mental representation are a hallmark of ED pathology. These deficits impede introspection, symbolic thinking, and verbal expression of emotions, often leaving patients reliant on action-based defenses such as restrictive eating, binging, purging, or self-harm. These behaviors serve as maladaptive mechanisms to regulate overwhelming emotional states.

Bateman and Fonagy (2004) link these deficits to early developmental disruptions in attachment and emotional attunement. They highlight the importance of caregivers naming and validating a child's emotional states, a process critical for fostering mentalization. When this early relational function is inconsistent or absent, the child may struggle to differentiate between internal and external experiences, leaving them vulnerable to emotional dysregulation and primitive defenses.

Common manifestations in ED patients

- *Alexithymia*: The inability to identify and articulate emotions (Meneguzzo et al., 2021).
- *Symbolization deficits*: A tendency to rely on concrete actions rather than symbolic or verbal expression to manage distress.
- *Discrepancies in communication channels*: As noted by Clarkin, Fonagy, and Gabbard (2010), ED patients often display misalignment between verbal statements, non-verbal behaviors, and countertransference reactions, reflecting their fragmented internal experience.

Structuring the therapeutic approach in MBT

MBT emphasizes the importance of creating a structured and predictable therapeutic environment, particularly for patients who struggle with representational deficits. Early in therapy, the clinician should clearly outline the goals, methods, and expectations of treatment. This approach:

- *Reduces anxiety*: By demystifying the therapeutic process, patients experience less fear of the unknown.
- *Enhances engagement*: Transparent communication fosters collaboration and agency.
- *Bridges representation gaps*: Structured explanations compensate for patients' difficulties in conceptualizing abstract processes.

Robinson, Skårderud, and Sommerfeldt (2019) highlight the need for simplicity and curiosity in interactions with ED patients. For example:

- *Speak in straight forward terms*: Avoid abstract language or metaphors that may confuse patients (Izydorczyk, 2022).
- *Show genuine curiosity*: Demonstrate an interest in understanding the patient's unique emotional experience.

Connecting actions to affects: A core principle of MBT

MBT seeks to help patients connect their behaviors to underlying emotional states, facilitating a shift from action-based defenses to reflective engagement. This focus on linking actions to affects is essential for helping patients mentalize their emotional triggers and relational patterns.

MBT emphasizes the development of reflective capacity and mentalization, making it particularly effective for ED patients with deficits in symbolic thought and emotional regulation. Key principles include:

- *Clarification*: Is a fundamental technique in MBT, aimed at helping patients with EDs gain deeper insight into the connections between their emotions, behaviors, and interpersonal dynamics.
- *Focus on affects*: Helping patients name and process their emotions within the therapeutic relationship.
- *Affect naming*: This intervention assists patients in identifying and labeling their emotions, which is crucial for emotional regulation. A therapist might observe, "It sounds like you might be feeling overwhelmed. Could that be part of what's going on?"
- *Bridging actions and affects*: Exploring the emotional triggers of ED behaviors, such as binging or restricting.
- *Non-regressive approach*: Avoiding interpretations that encourage regression, instead fostering growth in reflective functioning.

Affects, attachment, and food: Relational dynamics in EDs

Philippe Jeammet (1994) insightfully observed that ED patients relate to others as they relate to food. This dynamic is shaped by early attachment experiences:

- *Anorexia nervosa*: These patients often present themselves as emotionally impenetrable, mirroring their restrictive approach to food and relationships. They may isolate themselves to maintain control and avoid perceived intrusions.
- *Bulimia nervosa*: These patients often display relational voracity, paralleling their compulsive need to consume and expel. This binge-purge cycle reflects an unmet craving for emotional connection.

Gianna Williams (1997) described these dynamics as:

- No-entry defenses in AN: Patients construct impermeable emotional barriers.
- Porous membranes in BN: Temporary incorporation is followed by rapid expulsion, mirroring relational and emotional instability.

Therapeutic focus on affect

Focusing on affect is central to MBT's approach for ED patients. This includes:

- *Identifying predominant affects*: Recognizing which emotions dominate the patient's relational and behavioral patterns.
- *Tracing emotional triggers*: Linking specific emotions to ED-related behaviors (e.g., restrictive eating or binging).
- *Promoting mentalization*: Supporting the patient's ability to reflect on emotional experiences rather than reacting impulsively.

Petrucelli (2015) emphasizes the importance of understanding how affective triggers influence behaviors, such as the role of shame or anger in episodes of binging or purging.

Balancing challenge and support

Therapists in MBT must balance challenging maladaptive patterns with providing a safe, empathetic environment:

- *Challenge*: Confronting discrepancies in behavior or relational dynamics helps patients gain insight into their defenses.
- *Support*: Maintaining a consistent and empathetic presence ensures that patients feel secure enough to explore their vulnerabilities.

This balance enables patients to transition from action-based defenses to reflective functioning, marking a critical step toward emotional and relational growth.

Conclusion

Mentalization-Based Therapy (MBT) provides a structured and compassionate framework for addressing the representational deficits and emotional dysregulation prevalent in ED patients. By fostering connections between actions and affects, emphasizing curiosity, and creating a predictable therapeutic environment, MBT helps patients develop the reflective capacity needed for meaningful self-awareness and relational stability. This transformation not only enhances mentalization but also lays the foundation for enduring emotional and psychological growth.

Bibliography

Bateman, A. and Fonagy, P. (2004). *Psychotherapy for Personality Disorder: Mentalization-based Treatment*. New York: Oxford University Press.

Bateman, A. and Fonagy, P. (2019). *Handbook of Mentalizing in Mental Health Practice*. Washington DC: American Psychiatric Association Publishing.

Blatt, S. (1974). Levels of object representation in anaclitic and introjective depresion. *Psychoanalytic Study of the Child*, 29(1): 107–157.

Bond, M. P. (1995). The development and properties of the Defense Style Questionnaire. In H. R. Conte and R. Plutchik (eds.) *Ego Defenses: Theory and Measurement*. New Jersey: John Wiley & Sons, 202–220.

Bruch, H. (1978). *The Golden Cage: The Enigma of Anorexia Nervosa*. Cambridge, MA: Harvard University Press.

Clarkin, J., Yeomans, F., and Kernberg, O. F. (1999). *Psychotherapy for Borderline Personality*. New Jersey: John Wiley & Sons.

Clarkin, J. F., Yeomans, F., and Kernberg, O. F. (2006). *Psychotherapy for Borderline Personality: Focusing on Object Relations*. Washington DC: American Psychiatric Publishing.

Clarkin, J., Fonagy, P., and Gabbard, G. (2010). *Psychodynamic Psychotherapy for Personality Disorders: A Clinical Handbook*. Washington DC: American Psychiatric Publishing.

Corcos, M., and Jeammet, P. (2001). Eating disorders: Psychodynamic approach and practice. *Biomedicine and Pharmacotherapy*, 55(8): 479–488.

Farrel, E. (2000). *Lost for Words: The Psychoanalisis of Anorexia and Bulimia*. New York: Other Press.

Frosch, J. (1983). *The Psychotic Process*. New York: International Universitities Press.

Gratch, J. (2016). *El Estilo Defensivo en Pacientes con Trastornos de la Conducta Alimentaria: Una Revisión Bibliográfica*. Magister thesis in psychoanalysis. Buenos Aires: University La Matanza.

Green, A. (1999). *Narcisismo de Vida Narcisismo de Muerte*. Buenos Aires: Paidós.

Gunderson, J. (2000). Psychodynamic psychotherapy for Borderline Personality Disorders. In J. Gunderson and G. Gabbard (eds.) *Psychotherapy for Personality Disorders. Review of Psychiatry (19)*. Washington DC: American Psychiatric Press, 33–64.

Izydorczyk, B. (2022). *Body Images in Eating Disorders. Clinical Diagnosis and Integrative Approach to Psychological Treatment*. London: Routledge, Taylor& Francis Group.

Jeammet, P. (1992). *La Boulimie, Monographies Revue Francoise de Psychanalyse*. PUF. Spanish versión: Las conductas bulímicas como modalidad de acomodamiento de las disregulaciones narcisistas y objetales. *Psicoanálisis con Niños y Adolescentes*, 1993, (5): 44–63.

Jeammet, P. (1994). El abordaje psicoanalítico de los trastornos de las conductas alimentarios. *Psicoanálisis con Niños y Adolescentes*, 6: 25–42.

Kernberg, O. F. (1984). *Severe Personality Disorders*. New Haven, CT: Yale University Press.

Kernberg, O. F. (2004). A technical approach to eating disorders in patients with Borderline Personality Organization. In *Aggressivity, Narcissism, and Self-destructiveness in the Psychotherapeutic Relationships: New Developments in the Psychopathology and Psychotherapy of Severe Personality Disorders*. New Haven, CT: Yale University Press, 205–219 (chapter 13).

Kernberg, O. F. (2012). *The Inseparable Nature of Love and Aggression: Clinical and Theoretical Perspectives*. Washington DC: American Psychiatric Publishing.

Kernberg, O. F. (2018). *Treatment of Severe Personality Disorders: Resolution of Aggression and Recovery of Eroticism*. Washington, DC: American Psychiatric Association Publishing.

Kernberg, O. F., Selzer, M. A., Koenigsberg, H. W., Carr, A. C., and Appelbaum, A. H. (1989). *Psychodynamic Psychotherapy of Borderline Patients*. New York: Basic Books.

Kernberg, P. F., Weiner, A. S., and Bardenstein, K. K. (2000). *Personality Disorders in Children and Adolescents*. New York: Basic Books.

Koenisberg, H., Kernberg, O. F., Stone, M., Appelbaum, A., Yeomans, F., and Diamond, D. (2000). *Borderline Patients: Extending the Limits of Treatability*. New York: Basic Books.

Mahler, M. S. (1968). *On Human Symbiosis and the Vicissitudes of Individuation: Volume 1: Infantile Psychosis*. New York: International Universities Press.

Mahler, M. S., Pine, F., and Bergman, A. (1975). *The Psychological Birth of the Human Infant: Symbiosis and Individuation*. New York: Basic Books.

McWilliams, N. and Shedler, J. (2017). Personality syndromes P Axis. In V. Lingiardi and N. McWilliams (eds.) *Psychodynamic Diagnostic Manual Second edition PDM-2*. New York: The Guilford Press, 15–70.

Meneguzzo, P., Garolla, A., Bonello, E., and Todisco, P. (2021). Alexithymia, dissociation and emotional regulation in eating disorders: Evidence of improvement through specialized inpatient treatment. *Clinical Psychology and Psychotherapy*, 29(2): 718–724.

Perry, C. (1991). *The Defense Mechanism Rating Scales (DMRS)*, 5th ed. Cambridge, MA.

Perry, J. C., Kardos, M., and Pagano, C. (1993). The study of defenses in psychotherapy using the Defense Mechanism Rating Scales: The concept of Defense Mechanisms. In U. Hentschel, G. J. W. Smith, W. Ehlers, and J. G. Draguns (eds.) *Contemporary Psychology: Theoretical, Research and Clinical Perspectives*. New York: Springer, 122–132.

Persano, H. (1999). *La Historización durante el proceso psicoanalítico con pacientes de estructura fronteriza*. Desafíos Clínicos Actuales de la Psicoterapia al Psicoanálisis, APA XXVII Congreso Interno y XXXVII Symposium: "Desafíos Clínicos Actuales. De la Psicoterapia al Psicoanálisis"(2): 191–200. Argentine Psychoanalytic Association.

Persano, H. (2005). Abordagem psicodinâmica do paciente com trastornos alimentares. In C. Eizirik, R. Aguiar, and S. Schestatsky (eds.) *Psicoterapia de Orientação Analítica: Fundamentos Teóricos e Clínicos*. Porto Alegre: Artmed Ed., 674–688 (chapter 49).

Persano, H. (2006). Contratransferência em pacientes com transtornos alimentares. In J. Zaslavsky and M. J. dos Santos (eds.) *Contratransferência teoria e prática clínica*. Porto Alegre: Artmed ed., 150–166 (chapter 10).

Persano, H. (2019). Mecanismos de Defensa. In H. L. Persano (ed.) *El Mundo de la Salud Mental en la Práctica Clínica*. Buenos Aires: Akadia Ed., 319–338.

Persano, H. (2022). Self-Harm. *International Journal of Psychoanalysis*, 103(6): 1089–1103.

Persano, H. and Ventura, A. (2006). Contratransferência em pacientes com transtornos da personalidade borderline e narcisista. In J. Zaslavsky and M. J. dos Santos (eds.) *Contratransferência Teoria e Prática Clínica*. Porto Alegre: Artmed Ed., 103–124 (chapter 7).

Persano, H. L., Ventura, A., Buconic, F., Chertcoff, L., García Lizziero, E., García Méndez, C., Mayan, N., and Volpe, N. (2011). *Dependence relationship between eating disorders and borderline personality disorders through semi structured interview DIB-R*. 15th World Congress of Psychiatry Our Heritage and Our Future. Buenos Aires, 18–22 Sept. 2011. doi:10.13140/RG.2.2.29923.99364.

Persano, H. L., Chertcoff, L., Gutnisky, D. A., GarcíaLizziero, E., Ventura, A. D., and Cohen, D. (2016). *The Inventory of Personality Organization (IPO) in clinical (BPD-ED) and control samples.* 9th Joseph Sandler Conference: The Relationships between Psychoanalytic Research and Clinical Work. Buenos Aires, July 2016. doi:10.13140/RG.2.2.16904.44800.

Petrucelli, J. (2015) (ed.). *Body-States: Interpersonal and Relational Perspectives on the Treatment of Eating Disorders.* London and New York: Routledge.

Robinson, P., Skårderud, F., and Sommerfeldt, B. (2019). *Hunger: Mentalization-based Treatments for Eating Disorders.* Cham: Springer International Publishing.

Robinson, P. and Skårderud, F. (2019). Eating Disorders. In A. Bateman and P. Fonagy (eds) *Handbook of Mentalizing in Mental Health Practice.* Washington DC: American Psychiatric Association Publishing, 369–386 (2nd edition).

Selvini Palazolli, M. (1974). *Self-Starvation: From the Intrapsychic to the Transpersonal Approach to Anorexia Nervosa.* New York: Jason Aronson, (1978 edition).

Skårderud, F. and Fonagy, P. (2012). Eating disorders. In A. W. Bateman and P. Fonagy (eds.) *Handbook of Mentalizing in Mental Health Practice.* Washington DC: American Psychiatric Publishing, 347–383 (1st edition).

Tasca, G. (2010). Attachment and eating disorders: A research update. *Current Opinion in Psychology*, 25: 59–64.

Varela, B. (2016). Cómo integrar las defensas a la formulación de caso y a la determinación de los focos en psicoterapia. In R. Bernardi, B. Varela, D. Miller, R. Zytner, L. de Souza, and R. Oyenard (eds.) *La Formulación Psicodinámica de Caso: Su valor para la práctica clínica.* Montevideo: Grupo Magro Editores, 129–144.

Ventura, A. (2014). Psicoterpia de los trastornos de la personalidad. In *APSA, Proapsi Programa de actualización en Psiquiatría.* Buenos Aires: Ed. Panamericana.

Williams, G. (1997). Reflections on some dynamics of eating disorders "no entry" defences and foreign bodies. *International Journal of Psychoanalysis*, 78(5): 927–941.

Winnicott, D. (1949). Hate in the counter-transference. *International Journal of Psychoanalysis*, 30: 69–74.

Yeomans, F., Selzer, M., and Clarkin, J. (1992). *Treating The Borderline Patient. A Contract-Based Approach.* New York: Basic Books.

Yeomans, F., Clarkin, J., and Kernberg, O. (2002). *A Primer of Transference Focused. Psychotherapy for the Borderline Patient.* New Jersey: Jason Aronson.

Yeomans, F. and Diamond, D. (2010). Transference-focused psychotherapy and Borderline Personality Disorders. In J. Clarkin, P. Fonagy, and G. Gabbard (eds.) *Psychodynamic Psychotherapy for Personality Disorders: A Clinical Handbook.* Washington DC: American Psychiatric Publishing, 209–238.

Yeomans, F., Clarkin, J., and Kernberg, O. F. (2015). *Transference Focused Psychotherapy for Borderline Personality Disorder: A Clinical Guide.* Arlington, VA: American Psychiatric Publishing.

Zanarini, M. C., Gunderson, J. G., Frankenburg, F. R., and Chauncey, D. L. (1989). The revised diagnostic interview for borderlines: Discriminating BPD from other axis II disorders. *Journal of Personality Disorders*, 3(1): 10–18.

Zeeck, A., Endorf, K., Euler, S., Schaefer, L., Lau, I., Flösser, K. V., ... Hartmann, A. (2021). Implementation of mentalization-based treatment in a day hospital program for eating disorders—A pilot study. *European Eating Disorders Review*, 29: 783–801.

10 Beyond the individual

Sociocultural factors in eating disorders

Examining the role of societal pressures, media, and cultural expectations

Eating disorders (EDs), like certain personality disorders, are closely tied to the social constructs of their time. They are conditions deeply embedded in a complex network of relationships between the individual, their body, and the cultural meanings ascribed to them. These disorders do not exist in isolation; rather, they reflect the intricate ways in which the self, the body, and society are interwoven.

Social representations and the body as a cultural construct

In understanding EDs, we must consider the cultural shaping of ideals and the symbolic role that the body represents in contemporary society. Serge Moscovici (1961) introduced the idea of social representations, arguing that they go beyond traditional concepts of opinion and image to form a "complex web of beliefs, thoughts, and attitudes" (Farr, 1994). Social representations are more than opinions; they are cognitive systems, aesthetic in nature, with their own internal logic and language (Moscovici, 1961). In individuals with anorexia nervosa (AN) or bulimia nervosa (BN), these representations often manifest as deeply ingrained attitudes toward food and body image—attitudes that reflect their values, ideals, and relationships to their own and others' bodies.

These social representations illustrate how each society or culture creates unique interpretations of the body. However, in contemporary society, these representations are increasingly homogenized, with narrow ideals of beauty and body type dominating the cultural landscape. This "homogenization of social representations" places immense pressure on individuals to conform to a standardized body ideal. As Moscovici noted, social representations can shift personal opinions into public expectations, creating a universal standard that often feels inescapable to those affected (Moscovici, 1961).

DOI: 10.4324/9781032724997-10

The interplay of individual and culture in shaping pathology

This dynamic reveals a deep relationship between an individual's mental state and the inter-subjective fabric of society, in which they seek to align or distinguish themselves. Robert Farr (1993) described social representations as "cognitive systems with their own logic and language, systems of values, ideas, and practices". These representations serve a dual function: first, as an order that allows individuals to navigate their social and material world; second, as a framework for communication that defines social codes, enabling people to name and classify aspects of their world and group identities (Farr, 1993); (Mora, 2002).

EDs in contemporary society exemplify this concept. Those suffering from AN and BN form perceptions about body image rooted in these societal values, seeking to align with or challenge cultural norms. Social representations are a form of mental reconstruction of reality generated through the exchange of information between individuals (Mora, 2002). These representations function as systems that guide behavior and identity formation, influenced by the era's ideologies.

Social representation exists when several people come to share that representation by means of communicating and agreeing on similar beliefs. Social representation also refers to beliefs that are publicly displayed. Such beliefs, scripts, and implicit theories are structured by, and anchored on, ideological and value systems. Social representations address three core needs: to classify complex events, to justify actions (often against others), and to differentiate groups (Páez et al., 2012). This framework helps explain the pressure many feel to adhere to cultural body ideals. When an adolescent engages in restrictive eating or purging, they are not only responding to individual desires but also expressing a cultural narrative that equates physical appearance with self-worth and inclusion in society

Media influence and the transformation of body image

In the 20th century, the body, particularly the female body, became a focal point of mass media, which increasingly propagated specific aesthetic ideals—thinness chief among them. Media do not merely reflect social norms; they actively shape them. As Moscovici observed, social representations are not passive reflections but dynamic systems that guide behavior and communication in everyday life (Moscovici, 1988). As Mora (2002) further interprets, "social relationships require individuals to be capable of responding at any moment" to expectations shaped by cultural discourse. This constant pressure to meet a standardized ideal of beauty transforms the body into a public symbol, moving from private judgment to a socially defined image.

Technological advances have reinforced these pressures, creating illusions of omnipotent control over body shape, diet, and even caloric intake. Computerized diet plans, fitness apps, and specific surgical interventions have all promoted the idea that one's appearance can and should be meticulously managed. The human body, once nurtured through communal practices, has become an object for scrutiny, evaluated more on appearance than substance. Many individuals, even those with limited means, adopt costly diets lacking in nutritional value, driven by a cultural fixation on achieving an "ideal" appearance.

Social media significantly influences body image perceptions, often contributing to the development of EDs. Platforms such as Instagram, TikTok, and Facebook expose users—particularly adolescents and young adults—to idealized body types and lifestyles, fostering social comparison, internalization of thin or muscular ideals, and body dissatisfaction. These factors are recognized as key risk factors for EDs, including AN, BN, and binge-eating disorder (BED).

Research consistently underscores the connection between social media use, body image concerns, and disordered eating behaviors. A recent study by Dahlgren et al. (2024) specifically found a strong association between social media usage, eating disorder pathology, and appearance ideals among Norwegian adolescents. The study highlighted those platforms emphasizing visual content, such as Instagram and TikTok, exerted a particularly detrimental influence on adolescents' perceptions of their appearance, significantly contributing to elevated levels of eating disorder pathology (Dahlgren et al. 2024).

A study published in *PLOS Global Public Health* (Bhatia and Dane, 2023) analyzed evidence from 50 studies conducted across 17 countries. The authors concluded that social media usage contributes to body image concerns, EDs, and poor mental health by promoting mechanisms such as social comparison and the internalization of thin or fit ideals.

While social media often has detrimental effects on body image and eating behaviors, it also holds potential as a tool for positive interventions. Emerging research suggests that social media can be leveraged to provide support and disseminate recovery-oriented content for individuals affected by EDs. For example, Jordan reviewed how social networks could serve as valuable tools for professionals to engage with vulnerable groups and facilitate interaction and peer support among individuals diagnosed with EDs (Jordan et al., 2021). Such initiatives could transform social media into a space that promotes healing and community building.

In conclusion, social media plays a dual role in shaping body image and eating behaviors. On one hand, it often exacerbates risks by reinforcing unrealistic appearance ideals and promoting social comparison, contributing to body dissatisfaction and eating disorder pathology. On the other hand, with intentional and mindful usage, social media platforms can be repurposed as avenues for positive engagement, enabling professionals to reach at-risk individuals and fostering supportive networks for recovery. Harnessing its potential responsibly could mitigate its harms and amplify its capacity to support mental health and well-being.

Identity, autonomy, and the fragmented self

As women gained independence in the 20th century, their bodies increasingly became symbols of autonomy and rebellion against objectification. However, rather than achieving complete agency, many women found themselves subject to new and exacting aesthetic standards. The body, originally a medium of self-expression, often became ensnared by these externally imposed ideals. This dynamic is vividly illustrated in personal accounts from fashion models, who describe the relentless effort required to mold and maintain their bodies to meet industry expectations—standards that mirror broader cultural pressures.

This tension between autonomy and control encapsulates what some clinicians term a "clinic of emptiness" (Lutenberg, 2008), where individuals experience emotional voids that mirror an emptiness within the mind's structure. In this framework, the relentless demand to project a perfected image and remain constantly prepared to meet external expectations leave little space for genuine introspection or emotional grounding. The result is a profound disconnect, as individuals prioritize appearances over internal well-being.

The perpetual expectation to appear "ready", both physically and behaviorally, fosters a pervasive sense of internal emptiness. Mora (2002) describes this phenomenon as "a subjective expression of [the individual's] own perceived inadequacy", where the pursuit of perfection becomes a compensatory mechanism for deeper feelings of insufficiency. Far from empowering, this relentless quest for perfection transforms the body into a battleground for navigating societal pressures and cultural ideals.

In this context, the body shifts from a medium of self-expression to a vessel for meeting external demands, illustrating a paradox where the desire for autonomy and self-determination is overshadowed by conformity to societal expectations. This dynamic not only reflects individual struggles but also underscores broader cultural conflicts, where the pursuit of idealized standards perpetuates cycles of inadequacy and alienation.

The interplay between societal standards and the clinic of emptiness underscores a broader paradox. While these ideals often promise agency and self-determination, they simultaneously impose a framework that exacerbates feelings of inadequacy and alienation. This cycle reflects the profound impact of societal pressures on individual identity, making the body both a canvas for expression and a battleground for self-worth.

The cultural ideal of speed and instant gratification in bulimia nervosa

BN, with its cycles of binging and purging, reflects several key traits of contemporary culture: speed, impulsivity, and a relentless pursuit of instant gratification. The act of binge eating conveys an urgent attempt to fill an existential void, mirroring society's demand for immediacy and the constant consumption of experiences.

This urgency is perhaps best captured by the line from an Argentine rock song: *"No sé lo que quiero pero lo quiero ya"*, which translates to: *"I don't know what I want, but I want it now"*[1]. In this context, bulimic behaviors align with a cultural paradigm in which physical self-control becomes a substitute for self-worth, reinforcing unattainable ideals propagated by media and social expectations. Another powerful lyric from Argentine rock conveys this transitory, fast-paced ethos: *"Esas motos que van a mil, solo el viento te harán sentir, nada más, nada más"*[2] which translates to *"Those motorcycles going a thousand miles an hour, only the wind will make you feel—nothing more, nothing more"*. This line embodies the pursuit of intense, fleeting experiences to escape or feel alive, but ultimately reveals how these sensations are ephemeral, offering only brief relief before an inner emptiness returns. Like the impulsive and momentary satisfaction associated with binge eating, these behaviors are, in the end, as hollow as the thrill of speed—offering a temporary sense of fullness before the void inevitably resurfaces.

Lipovetsky argues that modern individuals navigate a world increasingly dominated by a sense of emptiness, a pervasive void that stems from the disintegration of stable structures and values in contemporary life (Lipovetsky, 1983). Within this context, BN serves as a striking metaphor and manifestation of this struggle, embodying a cyclical attempt to temporarily "fill" the emptiness. The act of consumption—both literal and symbolic—offers fleeting relief but ultimately reinforces the very void it seeks to address. This paradox highlights the deeper existential crisis faced by individuals caught in this pattern, where satisfaction is perpetually sought but never truly achieved.

This condition resonates with Zygmunt Bauman's concept of life in a "liquid modernity", a state characterized by constant flux, instability, and the erosion of traditional anchors of identity and meaning. In this liquid world, nothing remains fixed—relationships, goals, and even self-perception are transient and fluid. Individuals, therefore, find themselves in a relentless pursuit of meaning through ephemeral experiences and achievements, only to watch them dissolve as quickly as they are grasped (Bauman, 2000). This continuous striving for fulfillment mirrors the compulsive cycle of BN, where temporary gratification gives way to guilt, dissatisfaction, and an intensified sense of emptiness.

1   Song: "Lo quiero ya", SUMO Band, 1987.
2   Song "Seminare", Seru Giran Band, 1978.

Together, Lipovetsky's and Bauman's perspectives provide a powerful lens for understanding how modern societal conditions shape not only individual behaviors but also broader cultural patterns. The act of seeking fulfillment through transient means—whether through consumerism, social validation, or physical ideals—becomes emblematic of the broader existential struggle of modern life. This perpetual search for meaning in a world without fixed foundations underscores the psychological and emotional toll of navigating liquid modernity, where the very mechanisms meant to soothe often deepen the sense of disconnection and inadequacy.

The alienation of self and body in modern culture

In contemporary culture, individuals increasingly experience alienation, not only from their bodies but also from a deeper, meaningful sense of self. The pressure to conform to socially sanctioned images and ideals creates what Serge Moscovici terms "pressure to infer"—a societal demand for individuals to quickly adopt and express ready-made opinions, stances, and behaviors on matters of public interest. This expectation is particularly pronounced during adolescence, a formative stage when individuals are still developing their identities and worldviews. According to Moscovici, this "pressure to infer" forces individuals to prematurely adopt rigid beliefs about their bodies and identities, often before they have had the opportunity to fully explore or internalize these beliefs. He describes this phenomenon as "character rigidity", a condition that manifests clinically in disorders like AN, where inflexible attitudes about the body are coupled with similarly unyielding personality traits (Moscovici, 2014).

For adolescents, this rigidity presents significant challenges. As Mora explains, the developmental stage of adolescence is naturally marked by fluctuations—both physical and emotional. However, the cultural demand for fixed and definitive stances on body image conflicts with this inherent variability. Adolescents, pressured to solidify their self-perceptions prematurely, may find themselves locked into patterns of self-worth and identity that persist into adulthood. This inflexibility can hinder the natural evolution of self-image, constraining adolescents' capacity to adapt and grow in response to life's changes (Mora, 2002).

Jeammet and Bochereau, in *"La Souffrance des Adolescents"*, emphasize that much of adolescent suffering arises from this struggle for autonomy and self-definition in a culture that values instantaneous and unwavering adherence to social norms. Adolescents are caught between their need for self-exploration and the societal expectation to conform, leaving them vulnerable to feelings of inadequacy and alienation. The rigidity imposed by cultural standards exacerbates their struggle, fostering a disconnection from both their bodies and their authentic selves (Jeammet and Bochereau, 2007).

This alienation is not only a personal issue but a broader cultural phenomenon. The pervasive societal focus on appearances, quick judgments, and definitive stances leaves little room for the fluid, evolving nature of selfhood. As a result, individuals, particularly adolescents, may come to view themselves through the lens of societal expectations rather than their intrinsic qualities. This dynamic underscores the importance of fostering environments that allow for self-exploration and fluidity, helping individuals navigate the tension between societal pressures and their evolving sense of identity.

Sociocultural influences and the fragmented self

The fragmentation of the self in modern societies is deeply intertwined with social and cultural pressures, particularly those surrounding body image. Media, technology, and societal expectations create a complex landscape in which individuals are inundated with idealized portrayals of beauty and success. These external forces often distort how individuals perceive their own bodies and construct their identities, leading to a fragmented sense of self. EDs, especially AN and BN, expose this fracture, as they manifest the painful intersection between self-worth and societal ideals, where physical appearance becomes both a battleground and a prison.

In contemporary culture, the body is frequently commodified and reduced to a canvas for external validation, stripping it of its autonomy. For individuals with EDs, the body often ceases to be a personal space and instead becomes a reflection of collective ideals imposed by relentless aesthetic demands. As a result, EDs serve as maladaptive coping mechanisms, offering individuals a semblance of control in an environment that consistently undermines their sense of self. This dynamic aligns with what Zygmunt Bauman (2000) describes as the liquid nature of modern life, where identities are constantly shaped, dissolved, and reshaped in response to societal expectations, leaving individuals with a fragile and unstable sense of who they are.

The fragmentation is further exacerbated by technology and social media, which amplify aesthetic pressures and reinforce unrealistic body standards. The constant comparison enabled by these platforms creates a dichotomy between the "ideal self" portrayed online and the individual's lived reality. This dissonance fosters a disjointed identity, where individuals feel increasingly alienated from their authentic selves. As Serge Moscovici (2014) notes, the "character rigidity" that emerges from societal pressures further entrenches this fragmentation, as individuals are compelled to adopt inflexible beliefs about their bodies and identities to meet external demands.

True recovery from EDs and the associated fragmentation of self requires more than addressing disordered eating behaviors. It necessitates a holistic approach that dismantles the sociocultural influences tying self-worth to body image. This means challenging the pervasive narratives that equate physical appearance with value and fostering environments that promote self-acceptance and authenticity. As Jeammet and Bochereau (2007) emphasize, the journey toward healing must involve creating spaces where individuals can explore and redefine their identities without the burden of external pressures. Only by reclaiming both their physical selves and their intrinsic sense of identity can individuals move beyond the fractured self-imposed by modern society.

Impact of social and cultural factors on body image and disordered eating

Social and cultural factors play a profound role in shaping body image perceptions and influencing the development of disordered eating behaviors. These forces operate through societal norms, media portrayals, and cultural expectations, molding individuals' attitudes toward their bodies and eating habits in pervasive and often detrimental ways.

Mass media frequently promote narrow and unrealistic beauty standards, such as thinness for women and muscularity for men. Exposure to these ideals has been shown to contribute to body dissatisfaction and unhealthy eating behaviors. The mechanisms behind this influence include awareness, perceived pressures, and the internalization of these beauty standards, all of which are significantly associated with how individuals evaluate their bodies. Cultural norms further dictate acceptable body types, influencing self-perception and driving behaviors aimed at achieving these ideals. Western cultures, for instance, often idealize thinness, creating a cultural environment that fosters dissatisfaction and vulnerability to EDs. Meanwhile, non-Western cultures may emphasize different aesthetic ideals, though acculturation and socioeconomic status can mediate these influences, shifting perceptions of body size and weight.

The interplay between media and other socializing agents, such as parents and peers, reinforces these cultural standards. Media messages, absorbed and echoed in daily interactions, create a feedback loop that amplifies body image pressures. Parents and peers often serve as intermediaries, consciously or unconsciously transmitting societal beauty ideals and shaping how individuals internalize these standards. As Cash argues, the influence of cultural and personal meanings attached to physical appearance is universal, transcending gender, cultural boundaries, and the narrow focus on EDs that has historically dominated body image research. He emphasizes that "all people are embodied, and their lives are powerfully shaped by the personal and cultural meanings of their physical appearance" (Cash, 2005).

This highlights the importance of addressing body image issues in a broader, more inclusive framework. Researchers must move beyond the gender-biased, Western-centric, and eating disorder–driven perspectives that have dominated the field. Expanding body image research to account for diverse cultural, social, and individual experiences is essential for fostering a more holistic understanding of how physical appearance shapes one's identity and well-being. By challenging narrow beauty ideals and considering the broader cultural and social contexts, we can begin to address the deep-seated influences that contribute to body dissatisfaction and disordered eating, paving the way for healthier and more inclusive body image perceptions.

Social media, mirrors, and the self-creation of body image in eating disorders

The rise of social media has significantly intensified exposure to idealized body images, often contributing to body dissatisfaction and disordered eating behaviors. Platforms that emphasize visual content and encourage sharing of daily food intake, fitness routines, and physical transformations cultivate body aspiration rather than genuine food or health inspiration. This constant exposure can lead individuals to pursue unhealthy behaviors to mirror these curated, idealized images.

There is a pervasive tendency in today's digital age to shape our bodies according to personal fantasies, sculpting an image that aligns with a desired self-concept—yet this aspiration comes with real consequences. As Masson (2015) notes, *"The body of our dreams is a body without the 'body'"*, suggesting that the idealized form people chase is often devoid of the natural and imperfect realities of physical existence. In this sense, social media acts as a mirror not of our real selves but of a body stripped of its humanity, presenting an image that is ultimately unattainable.

This digital "mirror" fosters a form of self-construction centered on appearance rather than substance, cultivating an externalized self-concept that prioritizes physical presentation over intrinsic self-worth. Within this framework, individuals are driven to craft an illusion of perfection—a body meticulously edited, filtered, and curated to align with societal standards—while becoming increasingly disconnected from the body's authentic needs and lived experiences. Social media's constant feedback loop amplifies this process, reinforcing an identity tethered to appearance and intensifying cycles of body dissatisfaction and EDs.

In this sense, social media reflects an idealized, often distorted version of the self, pressuring individuals to conform to artificial standards. This mirror image propels a relentless pursuit of perfection, transforming the body into both a project and a prison—a site of conflict where self-worth clashes with physical reality. Ultimately, this form of self-creation elevates image over substance, leaving individuals trapped in a state of chronic dissatisfaction with their natural bodies (Persano, 2005).

Expanding body image ideals across genders and cultures

While body image studies have traditionally focused on women, societal pressures increasingly affect men, particularly in the pursuit of a hyper-muscular physique. Media portrayals of idealized, sculpted male bodies fuel issues like body dysmorphic disorder and muscle dysmorphia, with men striving to meet an ideal defined by strength and muscularity. These ideals are constructed and sustained by a dense web of social and economic forces, where economic interests heavily shape bodily ideals to sell products and lifestyles. The drive for a "perfect" body, then, is not only personal but a broader social construct, deeply embedded in cultural messages designed to sustain consumer demand.

Feminist theorists offer insight into the complexities underlying these pressures. Susie Orbach illustrates how self-starvation in women exists at the intersection of multiple, intersecting influences: the mother-daughter relationship, patriarchal societal structures, and women's basic needs (Hepworth, 1999). Susie Orbach has extensively explored the intricate relationship between women and their bodies. Her seminal work, *"Fat is a Feminist Issue"* (1978), delves into the psychological and societal factors influencing women's eating behaviors and body perceptions. Orbach argues that societal pressures and cultural norms often lead women to develop unhealthy relationships with food and their bodies, viewing fatness as a feminist issue intertwined with identity and self-worth (Orbach, 2016).

In her later book *"Bodies"* Orbach examines how contemporary culture shapes our understanding of the body. She discusses the impact of media portrayals, beauty standards, and the commodification of the body, highlighting how these factors contribute to body dissatisfaction and the pursuit of unattainable ideals. Orbach emphasizes that the body has become a measure of personal worth, leading to widespread issues such as EDs and body dysmorphia (Orbach, 2019).

Orbach's work underscores the importance of addressing the societal and cultural influences that affect women's body image. She advocates for a more compassionate and holistic approach to understanding the female body, one that recognizes the complex interplay between individual psychology and external pressures. By challenging prevailing beauty norms and promoting body acceptance, Orbach's contributions continue to inform discussions on feminism, body image, and mental health. Orbach and other feminist scholars argue that patriarchal society imposes a need to restrict women's "appetite"—not only for food but also for autonomy and sexuality—as a means of control. This suppression aligns with wider cultural pressures that seek to limit women's expression and agency, making the denial of physical nourishment a metaphor for the restriction of female desire and autonomy (Hepworth, 1999).

In multicultural societies, minority groups face additional complexities around body image, leading to unique, often underreported challenges.

Navigating body ideals that differ from those of the dominant culture complicates body image perceptions, sometimes deterring individuals from seeking support for EDs. Within these communities, the tension between maintaining cultural identity and assimilating dominant cultural standards further amplifies body image struggles, impacting how individuals perceive their bodies and access resources for support.

Addressing these influences requires a multifaceted approach that integrates media literacy, cultural sensitivity, and the promotion of diverse and inclusive body representations. Such an approach acknowledges the intricate intersections of media portrayals, societal expectations, and individual experiences, providing a more comprehensive lens through which to understand and support individuals grappling with body image issues and EDs. By recognizing these varying influences, we can move toward an understanding that transcends narrow, homogenous ideals and respects the diversity of body ideals across different cultures and gender expressions.

Existential fragility: Exclusion and marginality in modern societies

EDs, while not universally present across cultures, have significantly increased within contemporary societies, especially following globalization and the profound socio-economic shifts it has catalyzed. Since the 1970s, advances in technology have reshaped labor, social hierarchies, and governance structures, resulting in a reorganization of power and shifting patterns of social inclusion. Roberto Castel (1997) describes this new context as one marked by fragility in employment, social integration, and an increased risk of disconnection from meaningful social bonds. Over the last decade, the transformation of the job market and the fragmentation of traditional social ties have led to growing fear among many individuals of being left behind, deepening a pervasive gap between the individual and full participation in social life.

In this context, individuals with EDs often experience a heightened sense of exclusion. They may see their physical appearance and eating habits as ways to gain acceptance and inclusion within society's dominant standards. Yet, ironically, these efforts to align with societal body ideals often reinforce their exclusion by promoting isolation, both physically and emotionally. Their attempts to conform to the cultural model of the "ideal body" place them in a precarious position characterized by weak social ties, inadequate support networks, and fragile employment prospects, ultimately increasing their vulnerability. These conditions can lead to a tragic cycle of isolation and self-withdrawal, limiting opportunities for self-reflection, personal growth, and meaningful connections (Persano et al., 2003).

The result is a modern reality filled with pervasive unease. Individuals increasingly struggle to find a sense of identity and a meaningful place within society, often experiencing an inner emptiness that amplifies their feelings of alienation and vulnerability. This "existential fragility" fosters an externalized sense of violence and competition, reflecting both a lack of personal fulfillment and a collective inability to build cohesive social bonds (Osofsky, 1997).

As Persano et al. (2003) observe, the challenges faced by individuals in contemporary society are rooted in the absence of clear roles, weakening social bonds, and the scarcity of both material and symbolic resources. These conditions contribute to an environment where personal struggles, such as EDs, reflect larger societal issues and tensions. Central to this dynamic is the paradox of inclusion and exclusion within modern culture: individuals strive to meet societal ideals of the "perfect" body, seeking validation and a sense of belonging, yet often find themselves ensnared in a cycle that deepens feelings of isolation and marginality.

Eating disorders (EDs) vividly expose a profound cultural contradiction. On the one hand, individuals who conform to rigid aesthetic standards may achieve fleeting moments of societal approval or inclusion. On the other hand, this very conformity alienates them from their authentic selves and meaningful connections with others. The pursuit of perfection becomes a double-edged sword: a desperate bid for acceptance that paradoxically deepens feelings of exclusion due to the emotional and physical toll it exacts.

This relentless chase of an unattainable ideal reflects not only personal struggles but also the pervasive pressures of a culture that equates self-worth with appearance. Ultimately, individuals are left trapped in cycles of dissatisfaction and self-punishment, highlighting the destructive interplay between societal expectations and personal vulnerability.

This paradox underscores the urgency of addressing EDs not merely as individual psychological conditions but as phenomena deeply embedded within social and cultural contexts. The societal emphasis on perfection and conformity demands a systemic response, one that challenges the very ideals perpetuating this cycle. Interventions must extend beyond clinical treatment to include efforts to dismantle harmful norms, foster inclusive representations of bodies, and rebuild social bonds that offer genuine connection and support.

Ultimately, understanding EDs as reflections of broader societal tensions opens a pathway toward more holistic solutions. By addressing the cultural forces that shape and sustain these struggles, we can begin to mitigate their impact and create a society that values individuals for more than their ability to conform to narrow and exclusionary ideals.

The psychoanalytic perspective on societal influences and their implications for treatment

Freud's civilization and its discontents and the modern struggles of eating disorders

In *"Civilization and Its Discontents"* (Freud, 1930 [1929]), Sigmund Freud argues that life is unavoidably filled with "pain, disappointment, and insoluble tasks". To cope with this intrinsic suffering, he suggests that individuals turn to what he calls "auxiliary constructions"—powerful distractions like intoxicating substances or substitute satisfactions—that offer temporary escape from the hardships of social existence. These substitutes provide symbolic relief, allowing people to momentarily transcend the burdens of life by retreating into experiences that lessen their awareness of discomfort. Freud also points to art as a unique auxiliary construction, one that transforms suffering into a source of relief, pleasure, and creativity. Unlike other forms of escape, art does not simply distract but has the potential to transmute suffering, channeling it into expressions that enrich personal and cultural experience, offering a profound and more sustainable form of solace.

Freud elaborates that true well-being in society is not achieved through sustained happiness but through a "succession of contrasts" between pleasure and unpleasure. He suggests that human enjoyment depends more on these shifting intensities than on a static, continuous state of contentment, as it is in the movement between opposites that we experience the fullness of life's emotional range. For Freud, this contrast-driven pleasure reflects an intrinsic part of human psychology, where satisfaction is heightened by its relationship to preceding discomfort or deprivation (Freud, 1930 [1929])

In the case of individuals with EDs, however, these contrasts transform into a relentless cycle of suffering rather than a balanced rhythm of highs and lows. For those who struggle with patterns like binging and purging, the moments of relief they experience are often brief and come at significant physical and emotional cost. The temporary pleasure found in a binge is soon overshadowed by guilt, shame, and the compulsion to purge, which not only compounds their distress but leaves them emotionally and physically depleted. This cycle mirrors Freud's observation of civilization's inherent inability to provide lasting contentment, as each moment of gratification is quickly eroded by the inevitable return of dissatisfaction.

Moreover, in this context, the "succession of contrasts" that Freud (1930 [1929])views as vital to human satisfaction takes on a punishing quality. Rather than enhancing enjoyment, the contrasting experiences—of indulgence and deprivation, of control and loss of control—intensify the sense of suffering. For someone with an ED, the pleasure derived from food becomes entangled with self-punishment, blurring the line between relief and distress. Freud's insights suggest that, within the framework of modern societal expectations and pressures, these individuals experience not a healthy fluctuation but a distorted cycle of temporary relief and chronic dissatisfaction, exposing the limits of modern society's capacity to meet deep emotional needs and to foster genuine, sustainable well-being.

In modern societies, where media and cultural norms intensify pressures to attain idealized body images, individuals with EDs often turn to disordered eating to establish control and a sense of self-worth. Freud would recognize this behavior as a form of "substitute satisfaction", a coping strategy designed to manage the unrelenting pressures of social expectations. Many individuals with EDs withdraw from social interactions, seeking what Freud describes as "solitude as an immediate protection from the pains that society brings" (Freud, 1930 [1929]). This solitude becomes a refuge, providing temporary shelter from the perceived judgments of others. However, rather than resolving their suffering, this isolation can deepen their loneliness and exacerbate feelings of inadequacy, creating a cyclical pattern of self-deception that intensifies rather than alleviates distress.

Freud often explored themes related to human happiness, social structures, and the conflicts between individual desires and societal demands. In *Civilization and Its Discontents* (1930), he examines how civilization imposes restrictions on individuals to maintain social order, often at the expense of personal happiness. Freud generally held a more skeptical and ambivalent view of the possibility of universal happiness, given the inherent tensions between human nature and societal constraints.

Collective solutions, framed as an ideal of "working together for the happiness of all", could serve as a guiding intention for society. This vision of shared purpose sharply contrasts with the isolated paths often taken by individuals with EDs, who may avoid group interactions or support systems due to feelings of shame, self-judgment, or fear of exposure. The strong cultural emphasis on personal achievement and individual beauty fosters a sense of isolation, creating significant barriers to building supportive and healing communities.

This individualistic framework highlights the dynamics of societal alienation, revealing how individuals often abandon mutual support in favor of solitary, yet ultimately insufficient, coping mechanisms. The pursuit of personal ideals—intended to bring fulfillment—often results in a disconnection from the collective bonds that are crucial for lasting well-being. Shifting the focus from isolated striving to fostering shared support could enable society to create environments that promote both individual growth and communal flourishing. Such a transformation would address the deep psychological needs recognized as fundamental to human happiness and social harmony.

Modern society's emphasis on self-reliance and personal achievement intensifies the struggle for those with EDs, as body image is framed as an individual responsibility rather than a communal one. This cultural framework downplays the importance of shared mental well-being and promotes isolation over connection. Individuals facing EDs attempt to meet society's demanding image standards not through collective efforts but through self-punishment and internalized criticism. This relentless self-surveillance reflects what Freud would call "substitute satisfactions"— attempts to fill an internal void with behaviors that ultimately deepen suffering (Freud, 1930 [1929]).

Freud's insights offer a profound framework for understanding the psychological struggles faced by individuals with eating disorders (EDs), who often retreat from supportive relationships and isolate themselves to shield against societal judgment. This self-imposed solitude, meant to serve as a protective barrier, paradoxically exacerbates feelings of loneliness and inadequacy. Instead of providing relief, it creates a self-perpetuating cycle in which isolation deepens suffering. Psychoanalysis helps illuminate this dynamic, framing such isolation as a desperate yet ultimately ineffective refuge from the overwhelming pressures of society.

In contemporary culture, where individualism is often prioritized over community support, a psychoanalytic perspective suggests that healing from eating disorders (EDs) requires a shift from isolation and self-criticism to collective understanding and shared support. This transition is particularly challenging in a society that celebrates personal success and individual achievement, frequently at the expense of communal mental well-being.

For individuals struggling with EDs, psychoanalytic insights emphasize the importance of fostering a more inclusive approach—one that values mutual support over solitary coping mechanisms. By encouraging individuals to move beyond self-imposed isolation, this perspective highlights the potential of a community-oriented path to healing, where connection and shared experiences play a central role in recovery.

Alienation from collective values and modern strategies of escape

In today's globalized societies, where collective values often feel distant and impersonal, individuals increasingly experience a sense of alienation, struggling to find belonging within a culture that feels imposed upon them. In line with Freud's ideas in *"Civilization and Its Discontents"*, many attempt to escape the pressures of contemporary society by turning inward, resorting to behaviors that mimic the effects of "intoxicating substances" as temporary relief from cultural demands (Freud, 1930 [1929]). For some, this means withdrawing from social interaction, finding refuge in solitude as a shield against societal judgment. Others desperately strive to conform, adopting the ideals and behaviors they believe will secure acceptance, especially those that center on the "idealized body image" that culture relentlessly promotes.

Social representations, those shared beliefs and expectations society holds regarding individuals' appearance and behavior, play a crucial role in shaping these ideals. In contemporary culture, young people are often, even implicitly, encouraged to adopt extreme behaviors as a form of self-control and validation. For those with EDs, this can take on the form of self-harm, which, as expressed in online forums by individuals grappling with these issues, becomes a means to alleviate intense emotions. As one youth wrote:

Self-injury can help a person release intense feelings like anger, sadness, loneliness, shame, guilt, and emotional pain. Many people who cut do it to release all the emotions they're feeling inside. Others may feel so numb that seeing their own blood helps them feel alive because they often feel dead inside

In this context, self-injury becomes a means of making emotional suffering tangible and of expressing self-judgment and self-punishment. It reflects a desire to impose control over one's body, marking it with symbols of failure or self-loathing: "Some people feel such self-hatred for themselves and their bodies that they write insulting names on their bodies to remind themselves how terrible they are" (Persano, 2022).

Self-injury often serves as a coping mechanism for releasing intense emotions such as anger, sadness, loneliness, shame, guilt, and emotional pain. For many, the act of cutting or other forms of self-harm becomes a way to externalize and momentarily relieve the overwhelming emotions they feel internally. As some individuals describe, self-injury provides a release for pent-up emotions, while others, feeling emotionally numb, turn to it as a means of reconnecting with their bodies. Seeing their own blood, for instance, offers a visceral reminder of being alive in contrast to the emotional deadness they may experience (Persano, 2022).

This behavior underscores the complex interplay between emotional pain and physical expression, where the body becomes both a canvas and a battleground for unresolved feelings. Self-injury highlights a profound inner turmoil—a struggle to reconcile overwhelming emotions, feelings of worthlessness, and a deep need for control or expression. Understanding this dynamic is crucial for providing compassionate and effective support, helping individuals address the root causes of their distress and develop healthier ways of coping and expressing their emotions (Persano, 2022).

In these cases, self-harm becomes a culturally mediated form of self-expression, a way to give meaning to internal pain through physical action. Observing artistic representations of this phenomenon, one can see how the body becomes a site of cultural suffering, where individuals can share their distress in virtual, often anonymous, spaces. Sometimes, the body itself becomes a canvas for statements of personal defeat.

In one powerful image, an individual write, "They won", symbolizing how external societal pressures have invaded their sense of self, forcing them to turn this struggle into a message that can be shared with peers. This "thinking through action" reflects an effort to make sense of suffering and to validate it within a society that often overlooks inner pain in favor of outward conformity. It becomes, in effect, a visual language that expresses both resistance and submission, echoing Freud's view of how societal pressures shape individual coping mechanisms.

Psychoanalytic insights resonate strongly here, as the struggle to meet collective ideals often leads to extreme, isolating behaviors that underscore the tension between individual suffering and cultural expectations. Self-harm and other disordered behaviors reflect a desperate attempt to control and externalize internalized societal demands, reinforcing the disconnect between individuals and collective values in modern culture.

The cultural malaise of exclusion and self-destructive behavior

Freud posited that cultural malaise arises from the renunciation of our most primal drives—sexuality and aggression—to exist harmoniously within society (Freud, 1930 [1929]). Yet, in contemporary times, this malaise has evolved. Today's cultural discontent is deeply rooted in experiences of social exclusion and alienation, which have given rise to new forms of self-destructive behaviors, intensified by a pervasive pre-occupation with death. Such behaviors, including self-harm, EDs, and suicidal ideation, are not isolated or purely personal but are deeply inter-woven within a network of social relationships that create a sense of isolation in an ever-connected world. This paradoxical isolation fosters a belief in self-reliance, where individuals are pressured to resolve their place within society on their own, without communal support or shared understanding.

In many ways, EDs epitomize this modern cultural phenomenon. Those who suffer from AN, BN, and other forms of disordered eating often engage in severe self-maltreatment as they attempt to gain social acceptance and validation through adherence to rigid aesthetic ideals. This drive toward self-destruction reflects an implicit belief that bodily sacrifice—through starvation, purging, or extreme control—will grant a form of acceptance, yet this acceptance remains elusive. In these individuals, body harm becomes an attempt to manage inner pain and fulfill society's unattainable standards, reinforcing Freud's notion that such behaviors are deeply linked to unfulfilled social and cultural pressures.

In the context of modern culture, these self-destructive behaviors often represent a silent cry for inclusion. The individual's desperate attempts to meet idealized body standards and gain societal approval frequently manifest in behaviors that harm the body. Through starvation, purging, or excessive exercise, they attempt to suppress not only physical appetite but also deeper desires for acceptance, love, and connection. Freud's perspective on cultural malaise offers a lens through which to view this struggle: self-destructive actions are often the individual's reaction to a culture that provides little space for genuine fulfillment and meaningful human connection. The acts of self-starvation or bodily harm, then, serve as both rebellions against and submission to a society that demands conformity to narrow ideals of beauty and worth.

The tragic outcome for many individuals grappling with these disorders is a persistent flirtation with death, be it through the slow destruction of their bodies or the contemplation of suicide. The body, in its wounded state, becomes a battleground where the person both fights against and succumbs to societal pressures. In some cases, the ultimate culmination of this struggle is a life marked by perpetual cycles of self-harm, leading to physical degradation and, tragically, even death. As Freud might suggest, these individuals are seeking escape not only from their own inner turmoil but from a culture that seems to insist on perfection and beauty at any cost, pushing them toward self-erasure as the price of belonging.

In essence, the self-destructive behaviors exhibited by individuals with EDs reflect a broader cultural pathology—one in which societal pressures compel individuals to sacrifice aspects of themselves in the pursuit of acceptance. The irony, as psychoanalytic insights reveal, is that this relentless chase for societal ideals often results in deeper isolation, unfulfillment, and disconnection from meaningful relationships. Their suffering underscores the urgent need for a cultural shift: moving away from the isolating pursuit of perfection toward a framework of genuine inclusion—one that values individuals for more than their physical appearance and fosters connections built on empathy, acceptance, and mutual support.

Isolation and fragmentation in contemporary art and culture

Psychoanalytic insights into culture suggest that both art and solidarity can serve as powerful pathways for addressing the pervasive discontent that characterizes modern societies. Art, as a medium of expression, offers a unique avenue for individuals to convey their perceptions of the world, encapsulating both personal and collective experiences. Through its capacity to explore and reflect the complexities of human emotions and societal dynamics, art becomes a vital tool for fostering understanding and connection.

Argentine artist Berta Jakubowicz Teglio[3] offers a powerful exploration of this theme, reflecting the isolation and absence of genuine human connections within contemporary culture. Her piece *"Cada cual atiende su juego"* (2001), (*"Each Tends to Their Own Game"*) poignantly portrays this sense of detachment. It shows individuals caught in a network that appears to connect them but ultimately leaves them isolated, each within their own world. The intricate, almost mechanical nature of this "network" allows people to coexist, yet they remain separated, following isolated, parallel paths. The title itself suggests that everyone is confined to their own reality, moving in solitary directions—ascending or descending without intersecting with others. This imagery encapsulates the illusion of freedom that defines much of modern culture: a self-contained freedom without the richness of true human interaction and connection.

Jakubowicz Teglio deepens this theme in her work *"Rehén"* (2001), (*"Hostage"*) symbolizing how the contemporary cultural web not only

---

3   Berta Jakubowicz Teglio, born in Buenos Aires in 1950, is a distinguished textile artist known for her innovative contributions to contemporary art.

isolates individuals but entraps them. Here, the connections take on a suffocating quality, burdening people with overwhelming expectations and stifling genuine interaction. The art reflects a cycle in which the very connections that should empower and unite people instead reinforce their isolation and disconnection, underscoring a collective experience of entrapment.

In a world increasingly defined by the isolation and fragmentation captured in Jakubowicz Teglio's art, the need for self-validation through external image has become paramount. This cultural emphasis on outward appearance mirrors the pressures faced by individuals struggling with EDs. Their efforts to conform to societal ideals of beauty and body image reflect a broader cultural malaise—a quest for acceptance and recognition that often leads to intensified feelings of inadequacy and isolation. In this context, the body becomes not only a symbol of personal identity but also a battleground for societal approval. The relentless pursuit of cultural ideals creates a deep disconnection from oneself, where self-doubt and self-criticism replace self-acceptance (Personal Communication, *Sociologist* Delia Franco, 2007).

Many individuals in contemporary society grapple with a profound sense of confinement, a struggle often intensified by the pervasive pressures of societal beauty standards. For those suffering from EDs, this confinement is not merely abstract but deeply felt, as their lives are often shaped by rigid expectations surrounding appearance and self-control. Many channel these struggles into self-expressive works of art, creating pieces that poignantly reflect their internal battles and the external pressures they endure.

To explore these dynamics in a therapeutic context, art pieces by Jakubowicz Teglio were introduced to patients in the Day Hospital Unit's culture workshop. The workshop seeks to bridge patients' personal experiences with art, fostering connections that help expand their mental representations and provide relief from painful emotions. Within this setting, psychoanalytic approaches are seamlessly integrated with group art workshops, offering a pathway to healing where creativity and shared experiences promote self-understanding and cultivate collective support.

Art serves as both a mirror and a critique of modern society, embodying cultural norms and individual struggles while offering a space for reflection, healing, and transformation. The interplay between personal experiences and societal expectations is vividly illustrated in therapeutic and contemporary art practices, such as those seen in a workshop at the Day Hospital Unit for Eating Disorders and the works of textile artist Berta Teglio. Both provide unique lenses through which to understand the complexities of modern culture and its effects on individuals.

In the workshop, an individual (patient) created an artwork featuring interwoven lines forming a cage—a powerful metaphor for the entrapment within societal expectations. The piece reflects the constraints of cultural ideals, where the body becomes a contested space in the relentless pursuit of perfection. This visual narrative captures the internalization of societal pressures, leading to cycles of self-restraint, body control, and isolation. By externalizing these emotions, the individual transforms intangible struggles into a tangible form, bridging their personal pain with broader cultural critiques.

Similarly, Berta Teglio's textile art engages with themes of modern society and culture, often exploring the symbolic and emotional weight of entanglement, structure, and fragmentation. Teglio's works, such as her use of interwoven materials and abstract forms, evoke a dialogue about the interplay between the individual and collective, the fragile and the enduring. Her art often reflects the pressures and complexities of contemporary life, inviting viewers to question the cultural norms and systems that shape their identities and relationships. The physicality of her medium—textile—underscores themes of interconnectedness and constraint, resonating with the cage imagery from the therapeutic workshop.

Both the workshop piece and Teglio's art highlight how art can serve as a means of exploring and critiquing the pervasive constraints of modern society. They reveal how cultural pressures—whether through ideals of beauty, success, or conformity—manifest in personal experiences of entrapment and alienation. At the same time, they demonstrate the transformative potential of art as a pathway for recovery and understanding. By externalizing these struggles, both artists and individuals in therapeutic settings can challenge the societal norms that perpetuate cycles of control and dissatisfaction.

Moreover, when such artworks are shared within communities, whether therapeutic or artistic, they foster collective reflection and solidarity. Teglio's art invites societal critique, just as the cage imagery in the workshop promotes connection among individuals facing similar challenges. Together, these works exemplify how art can transcend personal expression to address universal themes, making visible the often-hidden tensions between individuality and cultural expectations.

In this way, art becomes a vital tool for navigating the complexities of modern culture. It allows individuals to process and express their struggles, fosters dialogue about societal pressures, and creates a space for imagining alternative narratives that prioritize authenticity and connection over conformity and control. Through the convergence of therapeutic practices and contemporary art, the transformative power of creativity becomes a beacon for self-discovery and collective healing.

This collective aspect fosters connection and solidarity among those affected, creating a space where individuals can begin to challenge the societal ideals that contribute to their sense of confinement. Through shared artistic expression, they find a way to articulate the unspeakable, transform personal pain into communal understanding, and explore pathways to reclaim their autonomy and sense of self. Such works not only reveal the impact of societal pressures but also serve as a powerful reminder of the resilience and creativity of those who navigate these challenges.

Eating disorders (EDs), as manifestations of cultural malaise, serve both as symptoms of and responses to the broader societal forces that prioritize individualism, superficial validation, and isolation. The relentless pressure to seek validation by conforming to external ideals often traps individuals in a cycle of self-deception, where public image takes precedence over authentic human connection. Drawing from psychoanalytic and philosophical perspectives, the remedy for this suffering lies in shifting from isolation toward collective solidarity. In such a framework, individuals are valued not for their adherence to unattainable standards, but for their shared humanity—acknowledged and celebrated through genuine, mutual connections that foster empathy and belonging.

The new cultural malaise: Hegemonic image and hyperreality

Freud's concept of cultural malaise, which originally centered on the repression of instinctual drives to conform to societal norms, has taken on new dimensions in contemporary culture. In today's world, this malaise extends to what can be described as "the violence of detachment", a phenomenon marked by the erosion of protective cultural structures and the growing dominance of idealized, hyperreal images. These images blur the boundaries between reality and the culturally constructed ideals of perfection, creating an environment where the pursuit of these unattainable standards becomes a source of profound psychological distress.

This evolution of cultural malaise is particularly evident in the experiences of younger generations. As Osofsky (1997) highlights in "*Children in a Violent Society*", while direct violence may not always be present, indirect violence permeates the lives of children in modern societies. This indirect violence manifests through societal pressures, the hyper-commercialization of identity, and the omnipresence of unattainable ideals. The result is a subtle but pervasive harm that impacts their ability to develop a stable sense of self and security.

In this context, the "violence of detachment" refers to the disconnection individuals feel from authentic experiences, community support, and personal identity. The hyperreal images promoted by media and cultural norms replace genuine human connection with a relentless drive for perfection, fostering alienation and dissatisfaction. These idealized images attain a life of their own, becoming more real than reality itself—a phenomenon Baudrillard described as the "hyperreal" (Baudrillard, 1998). This disconnects between the real and the ideal exacerbates the sense of cultural malaise Freud originally described, now compounded by modern technologies and media saturation.

Thus, contemporary cultural malaise is no longer solely about the repression of drives but also about the psychological consequences of living in a society dominated by unattainable ideals and indirect violence. Addressing this malaise requires a re-evaluation of societal priorities, focusing on fostering genuine connections, challenging unrealistic standards, and rebuilding cultural structures that protect and nurture rather than isolate and harm.

In this hyperreal environment, the physical body, with its natural imperfections, contrasts starkly with the culturally sanctioned "legitimate" body—an idealized form influenced by complex social pressures. Pierre Bourdieu (1987) describes this body as "more spoken about than speaking", meaning it functions not as a natural expression of identity but as an object shaped by societal norms and expectations. In modern culture, attributes like youth, beauty, and thinness are no longer seen as merely personal traits but have become aestheticized markers of worth and social acceptance (Bourdieu, 1987). They function as "commodifiable signs" within a consumer-driven society, reinforcing a hierarchy where "youth-signs" and other markers of desirability can be bought, sold, and used to confer social legitimacy and status.

This shift intensifies the cultural malaise Freud identified by embedding individuals in a world where personal value is closely tied to an idealized appearance that is almost impossible to achieve. In this landscape, the body is less an expression of individual identity and more a product shaped to meet society's hyperreal standards. The resulting disconnect between individuals' authentic selves and society's expectations can deepen feelings of inadequacy and alienation, reinforcing the cycle of cultural malaise Freud warned against.

Eating disorders and their relationship with culture: Collages of contemporary culture

Contemporary culture defies linear interpretation, manifesting itself as a complex web of intersecting patterns that both shape and bind individuals within it. This network of influences is vividly captured in what Ulloa describes as the "culture of mortification", a social phenomenon marked by:

> a lifeless quality, lacking strength, dim, and devoid of vitality... Once it takes root, the individual is restrained, on the verge of suppression as a thinking being... In these conditions, critical action diminishes, even self-criticism fades away. Instead, a persistent complaint emerges—one that never rises to the level of protest, as if the individual relies on their own weaknesses to seek the pity of those who oppress them
>
> (Ulloa, 1995).

Within this "culture of mortification", individuals become trapped in a passive state, where cultural expectations and ideals suppress autonomy and the ability to self-define. EDs illustrate how deeply these constraints can permeate personal experiences, as they often embody an individual's attempt to comply with societal standards, only to become more entrenched in self-criticism and diminished self-worth. Rather than empowering individuals, the cultural emphasis on image and self-control reinforces dependency on external validation, suppressing true self-expression.

This framework of passive compliance can be observed in the behaviors associated with EDs, where individuals internalize cultural ideals, yet feel unable to voice dissent or break free from the cycle of self-regulation. Bound by a pervasive sense of inadequacy, they may seek solace in meeting narrow standards of beauty, only to find themselves further distanced from their authentic selves. In a culture that subtly favors compliance over critical agency, the struggle of individuals with EDs reveals the broader impact of the "culture of mortification", a cultural force that prioritizes appearance and self-regulation over genuine empowerment and self-discovery.

By highlighting this complex cultural context, Ulloa's (1995) insights offer a deeper understanding of how modern society's web of expectations can stifle the individual, rendering autonomy and genuine self-expression elusive for those who, in striving to fit societal molds, are often left feeling both controlled and disconnected.

Media and the universality of bodily standards

Mass media is a primary force that propagates and universalizes ideals of "desirable bodies", reinforcing stereotypes of what constitutes a "legitimate" appearance. This constant reinforcement shapes perceptions of self-worth and identity according to socially constructed standards, leading individuals—particularly those vulnerable to EDs—to internalize an unattainable aesthetic ideal. The pervasive reach of media goes deep into individual psyches, embedding these ideals as benchmarks for personal value and acceptance.

This effect aligns with characteristics of the current era described by certain scholars: "By encouraging excessive ambitions and making their fulfillment impossible, the narcissistic society promotes self-denigration and self-contempt" (Lipovetsky, 1983). As this societal model destabilizes traditional frameworks, it further disorganizes values around food and body image. In affluent societies, where the abundance of choices creates a sense of overload, people experience what Guillemot (Guillemot and Lazenaire, 1994) terms "gastro-anomie". Drawing on Emile Durkheim's concept of "anomie" (1987), this state reflects a lack of guiding norms to regulate social behavior, leading to feelings of fragmentation, disintegration, and confusion around food choices.

This sense of fragmentation often becomes manifest on the body itself through self-inflicted wounds, where physical scars express internal chaos and a lack of containment. For some, self-harm provides a fleeting sense of relief or calm; for others, it acts as a form of self-punishment for failing to meet an impossible cultural ideal. In this way, the body becomes a canvas of both social critique and self-judgment, symbolizing a painful struggle with societal expectations.

Addressing these urgent, evolving forms of suffering requires a perspective that recognizes science and culture as active, interconnected processes shaped by social dynamics. Discourses, social practices, and language are not passive tools, they are active constructs that must be deconstructed, examined, and questioned. A productive approach to understanding and addressing EDs must embrace this complexity, viewing the causal chains of suffering not as isolated occurrences but as part of a shared cultural landscape.

How psychoanalysis can help: From individual to social cure

Psychoanalysis offers a unique lens for understanding the complex interplay between individual psychology and social context in the treatment of EDs. This approach is exemplified in the case of a young woman who joined our therapeutic program after hospitalization for a severe electrolyte imbalance, a consequence of frequent vomiting used to maintain her weight.

During her initial interview, she remarked:

> What bothers me is not knowing how I am right now. Physically, on the outside—I'm great! at a competitive level, in the market, let's put it that way; because that's how clothes are, that's what sells. If a shirt doesn't fit, or if there's a visible roll, you're just out.

Her words reveal an acute awareness of social expectations and the powerful influence of image as a determinant of worth. She expressed her belief that her physical appearance allowed her to "fit in", enabling her to meet the approval of her social circle and society at large.

Yet she went on to acknowledge the discrepancy between this image and her actual health:

> Outwardly, I'm supposedly a ten out of ten. Physically, my body isn't a ten—I have multiple complications: organ damage, heart arrhythmia, I'm low on sodium and potassium, I have gastritis....

This stark contrast between her image and her reality exposes a profound inner confusion:

> I don't even know how I really am!

In her case, BN provided a means to secure a place in society and a sense of belonging, albeit through the painful compromise of splitting herself into an outward "perfect" body and an inwardly struggling one. This fragmentation reflects a fractured identity and points to the broader cultural conditions that reinforce such divides.

Integrating individual and cultural healing in the "culture workshop"

To guide treatment at the specialized unit for EDs and establish meaningful goals for healing, we propose a methodology that positions all participants as co-researchers collaboratively addressing a shared challenge. This model emphasizes a transformative, interdisciplinary approach that transcends the limitations of traditional, hierarchical structures. By fostering collaboration, it ensures that diverse sources of knowledge are preserved and actively expanded, valuing each participant's unique insights as essential to a comprehensive understanding of the problem. Through this collective commitment to healing and understanding, an inclusive environment is created where genuine and lasting progress becomes possible.

This vision came to life at the "Day Hospital Unit for Eating Disorders" at the José T. Borda Hospital in Buenos Aires City through the creation of the innovative "Culture Workshop." Developed in collaboration with the Gino Germani Institute of the Faculty of Social Sciences at the University of Buenos Aires and under the leadership of sociologist Delia Franco, the workshop integrates the cultural dimension into the treatment of EDs. It acknowledges that these disorders are not merely individual psychological conditions but are deeply interwoven with societal and cultural pressures.

The "Culture Workshop" provides a transformative space where participants can critically examine and redefine the influences that shape their experiences. By addressing the cultural narratives and expectations that contribute to body dissatisfaction and disordered eating, the workshop moves beyond traditional clinical approaches. It fosters an environment of collective inquiry and reflection, enabling participants to unpack how societal ideals impact their self-perception and behavior. Through this process, the workshop helps participants gain new insights, empowering them to challenge and reframe the cultural forces contributing to their struggles.

Rooted in interdisciplinary collaboration, the "Culture Workshop" encourages participants to examine the interplay between personal experiences and societal expectations, uncovering the cultural forces that shape their lives. This approach reflects the therapeutic potential of art as both a medium for critique and a pathway to healing. For instance, artwork created during the workshop, such as a piece depicting interwoven lines forming a cage, vividly captures the sense of entrapment imposed by societal ideals. This imagery echoes the themes explored by artists like Berta Teglio, whose textile art delves into notions of entanglement, constraint, and the tension between individuality and collective norms.

By drawing parallels between the therapeutic process and Teglio's art, the workshop underscores how cultural pressures become internalized and manifest as personal struggles. Both the participants' creations and Teglio's works serve as powerful tools for reflection, illustrating the profound impact of societal ideals and offering new perspectives for understanding and addressing these challenges.

The collaborative framework of the workshop aligns with the principles of co-research, where participants, clinicians, and researchers collectively unpack the cultural narratives that perpetuate cycles of control and dissatisfaction. By fostering dialogue and exploration, the workshop not only facilitates individual recovery but also promotes a deeper cultural understanding. This approach ensures that healing transcends the clinical setting, addressing the societal roots of EDs and fostering resilience against cultural pressures.

Ultimately, the "Culture Workshop" demonstrates the power of integrating therapeutic practice with cultural critique. By creating a space where individuals can explore their struggles within a broader cultural context, it empowers participants to reclaim their narratives and challenge the societal expectations that shape their experiences. Through this interdisciplinary and collaborative approach, the workshop exemplifies how collective inquiry, and creativity can serve as pathways to healing, understanding, and cultural transformation.

The workshop's discussions focus on two central themes:

1   *Culture as imposition*: Culture is explored as a dominant force that normalizes suffering by creating standards and expectations that infiltrate and shape the body's meaning. This "cultural imposition" is seen as a power dynamic that not only frames how bodies are perceived but also defines the terms of social belonging.
2   *Culture as construct*: Culture is also viewed as an ongoing process, continuously drawing boundaries yet offering the potential to bridge different types of knowledge. This perspective allows for a dynamic interpretation of culture as a shared construction that can be redefined collaboratively.

In this therapeutic and investigatory space, individuals engage with their cultural landscapes, expressing their interpretations and personal experiences. This dialogue often leads to creative works that reflect their evolving understanding of the cultural expectations surrounding body image and self-worth. By discussing and co-producing these representations with therapists and sociologists, patients begin to reconstruct their relationships with their bodies and culture, with the potential to create new, more empowering social representations.

Collaborative creation: Bridging individual and social healing

The workshop invites patients to engage in various forms of creative expression, producing collective works that reflect their experiences with culture and body image. This creative process enables participants to delve into and articulate both the psychological and cultural dimensions of their eating disorder patterns. By positioning patients, staff therapists, and sociologists as co-creators, the workshop fosters active engagement with their condition, cultivating a sense of agency and shared purpose. In a symbolic act of reclamation and redefinition, participants renamed the "Day Hospital" as "Life's Hospital," signifying their collective desire for transformation and renewal.

These collaborative artworks serve a dual purpose: they are both therapeutic and investigative. On one level, they provide a means for participants to externalize and process their emotions, while on another, they offer profound insights into how cultural forces influence individual suffering. By encouraging shared creativity, the workshop dismantles the traditional hierarchical structure of therapeutic settings. This approach softens the boundaries between therapist and patient, creating a space for authentic and mutual exploration. Through this dynamic, participants transition from isolation to connection, and from suffering to understanding, as they work together to challenge the cultural frameworks that contribute to their struggles.

In sum, the workshop represents a psychoanalytic and cultural approach that acknowledges healing from EDs requires more than addressing individual symptoms. It reframes the therapeutic process as a co-investigation, empowering participants to confront and reshape the cultural narratives that underlie their disorders. By positioning psychoanalysis as both a tool for personal insight and a means for collective transformation, the workshop shifts the focus from isolated self-worth to a collaborative exploration of shared cultural dynamics. This innovative methodology highlights the potential for healing through connection, creativity, and a reimagining of cultural values, demonstrating the profound impact of integrating art and culture into therapeutic practices.

Understanding eating disorders through a socio-cultural lens

Viewing EDs through a socio-cultural lens allows us to see these conditions as complex, multidimensional phenomena shaped by contemporary social and cultural forces. These disorders do not arise in isolation; they are deeply intertwined with broader socio-cultural dimensions that have been transformed by macro-social changes over recent decades. This perspective challenges conventional mental health paradigms and calls for an expansion in both theory and intervention to address these disorders holistically.

EDs, from this view, cannot be fully understood or addressed by focusing on the individual alone. Rather, they must be situated within the wider social context that shapes and influences personal identity, self-worth, and behaviors. These social and cultural dimensions should therefore be integral to both our understanding and intervention efforts, targeting not only the individual symptoms but also the broader socio-cultural factors that contribute to the experience of suffering.

The "Culture Workshop", developed within the therapeutic framework at the Day Hospital Unit, illustrates the potential for a socio-cultural approach to foster healing. As described by Ulloa, it aims to cultivate "psychological security", a group atmosphere where members' experiences resonate with one another, creating "an emotional resonance that fosters intimacy and reduces intimidation" (Ulloa, 1995). The collaborative process dismantles hierarchical structures, repositioning each participant—whether patient, therapist, or researcher—as a co-investigator in exploring and addressing their condition. What began as a discovery space evolved into a source of well-being, shifting the focus from merely treating symptoms to addressing the root unease and blockages. In this collective space, shared understanding and wisdom flourish, creating a more communal, inclusive approach to knowledge and healing.

Although EDs have ancient origins, they are also products of the specific social and cultural pressures of our time. In both the visual expressions created by patients in the workshop and in contemporary art, we observe recurring themes of fragmentation, fragility, and isolation. These themes reflect not only individual experiences but also the pervasive cultural environment that often fails to listen to or fully understand the suffering behind these conditions.

Conclusion

To address EDs effectively, it is crucial to integrate both individual and socio-cultural perspectives, recognizing these disorders as symptomatic of a broader cultural malaise. This approach requires moving beyond traditional, individual-focused treatments to encompass collective strategies that address the cultural and societal influences underlying the disorder. By fostering environments of shared inquiry and mutual support, such as those provided by the "Culture Workshop", we can work toward interventions that promote understanding, empowerment, and healing not only for the individual but also within the social fabric that surrounds them. This shift from isolated treatment to a more communal and inclusive approach offers a pathway to a more holistic and sustainable cure for those grappling with EDs in our contemporary world.

Bibliography

Baudrillard, J. (1998). Simulacra and Simulations. In M. Poster (ed.) *Jean Baudrillard, Selected Writings*. Stanford, CA: Stanford University Press, 166–184.

Bauman, Z. (2000). *Liquid Modernity*. Cambridge: Polity Press in association with Blackwell Publishing Ltd.

Bhatia, K. and Dane, S. (2023). The social media diet: A scoping review to investigate the association between social media, body image and eating disorders amongst young people. *PLOS Global Public Health*, 3(3).

Bourdieu, P. (1987). Notas provisorias sobre la percepción social del cuerpo. In *Materiales de Sociología Crítica*. Buenos Aires: Ed. La Piqueta.

Cash, T. F. (2005). The influence of sociocultural factors on body image: Searching for constructs. *Clinical Psychology: Science and Practice*, 12(4).

Castel, R. (1997). La sociedad salarial. In *Las Metamorfosis de la Cuestión Social*. Buenos Aires: Paidós, 438–442.

Dahlgren, C. L., Sundgot-Borgen, C., Kvalem, I. L., Wennersberg, A. L., and Wisting, L. (2024). Further evidence of the association between social media use, eating disorder pathology and appearance ideals and pressure: a cross-sectional study in Norwegian adolescents. *Journal of Eating Disorders*, 12(1): 34.

Durkheim, E. (1987). *La División del Trabajo Social. (Vol. 39)*. Buenos Aires: Ediciones Akal.

Farr, R. M. (1993). Common sense, science and social representations. *Public Understanding of Science*, 2(3): 189–204.

Farr, R. M. (1994). Attitudes, social representations and social attitudes. *Papers on Social Representations*, 3(1): 30–33.

Freud, S. (1930) [1929]. Civilization and Its Discontents. *The Standard Edition of the Complete Psychological Works of Sigmund Freud, (21)*. London: The Hogarth Press, 59–145 (1991 edition).

Guillemot, A., and Laxenaire, M. (1994). *Anorexia Nerviosa y Bulimia: El Peso de la Cultura*. Barcelona: Masson.

Hepworth, J. (1999). *The Social Construction of Anorexia Nervosa. Inquiries in Social Construction*. London: Sage Publishing.

Jeammet, P., and Bochereau, D. (2007). *La Souffrance des Adolescents*. Paris: La Découverte.

Jordan, G. L., García, M. D., Cano, M. M., Cubo, M. J., Díez, B. L., Martín, A. S., … and Ayesa-Arriola, R. (2021). Can social media be beneficial for eating disorders? *European Psychiatry*, 64(1): S703.

Lipovetsky, G. (1983). *La Era del Vacío: Ensayos Sobre el Individualismo Contemporáneo*. Barcelona: Anagrama.

Lutenberg, J. (2008). El vacío mental estructural y el vacío emocional. *Revista de Psicoanálisis*, 65(4): 829–850.

Masson, C. (2015). Modified images of the Body. In E. Sukhanova and H. Thomashoff (eds.) *Body Image and Identity in Contemporary Societies: Psychoanalytic, Social, Cultural and Aesthetic Perspectives*. London: Routledge, 95–103 (chapter 12).

Mora, M. (2002). *La Teoría de las Representaciones Sociales de Serge Moscovici*. Mexico: Athenea digital.

Moscovici, S. (1961). *La Psychanalyse son Image et son Public: Et de sur la Representation Sociale de la Psychanalyse*. Paris: Press Universitaires de France.

Moscovici, S. (1988). Notes towards a description of social representations. *European Journal of Social Psychology*, 18(3), 211–250.

Moscovici, S. (2014). The new magical thinking. *Public Understanding of Science*, 23 (7):759–779.

Orbach, S. (2016). *Fat is a Feminist Issue*. London: Random House.

Orbach, S. (2019). *Bodies*. London: Profile books.

Osofsky, J. D. (1997). *Children in a Violent Society*. New York: Guilford Press.

Páez, D., Ubillos, S., Zubieta, E., and Marques, J. (2012). AIDS' social representations: Beliefs, attitudes, memory and social sharing of rumours. In A. Silvana de Rosa (ed.) *Social Representations in the 'Social Arena'.* London and New York: Routledge, 166–175.

Persano, H. L. (2005). Abordagem psicodinâmica do paciente com trastornos alimentares. In C. L. Eizirik, R. W. Aguiar, S. S. Schestatsky(eds.) *Psicoterapia de Orientação Analítica: Fundamentos Teóricos e Clínicos.* Porto Alegre: Artmed, 674–688 (chapter 49).

Persano, H. L. (2022). Self-harm. *The International Journal of Psychoanalysis,* 103 (6):1089–1103.

Persano, H. L., Bialakowsky, A., Franco, D., Cuesta, M.and Patrouilleau, M. (2003). Exclusión social y nuevos padecimientos en la cultura contemporánea, Abordaje Interdisciplinario en Dispositivos Colectivos. In X *Jornada Psicoanálisis y Comunidad: Angustia Social e Incertidumbre: Fragilización Existencial, Exclusión y Marginalidad, September 2003.* Buenos Aires: APA.

Ulloa, F. (1995). *La Clínica Psicoanalítica. Historial de Una Práctica.* Buenos Aires: Paidós.

11 Integration and future directions

Introduction: The complexity of eating disorders and psychoanalytic contributions

Extending Psychoanalysis beyond the couch: A holistic approach to complex disorders

No simple solution exists for problems as intricate and multifaceted as eating disorders (EDs). Achieving meaningful and lasting transformation requires an in-depth understanding of the dynamics underlying these conditions. Therapeutic goals must not merely address symptoms but aim for deeper psychic stability, requiring the individual to acknowledge their condition and actively engage as a suffering subject in the healing process. Psychoanalysis offers a profound framework for exploring the roots of suffering, fostering self-awareness, and promoting active participation in recovery.

Approaches that alienate individuals from understanding their suffering or promise external solutions detached from the patient's subjective experience are often doomed to fail. Such methods risk perpetuating psychic splitting—a defense mechanism that fragments the self and reinforces the symptomatic cycles characteristic of EDs. This splitting exacerbates suffering and significantly increases the risk of severe complications, including chronic conditions and even death. A comprehensive treatment strategy must integrate psychoanalytic insight with multidisciplinary and interdisciplinary approaches to address the full complexity of EDs.

Expanding psychoanalytic reach beyond the individual arena

Traditional psychoanalytic practice often unfolds within the confines of the "couch"—a one-on-one, introspective therapeutic relationship. However, the complexity of disorders like EDs necessitates a broader application of psychoanalytic principles, extending its reach into institutional, academic, and public health domains. This expansion reflects psychoanalysis' adaptability and its capacity to enrich approaches beyond individual clinical settings (Persano, 2014); (Schwartz, 2022).

DOI: 10.4324/9781032724997-11

Psychoanalysis in institutional settings

- In institutional contexts, psychoanalytic principles can be applied to therapeutic community models, day hospitals, and group therapy programs. Here, psychoanalysis helps create spaces where patients can explore their experiences collectively, fostering new relational dynamics and a sense of belonging. These settings allow psychoanalytic insights to inform the design of treatment programs, emphasizing the importance of containment, transference dynamics, and the therapeutic milieu.
- By working within multidisciplinary teams, psychoanalysts contribute a deep understanding of unconscious processes, enabling more nuanced interventions that address the psychological roots of disorders. This collaboration also helps bridge the gap between traditional psychoanalysis and more pragmatic, symptom-focused treatments, offering patients a comprehensive framework for recovery.

Academic integration

- Psychoanalysis has a vital role to play in academic settings, shaping the education and training of mental health professionals and health care. Its theoretical insights provide a rich foundation for understanding the unconscious mechanisms at play in EDs and other complex disorders. By integrating psychoanalytic concepts into curricula for psychology, psychiatry, and social work, academic institutions ensure that future practitioners are equipped with a deeper understanding of the human psyche.
- Additionally, psychoanalytic research can contribute to the development of innovative treatment models, exploring the intersections of body, mind, and culture. This research fosters dialogue between psychoanalysis and other disciplines, such as neuroscience, sociology, and public health, enriching the broader understanding of mental health conditions.

Public health and policy development

- Perhaps the most transformative potential of psychoanalysis lies in its ability to inform public health strategies and policies. By addressing the societal and cultural factors that contribute to EDs—such as unrealistic beauty standards, trauma, and social isolation—psychoanalytic insights can shape prevention programs and community interventions.
- Public health campaigns informed by psychoanalytic perspectives can challenge societal norms that perpetuate psychic suffering, promoting awareness and early intervention. Furthermore, psychoanalysis can

guide the design of policies that prioritize mental health services, ensuring equitable access to care and fostering collaboration between healthcare systems and community organizations.

Psychoanalysis as a bridge to comprehensive care

By extending its reach beyond the individual therapeutic setting, psychoanalysis demonstrates its relevance and adaptability in addressing complex modern disorders. It provides a framework for understanding not only individual suffering but also the systemic and cultural forces that shape mental health. Whether in institutional environments, academic research, or public health initiatives, psychoanalysis offers tools to address the intricate interplay of mind, body, and society.

Through its integration with multidisciplinary and interdisciplinary approaches, psychoanalysis transcends its traditional boundaries, enriching collective efforts to transform suffering into healing. This expanded role ensures that psychoanalysis remains a cornerstone of mental health care, offering profound insights and practical strategies for addressing the most challenging conditions in both clinical and societal contexts.

Integrating multidisciplinary and interdisciplinary approaches to eating disorders

EDs are among the most complex and multifaceted conditions in mental health, requiring a comprehensive and collaborative response. Both multidisciplinary and interdisciplinary approaches are essential for addressing the intricate physical, psychological, and social dimensions of these disorders, yet they serve distinct purposes and must work in tandem to achieve meaningful outcomes.

The multidisciplinary approach: A collaborative imperative

A multidisciplinary approach is foundational to effective treatment, necessitating the coordinated efforts of a diverse team of professionals. Psychiatrists, psychologists, nutritionists, clinical physicians, pediatricians, adolescent specialists, nurses, occupational therapists, social workers, gynecologists, endocrinologists, and odontologists must collaborate to address the wide-ranging needs of patients with EDs. Each discipline contributes unique expertise, from managing medical complications and nutritional rehabilitation to supporting emotional recovery and addressing underlying psychological factors.

However, assembling a diverse team is only the first step. True multidisciplinary care transcends the coexistence of different fields. It requires meaningful collaboration, shared treatment goals, and continuous communication among team members. Without this integration, treatment risks becoming fragmented, with professionals working in silos and failing to deliver cohesive care. The multidisciplinary model emphasizes the need for dynamic interplay among disciplines to provide a comprehensive and unified approach that supports effective and lasting recovery.

The interdisciplinary approach: Bridging boundaries

Interdisciplinary work goes beyond the collaboration of multiple fields; it fosters a deeper integration of methodologies and perspectives. Interdisciplinarity represents not just a convergence of knowledge but also a boundary that reveals the limitations of individual disciplines. This boundary compels professionals to engage with one another's expertise, creating a shared understanding of the complex interplay between biological, psychological, and sociocultural factors in EDs (Persano, 2014).

Such interdisciplinary dialogue is both challenging and indispensable, requiring continuous efforts to bridge diverse methodologies and epistemologies. Psychoanalysis, for example, offers invaluable insights into the unconscious mechanisms underlying EDs, providing a profound understanding of mental dynamics and the formation of the psyche.

However, as Persano et al. (2003) note, "the application of psychoanalysis in institutional contexts often diverges from its classical techniques". This evolution is captured in Racamier's (1970) concept of the "psychoanalyst without a couch", emphasizing the adaptations required for psychoanalytic work within collaborative institutional frameworks.

Building on this foundation, Birot, Chabert, and Jeammet, (2006) present an important exploration of psychoanalysts working with patients suffering from EDs in hospital settings, further enriching this dialogue. Similarly, Schwartz (2022) contributes significantly to the field by examining the application of psychoanalysis within the broader context of medical care.

Bringing multidisciplinary and interdisciplinary together

While the multidisciplinary approach ensures that diverse aspects of EDs are addressed by specialists from various fields, the interdisciplinary approach fosters a cohesive integration of these perspectives. Both models are necessary: the multidisciplinary team brings breadth and scope, while interdisciplinary dialogue ensures depth and integration. Together, they form a robust framework capable of addressing the multifaceted nature of EDs.

By fostering collaboration and mutual respect among disciplines, these approaches ensure that patients receive comprehensive care tailored to their unique needs. Recovery from EDs is not achieved through isolated interventions but through a dynamic, collective effort that unites diverse expertise with a shared understanding of the patient's experience. This holistic integration of multidisciplinary and interdisciplinary efforts offers the depth, breadth, and cohesion required to support long-term healing and transformation.

Some epidemiological data on eating disorders

Prevalence and incidence of eating disorders

EDs, encompassing anorexia nervosa (AN), bulimia nervosa (BN), and binge-eating disorder (BED), are significant public health concerns worldwide. They not only impose a substantial psychological burden on individuals but also impact physical health, relationships, and social functioning. The World Health Organization (WHO, 2022) identifies eating disorders (EDs) as a growing public health concern within the broader field of mental health, emphasizing their increasing global prevalence, early age of onset, and significant long-term consequences. EDs are not only associated with elevated rates of comorbidity—such as anxiety, depression, and substance use—but also with some of the highest mortality rates among psychiatric conditions. The WHO stresses the need for early detection, integrated care, and culturally sensitive prevention strategies, particularly among adolescents and young adults, where the burden of these disorders is rapidly rising.

Global impact

Globally, EDs affect millions of people across different age groups and socio-economic backgrounds. They are particularly prevalent among adolescents and young adults, often emerging during critical developmental periods such as puberty and young adulthood. These disorders also disproportionately impact women, although men are increasingly recognized as being affected, albeit often underdiagnosed.

Lifetime prevalence

International research reports a combined prevalence of EDs of 13.1% among young women (Gómez-Candela et al., 2016); (Stice, Marti, and Rohde, 2013). Furthermore, according to the consensus on the "Evaluation and Nutritional Treatment of Eating Disorders" from the Spanish Society of Clinical Nutrition and Metabolism (SENPE), the prevalence of AN ranges between 0.5–1%, and that of BN is estimated at 2–4%. Among adults, the most prevalent ED is BED, with a prevalence of 2–5%, which increases significantly among individuals enrolled in weight loss programs, reaching 19–30% (Gómez-Candela et al., 2016).

A comprehensive systematic review by Hoek and van Hoeken (2003) remains a cornerstone in understanding the epidemiology of EDs. Their findings revealed the following:

1 *Anorexia nervosa:*

- Lifetime prevalence in women: 0.9%
- Lifetime prevalence in men: 0.3%
- Characterized by an intense fear of weight gain and a distorted body image, AN lead to severe physical complications, including cardiovascular problems, osteoporosis, and organ failure.

2 *Bulimia nervosa:*

- Lifetime prevalence in women: 1.5%
- Lifetime prevalence in men: 0.5%
- Marked by recurrent binge-eating episodes followed by compensatory behaviors (e.g., vomiting, laxative use), BN is associated with electrolyte imbalances, gastrointestinal issues, and significant psychological distress.

3 *Binge-eating disorder:*

- Although not included in the Hoek and van Hoeken study, more recent data indicate that BED affects 2–3% of the general population, making it the most common ED. Unlike BN, it lacks compensatory behaviors, leading to a higher risk of obesity and related health complications.

However, when examining adolescents and young adults—the age groups most affected by EDs—the prevalence rises significantly, highlighting their heightened vulnerability. Among young females, particularly in early adolescence, EDs constitute a primary reason for seeking care in mental health services. As mentioned earlier, the prevalence of EDs varies depending on several factors, including the population studied. These disorders are predominantly concentrated in young populations aged 15 to 24 years and are more common among females, with a female-to-male ratio of 10:1 (Pérez et al., 2017).

The hidden burden

The true prevalence of EDs is likely underestimated due to:

- *Underdiagnosis*: Many individuals, particularly men and older adults, go undiagnosed due to societal stigma and a lack of awareness among healthcare providers.
- *Subclinical Cases*: Disordered eating behaviors that do not meet full diagnostic criteria can still cause significant distress and impairment.

Comprehensive multilevel approach to eating disorders treatment: Integrating prevention, intervention, and rehabilitation

Effectively addressing EDs requires a multilevel healthcare approach that integrates primary, secondary, and tertiary strategies. Each level serves a distinct and essential purpose: from prevention at the community level to targeted interventions and comprehensive rehabilitation programs. Therapeutic community models play a pivotal role across these stages, offering significant benefits by fostering collective recovery, reducing stigma, and ensuring accessibility.

The framework for these multilevel interventions was developed during my tenure as General Director of Mental Health Services at the Ministry of Health in the City of Buenos Aires and through my role as head of *The Network on Eating Disorders* within the same Ministry. These roles provided the foundation for designing and implementing a system that integrates diverse levels of care while emphasizing collaboration among public health services, therapeutic networks, and specialized programs (Persano, Rodríguez, and Salusky, 2021).

This networked approach optimizes public resources by enabling facilities to support one another through consultations and referrals. As a referral center, we receive patient transfers from both the network and programs, while also directing cases beyond our capacity to other networked facilities. This collaborative model ensures more efficient resource utilization and improves patient outcomes by leveraging the combined strengths of multiple centers (PAHO/WHO, 2010).

Although this book does not focus specifically on these multilevel interventions, it is important to briefly describe them to contextualize the broader discussion. The integration of primary prevention strategies, early intervention at the secondary level, and specialized rehabilitation at the tertiary level underscores the necessity of a coordinated, holistic approach. This system ensures that individuals with EDs receive the comprehensive care they need at every stage of their journey, from risk mitigation to long-term recovery and reintegration into their communities.

Primary level: Prevention strategies

At the primary level, prevention efforts focus on reducing risk factors and promoting protective factors for eating disorders. Public health campaigns, school-based programs, and community education initiatives aim to address societal pressures related to body image, promote healthy eating habits, and encourage early awareness of ED symptoms. These strategies target broad populations to mitigate the cultural and psychological factors that contribute to the development of EDs. Integrating therapeutic community models within this stage can foster environments of support and inclusion, reducing stigma and creating spaces for open dialogue about mental health and body image.

Secondary level: Early intervention

Secondary-level approaches focus on the early identification and intervention for individuals at risk of developing eating disorders (EDs) or presenting with early symptoms. Services at this level include screening in primary care settings, outpatient programs, and targeted interventions such as counseling and nutritional guidance. Specialized teams enhance secondary care by providing structured environments where patients can access group therapy, peer support, psychopharmacological treatments, psychotherapy, and brief hospitalizations when needed. These collaborative settings foster early engagement, effectively addressing symptoms and reducing the likelihood of progression to more severe stages, thereby minimizing the need for intensive care.

Tertiary level: Specialized treatment and rehabilitation

Tertiary-level care focuses on individuals with established EDs, providing specialized treatments and long-term rehabilitation programs. Day hospital programs and residential treatment centers are pivotal at this stage. Therapeutic community models, particularly within day hospital settings, have demonstrated significant benefits in optimizing healthcare resource utilization and enhancing accessibility. A systematic review by Zipfel et al. (2002) highlighted the advantages of day hospital programs for EDs in Toronto and Munich, noting better resource allocation and improved patient outcomes compared to inpatient care. These programs employ multidisciplinary teams to deliver comprehensive medical, psychological, and nutritional support tailored to each patient's unique needs.

Rehabilitation efforts at this level aim to reintegrate patients into society, address comorbid conditions, and reduce relapse risks. For chronic cases, full residential programs offer intensive care for ED patients. However, such facilities are currently unavailable in Argentina, posing challenges to the long-term management of these patients.

Economic and public health benefits of networks and programs with therapeutic communities in eating disorder care

Effective care for EDs requires not only multidisciplinary and interdisciplinary collaboration but also robust networks and therapeutic community models that enhance accessibility, efficiency, and equity in healthcare. Networks of care and therapeutic communities offer significant economic and public health advantages, particularly within public healthcare systems.

By providing group-based care, therapeutic communities enable a greater number of patients to access treatment compared to individual therapy models, which can be cost-prohibitive or restricted by insurance limitations. These communities ensure equitable access to care, reaching individuals across diverse socioeconomic backgrounds. Importantly, they foster environments that reduce stigma, promote peer support, and encourage a sense of shared purpose in recovery, elements critical to the long-term success of ED treatment (Persano, 2014).

The role of working networks in ED care

Working networks—comprising healthcare providers, community organizations, and public health systems—play a crucial role in creating cohesive pathways for ED care. These networks facilitate communication and collaboration between primary care, specialist services, and community resources, ensuring seamless transitions for patients across different stages of care. By linking prevention, intervention, and rehabilitation efforts, networks can address EDs comprehensively, providing patients with continuous and integrated support throughout their recovery journey (Persano et al. 2021).

Additionally, networks strengthen the reach and effectiveness of therapeutic community models by connecting these programs to broader public health strategies. They enable knowledge-sharing among professionals, ensure consistency in care standards, and adapt services to meet the unique needs of local populations.

Integrating therapeutic communities' programs across levels of ED care

The flexibility of therapeutic communities makes them highly adaptable across the three levels of care for EDs:

- *Primary level (Prevention)*: Therapeutic communities can be embedded in prevention programs to build supportive networks that promote awareness, reduce stigma, and foster early detection of ED risk factors.
- *Secondary level (Early intervention)*: These communities provide cost-effective and accessible settings for early intervention, offering structured group therapy, psychoeducation, and peer support that address ED symptoms before they escalate.
- *Tertiary level (Specialized treatment and rehabilitation)*: At the tertiary level, therapeutic communities provide structured environments for intensive treatment and long-term rehabilitation. By emphasizing collective recovery and community reintegration, they reduce the burden on inpatient facilities and help patients transition more smoothly to everyday life.

Holistic benefits of integrating networks and specialized programs in eating disorder care

The integration of therapeutic communities within well-structured care networks significantly enhances the efficiency and effectiveness of health-care systems. By optimizing resources, improving treatment outcomes, and ensuring accessible, equitable care, these networks enable a comprehensive approach to ED management. Through coordinated efforts, patients receive not only clinical treatment but also support that addresses the social, cultural, and emotional dimensions of recovery.

Networks act as vital connectors, ensuring that specialized programs and therapeutic communities are part of a seamless continuum of care. This interconnected system supports patients through every stage of their journey, from prevention to intervention and rehabilitation, promoting long-term recovery. Day hospitals and specialized programs provide safe and collaborative spaces for peer support, new healthy experiences, and collective recovery—key components for addressing the multifaceted nature of EDs.

This integrated approach also highlights the critical role of networks as public health tools. By pooling shared resources and fostering collaboration among multidisciplinary teams, networks create sustainable models of care. They prioritize early detection, comprehensive interventions, and holistic rehabilitation strategies, addressing EDs not only as individual clinical challenges but also as broader public health concerns.

The synergy between specialized day hospitals for EDs and specialized programs with robust networks fosters resilience, equity, and inclusivity within ED care. These systems help bridge gaps in access to care, reduce stigma, and provide a patient-centered framework that supports individuals in rebuilding their lives. By leveraging collective expertise and innovative care models, healthcare systems can pave the way for more sustainable and effective solutions, ensuring that no one is left without the support they need for recovery.

Integrating psychoanalytic approaches in the intensive care day hospital for eating disorder patients

Therapeutic services: Facilitating psychic change and transformation

The primary aim of the therapeutic services within our intensive care program is to support a comprehensive treatment strategy that fosters profound psychic change. This process represents a journey from suffering to transformative life change, emphasizing the verbalization of conflicts and the integration of fragmented aspects of the psyche.

For patients with severe characterological disturbances, these therapeutic interventions offer a space to process conflicts through verbal discourse, thereby expanding their capacity for pre-conscious verbal representations. By engaging patients in the exploration of deeply ingrained identifications tied to oppressive ideals or maladaptive behaviors, the program fosters a gradual integration of split psychic elements. This process often involves the emergence of archaic object relations in the therapeutic setting, providing a unique opportunity to examine and reconstruct these dynamics both intrapsychically and interpersonally (Persano, 2005).

The three topics are important: therapeutic community framework, milieu therapy environment, and embodiment experiences.

Therapeutic communities: A model for collaborative mental health care and recovery

Day hospital intensive care for patients with EDs draws conceptual inspiration from the therapeutic community model developed in post-World War II Great Britain—a pioneering framework that emphasizes collaborative, community-driven mental health care (Jones, 1953). At the core of this model is a profound principle regarding the interplay between society and mental health: if societal structures can contribute to the emergence of mental health disorders, they can also, through community-based interventions, become powerful tools for recovery and healing. This approach underscores the potential of group and community dynamics to foster individual well-being by creating supportive environments where collective care replaces isolation and alienation.

Although therapeutic community models have declined under contemporary pressures—such as fragmented information systems, increasing individualism, and the dominance of biomedical approaches—their principles remain highly relevant. These models counteract the alienation and burnout often experienced by health professionals working in siloed, discipline-specific settings by promoting teamwork, interdisciplinary collaboration, and shared problem-solving. They emphasize co-thinking and collective responsibility, creating spaces where both patients and professionals actively contribute to the healing process.

Community as a catalyst for recovery

García Badaracco (1990) expands the therapeutic community model by integrating multifamily-focused treatment, emphasizing its dual role: while societal factors often contribute to the development of mental health disorders, they can also be transformed into pathways for recovery. In this approach, therapeutic communities are intentionally designed to challenge and counteract the societal pressures that perpetuate conditions such as eating disorders. By fostering shared experiences, collaboration, and mutual understanding—not just among individuals but also within family systems—these communities create spaces for healing that are deeply rooted in connection and support. This multifamily dimension strengthens the community's capacity to address the complex relational dynamics often at the heart of these disorders, promoting a holistic recovery process.

A central element of this approach is the shift from symptomatic enactments to the verbal expression of emotions. This principle resonates with Freud's assertion that no one should be judged "in absentia or in effigy" (Freud, 1912). Therapeutic communities provide a structured and supportive space where symptom-driven behaviors can be safely contained and explored. Through this process, participants are encouraged to uncover and understand the origins of their distress. This exploration not only deepens insight but also ensures emotional safety and containment, enabling patients to process their experiences without fear of judgment or rejection.

Relevance in contemporary mental health care

Therapeutic communities remain a powerful response to the fragmented, often impersonal nature of modern healthcare. By integrating the principles of collaborative care and psychoanalytic exploration, they address the root causes of mental health disorders while creating spaces for connection and transformation. These communities exemplify the idea that healing is not a solitary endeavor but a collective process, rooted in the shared efforts of individuals and their communities.

This model underscores the potential for mental health care to be both innovative and deeply human, offering a vision of recovery that prioritizes not just the alleviation of symptoms but the restoration of individuals within their social and emotional contexts. Through these principles, therapeutic communities continue to serve as a blueprint for addressing complex mental health challenges, including EDs, in ways that are both effective and profoundly meaningful.

Horizontal structure and the integral role of nursing professionals in therapeutic communities

As Maxwell Jones (1953) emphasized, the success of the therapeutic community model lies in its horizontal structure, where hierarchical power dynamics are minimized, fostering an egalitarian environment that values the contributions of all team members. This approach promotes collaboration, mutual respect, and shared responsibility—key elements for the complex and multifaceted process of mental health recovery. Within this framework, nursing professionals play an integral and irreplaceable role, acting as a vital bridge between patients and the broader therapeutic team.

Nurses, by virtue of their continuous and direct contact with patients, are uniquely positioned to observe and interpret subtle fluctuations in mood, behavior, and resistance to therapy. Their proximity to patients allows them to detect nuances that might otherwise go unnoticed, providing critical insights into patient progress and challenges. These observations not only inform treatment strategies but also contribute to a deeper understanding of the patients' evolving needs.

The significance of integrating nurses' experiential knowledge into the therapeutic process was emphasized in a study on the co-production of knowledge conducted by sociologists in collaboration with a nurse's team (Bialakowsky et al., 2009). This research underscored how the informal, hands-on expertise of nurses serves as a valuable complement to formal clinical knowledge, thereby enriching the multidisciplinary team's approach to patient care. By sharing their daily observations and practical insights, nursing professionals play a crucial role in enhancing the team's capacity to adapt effectively to the complex dynamics of the therapeutic community.

To facilitate this integration, the nursing office is strategically located at the core of the intensive care day hospital for EDs. This central positioning ensures that nurses are the first point of contact for patients seeking care, enabling them to manage daily physical assessments, distribute medications, and address immediate patient concerns. Its placement is pivotal to the smooth functioning of the therapeutic community, serving as a hub where patients feel supported, and the team remains informed. This strategic design underscores the essential role of nursing staff in fostering both the operational efficiency and the therapeutic ethos of the community.

By embracing the principles of horizontal structure and actively leveraging the expertise of nursing professionals, therapeutic communities create a dynamic and inclusive environment that supports both patients and staff in the shared journey of mental health recovery.

The evolving role of staff in therapeutic communities: Cultivating stability and collaboration in changing times

In a true therapeutic community, every interpersonal interaction contributes to the healing process. This principle extends beyond clinical staff to include all individuals involved in maintaining the environment, from receptionists to cleaning staff. These roles, often overlooked, are critical in identifying subtle symptoms and maintaining a therapeutic milieu. For instance, a housekeeper noticing frequent bathroom visits might alert the team to possible purging behaviors, saying, "I think this patient is going to the bathroom too often—could they be vomiting again?" Such observations, when integrated into the care team's discussions, enhance the community's ability to respond holistically to patient needs.

Recognizing non-clinical staff as health agents rescues them from the alienation that repetitive work can impose. It also underscores the therapeutic community's ethos of inclusion and shared responsibility. For example, one young team member, initially part of an external service provider, has been with the program for over a decade and is regarded as an integral part of the therapeutic team. Her stability and commitment stand as a valuable counterpoint to the instability and fragmentation typical of what Zygmunt Bauman (2013) termed "liquid modernity".

In an era where roles and structures often feel transient, the therapeutic community's horizontal model stands out by emphasizing stability, collaboration, and a shared sense of purpose. In this model, nursing professionals and non-clinical staff play central roles in the therapeutic process. They are not only key observers of patient behavior but also active contributors to creating an emotional and physical environment conducive to healing. Their involvement extends beyond routine tasks to include participation in workshops and facilitating simple yet meaningful interventions within the psychological domain, reinforcing the community's collective commitment to recovery and well-being.

Daily case discussions provide a platform for articulating the informal and formal knowledge brought by all staff, ensuring that each voice contributes to patient care. This inclusion fosters a culture of respect and value, breaking down hierarchical barriers and enhancing the therapeutic potential of the community.

By embracing this horizontal structure, therapeutic communities not only improve outcomes for patients but also create an environment where every member of the team feels empowered and integral to the mission of care. This collective approach ensures that healing is not an isolated clinical endeavor, but a shared journey supported by a dynamic and inclusive community.

Bridging Psychoanalysis and therapeutic communities

By integrating psychoanalytic principles with the therapeutic community model, our program seeks to create a dynamic environment where symptoms are not merely managed but understood and transformed. The therapeutic community facilitates collective reflection and the co-creation of meaning, while psychoanalytic frameworks delve into the unconscious mechanisms driving disordered eating behaviors. Together, these approaches provide a robust structure for addressing the complex interplay of individual, interpersonal, and societal factors in eating disorders.

This integrated model not only promotes recovery but also empowers patients to move beyond symptomatic relief, fostering the development of a more cohesive, resilient sense of self. Through this synergy of psychoanalysis and therapeutic community principles, we aim to achieve lasting psychic transformation and a renewed capacity for meaningful engagement with life.

Transforming spaces for eating disorder treatment: The role of milieu therapy

The therapeutic environment as an active agent

Milieu therapy emphasizes the therapeutic environment as a dynamic and integral component of the healing process, particularly for individuals with eating disorders (EDs). Rather than serving merely as a backdrop, the milieu actively facilitates introspection, emotional growth, and gradual detachment from suffering. For patients with EDs, the environment must encourage shifts in attitudes toward food, body image, and social relationships, seamlessly integrating daily experiences into the therapeutic framework.

As Ammon (1995) noted, the therapeutic milieu fosters transient object cathexes, where meaningful connections to the surroundings play a pivotal role in the patient's recovery. These connections anchor individuals as they navigate complex emotional and behavioral challenges, offering stability and engagement throughout their journey.

The transformative power of physical space

The physical space where treatment occurs is a crucial factor in enabling therapeutic transformation. For individuals with EDs, the environment must foster safety, accessibility, and belonging, ensuring emotional security and support. A thoughtfully designed space can encourage reflection, emotional processing, and behavioral change, transforming the setting into an active participant in the therapeutic process.

Our work demonstrates this principle through the transformation of an outdated inpatient facility originally designed for individuals with chronic psychosis, such as schizophrenia. This renovation extended beyond aesthetics and functionality to create a space that symbolized care, renewal, and adaptability, specifically tailored to adolescents and young adults with EDs.

By embedding the principles of milieu therapy into the design, the reimagined facility became more than a setting; it became a therapeutic tool. The new environment fostered introspection and change, enabling patients to navigate their recovery journey with greater ease and support.

Integrating the milieu and space in ED treatment

The integration of milieu therapy and the transformative power of space highlights the interplay between environment and treatment in EDs recovery. A well-structured milieu supports patients by fostering new ways of relating to themselves and others. Simultaneously, a carefully designed physical space embodies the care and adaptability necessary to sustain this therapeutic process.

This dual focus addresses the unique needs of individuals with EDs, creating an environment that nurtures gradual growth and bridges the gap between suffering and healing. By prioritizing both relational and spatial dimensions of care, the therapeutic process becomes holistic and deeply rooted in the lived experience of recovery.

Interdisciplinary collaboration in space design

Transforming therapeutic spaces required a collaborative dialogue between healthcare professionals and architects to ensure the physical environment met the needs of both patients and staff. This process involved in-depth discussions about how therapeutic practices could inform architectural decisions throughout the building process. Architect Erik Guth encapsulated this approach with a pivotal question: *"Tell me how you work, and I will translate your needs into construction plans"* (Personal communication, *Architect* Eric Guth, 2004).

These discussions informed the design of spaces that allowed various disciplines to function effectively:

- *Therapeutic spaces*: Dedicated areas for group therapy, individual counseling, and nutritional education foster collaboration among psychologists, psychiatrists, and nutritionists.
- *Activity zones*: Spaces for art therapy, occupational therapy, and relaxation techniques provide creative and emotional outlets for patients.
- *Shared community areas*: Communal dining spaces and lounges promote positive social interactions and gradual exposure to food in a supportive setting.
- *Staff collaboration areas*: Offices and meeting rooms are tailored to facilitate interdisciplinary teamwork, ensuring seamless communication among professionals.

The impact of space on healing

The new therapeutic environment transcends its role as a treatment facility, embodying a vision of recovery and possibility. Natural light, open layouts, and welcoming colors create a sense of warmth and safety, reducing anxiety and encouraging emotional openness. Spaces that balance structure and flexibility allow patients to engage with treatment at their own pace while supporting staff in delivering personalized care.

The therapeutic milieu as a catalyst for recovery

The transformation of therapeutic spaces demonstrates the convergence of architectural design and treatment philosophy to create environments conducive to healing. For patients with EDs—who often grapple with control, self-perception, and interpersonal dynamics—the therapeutic milieu fosters introspection, connection, and gradual change. By integrating therapeutic principles into architectural design, these spaces not only meet clinical needs but also inspire hope, connection, and transformation for patients and professionals alike.

This process underscores the importance of collaboration, where the intersection of disciplines—architecture, healthcare, and psychoanalysis—creates spaces that truly support the journey from suffering to recovery. Within this milieu, the transformation of incidental interventions into structured therapeutic processes is emphasized through rigorous training and supervision, ensuring that all elements of care contribute meaningfully to patient outcomes.

Mentalizing and embodiment experiences in day hospital intensive care

The interplay between mentalizing processes and embodiment experiences is central to understanding and treating EDs. These dimensions, while closely related, are distinct. Traditional psychoanalytic approaches, such as "on the couch" therapy, focus on transforming the representational world through reflective processes. However, embodied memories—rooted in early relational and sensory experiences—require new embodied interactions for integration and healing. Consequently, day hospital programs that provide opportunities for new, healthy interpersonal and environmental experiences are crucial to therapeutic progress.

Mentalization theory and its relevance in eating disorder treatment

Mentalization theory provides critical insights into the psychological functioning of patients with EDs. As Peter Fonagy highlights, individuals with EDs, particularly those with AN, often face profound difficulties in the mentalizing process (Skårderud and Fonagy, 2012). This impairment hinders their ability to understand and interpret internal experiences as mental states—such as thoughts, feelings, or perceptions—resulting in a predominance of emotional expression through somatic channels. For instance, rather than identifying emotions like sadness or fear cognitively, patients may report vague bodily sensations such as feeling "empty" or "heavy," thereby translating affective distress directly into physical experience (Fonagy and Bateman, 2007).

Group approaches to enhance mentalizing

Group-based interventions play a pivotal role in addressing these deficits. According to Persano (2022), group therapy offers a dynamic space where patients can engage with others' perspectives, allowing them to listen to new words, experiences, and interpretations. This interaction fosters the development of new object representations and enhances the patient's mentalizing capacity. By participating in a shared therapeutic environment, patients begin to:

- Recognize and articulate their internal states.
- Develop empathy by understanding the mental states of others.
- Expand their capacity to symbolize and reflect on their experiences rather than expressing them solely through somatic symptoms.

Mentalization-based treatment (MBT)

Mentalization-Based Treatment (MBT), as described by Fonagy and Bateman (2007), is particularly well-suited for ED patients due to its focus on enhancing the ability to think about and regulate mental states. Key features of MBT include:

- *Improving emotional awareness*: Helping patients identify and label emotions rather than somatizing them.
- *Strengthening reflective functioning*: Encouraging patients to explore how their thoughts and feelings influence their behaviors and relationships.
- *Fostering relf-regulation*: Supporting the development of strategies to manage distress without resorting to disordered eating behaviors.

Integration of mentalization into EDs treatment

By incorporating mentalization principles into both group and individual therapeutic settings, treatment programs can address the core difficulties that perpetuate ED symptoms. Through this approach, patients gradually transition from experiencing emotions as physical sensations to understanding them as part of their psychological world. This shift not only improves their relationship with their bodies but also enhances their overall psychological resilience and interpersonal functioning.

Mentalization theory, therefore, provides a powerful framework for treating ED patients, offering a pathway to greater self-awareness, emotional regulation, and meaningful recovery.

This mentalizing deficit is closely linked to early attachment disruptions, which hinder the development of symbolization and self-representation. As Skårderud and Fonagy (2012) note, ED patients often describe distorted body image as visceral sensations tied to fear, anger, or sadness. These feelings, however, are experienced in the body rather than processed in the mind, leading the body to take on an exaggerated role in maintaining the sense of self (Morando et al., 2023).

Patients often treat their bodies as physical objects, devoid of psychological meaning. Fonagy et al. (2002) describe this phenomenon as a reliance on external validation to sustain identity, where the self is experienced as tangible rather than symbolic.

Philippe Jeammet's perspective: Defensive mechanisms and treatment approaches in eating disorders

Philippe Jeammet provides a valuable complement to Peter Fonagy's perspective by framing eating disorders (EDs) not merely as deficits in mentalization but as active defensive mechanisms. For Jeammet (1984), EDs represent a withdrawal from reality, where patients defensively detach affect from representations to shield themselves from overwhelming perceptions of their body image. This withdrawal, while protective, comes at the expense of symbolic and emotional processing, further entrenching the disorder.

Jeammet situates EDs within the broader framework of psychosomatic pathology, linking them to early failures in the structuring of the self (*Moi*). These early disruptions hinder personality development, resulting in a fragile self-concept and a persistent difficulty in integrating the physical and psychological aspects of the self. The body becomes the focal point for managing unprocessed emotions, leading to the symptomatic behaviors observed in EDs.

In addition to his theoretical contributions, Jeammet emphasized the importance of group settings in the initial stages of treatment. According to him, beginning treatment within a peer group rather than an individual framework helps to reduce resistance and creates a "plastic mind" more open to new ideas and relational experiences (Jeammet, 1984). This approach fosters a supportive environment where patients can engage with others facing similar struggles, providing a foundation for mutual understanding and change.

Inspiration for the day hospital program in Buenos Aires

Jeammet's insights significantly influenced the design of the Day Hospital Program for ED patients in Buenos Aires. During a personal discussion with Jeammet in 1998, he highlighted the value of integrating peer dynamics into therapeutic structures, as demonstrated in his work with hospital treatments in Paris. This exchange proved instrumental in shaping the framework of the Buenos Aires program, aligning it with his emphasis on the therapeutic potential of group settings (Personal communication, Philippe Jeammet, 1998).

Inspired by Jeammet's ideas, the Day Hospital Program prioritized group-based interventions that encouraged patients to confront their experiences within a collective context. This design sought to create an environment where patients could benefit from shared experiences, reducing isolation and resistance while promoting openness to new perspectives. The program integrated these principles into its therapeutic milieu, ensuring that group dynamics played a central role in facilitating emotional processing, symbolic integration, and recovery.

Jeammet's contributions underscore the importance of viewing EDs as complex phenomena that require both theoretical and practical innovation. His framing of EDs as defensive mechanisms highlights the interplay between early developmental failures and the body's role in managing unresolved emotions. Equally, his advocacy for group-based treatment emphasizes the need for relational contexts that foster connection, reduce resistance, and open pathways for psychological growth.

These ideas continue to resonate in contemporary ED treatment, offering valuable guidance for creating programs that address the intricate relationship between the self, the body, and interpersonal dynamics. Through their application in settings such as the Day Hospital Program in Buenos Aires, Jeammet's concepts remain a cornerstone of innovative and effective approaches to ED care.

The embodiment concept in EDs

Marianne Leuzinger-Bohleber further illuminates the role of embodiment, describing how environmental and relational factors shape and modify embodied self-representations. Early interactions between infants and caregivers play a pivotal role in constructing body images and the sense of self, while later social interactions contribute to their deconstruction and reconfiguration (Leuzinger-Bohleber, 2015).

For EDs patients, embodiment often reflects aggression internalized from traumatic early experiences. This embodiment manifests in self-harming behaviors, suicide attempts, or multi-impulsive actions such as substance abuse, which are attempts to numb or escape painful feelings. In these patients, the body becomes an externalized object subject to destruction, requiring specialized frameworks to contain and transform these destructive tendencies.

Embodiment and mentalization in day hospital programs

Day hospital programs provide an ideal setting to address the embodiment challenges and mentalizing deficits in ED patients. These programs offer structured opportunities for patients to rebuild connections between their physical sensations and mental representations through safe, healthy interpersonal and sensory experiences.

- *Peer group interactions*: Interaction within peer groups fosters a sense of belonging and enables patients to reflect on shared experiences, promoting relational and emotional growth.

- *Creative and therapeutic activities*: Group therapy, art therapy, and other creative outlets provide spaces where patients can symbolically express and process embodied trauma.
- *Healthy relational dynamics*: Engagement with staff and peers creates new relational templates, allowing patients to reconstruct their sense of self through positive and supportive encounters.

The goal is to transform painful embodied histories into new, healing experiences. By facilitating meaningful interactions and creating an environment where the body is valued and respected, these programs enable patients to recover from early aggression and maltreatment, reclaiming their bodies as integral and healthy aspects of their identity.

A unified approach to mentalization and embodiment

The treatment of EDs requires an integrated approach that addresses both the mentalizing deficits and the embodied experiences of patients. Fonagy's emphasis on mentalizing challenges, combined with Jeammet's framing of defensive withdrawal, highlights the interplay between early attachment disruptions, symbolization deficits, and psychosomatic pathology.

Leuzinger-Bohleber's focus on embodiment underscores the importance of environmental and relational factors in reshaping self-representations. Together, these perspectives inform the design of day hospital programs that provide a dual focus: fostering mentalizing capacities and facilitating the reconstruction of embodied experiences (Leuzinger-Bohleber, 2015).

Through a combination of psychoanalytic principles and experiential interventions, day hospital programs offer patients a pathway to reconnect body and mind, transform trauma into growth, and develop a cohesive and resilient sense of self. These spaces become more than treatment centers—they are environments where healing, transformation, and reintegration are actively nurtured.

Day intensive care for patients with eating disorders

Since 1999, the day hospital intensive care of "The Mental Health Unit for Eating Disorders" at the José T. Borda Hospital in Buenos Aires has implemented group-based methodologies, such as psychoanalytic group psychotherapy and thematic workshops, to address the complex nature of EDs. These group settings provide patients with a unique opportunity to confront their struggles collectively, creating a therapeutic environment of shared understanding and mutual support.

Group interventions actively challenge the isolating tendencies imposed by societal and cultural pressures, offering patients a space to explore and question the sociocultural norms that contribute to their disorders. By focusing on the shared dynamics that underpin EDs, these methodologies shift the emphasis from isolated symptom management to a broader exploration of the societal factors driving the behaviors.

Through fostering connection, empathy, and critical reflection, the program promotes a deeper understanding of EDs as disorders influenced by both individual psychology and the broader cultural framework, paving the way for more meaningful and lasting recovery.

Admission process for a day hospital intensive care: A comprehensive, interdisciplinary approach

The admission process for a therapeutic community reflects the interdisciplinary nature of the program, ensuring a holistic evaluation of each patient. This approach integrates assessments from six key disciplines—Psychiatry, Clinical Medicine, Nutrition, Psychology, Occupational Therapy, and Nursing—providing a thorough understanding of the patient's condition and needs. Each prospective patient undergoes interviews with healthcare professionals from these areas (Persano, 2014). Below is a detailed outline of the evaluation components:

Psychiatric evaluation

Psychiatrists focus on diagnosing and assessing the patient's clinical condition, including associated and differential diagnoses, as well as the need for psychotropic medication. Key areas of evaluation include:

- Personality functioning and structural personality assessment.
- Mood and cognitive functioning.
- Impulsivity patterns and potential risks of self-harm or life-threatening behaviors.

Clinical medical evaluation

It is essential that the same physician consistently follows the patient over time, rather than being frequently replaced by different professionals. This continuity allows for the development of trust, facilitates the detection of subtle changes in physical health, and enhances clinical decision-making. A stable physician evaluates the patient's overall physical health, focusing on:

- Clinical complications and risks, including cardiac and metabolic functions.
- Identification of differential diagnoses and associated medical conditions that may influence treatment.

Nutritional evaluation

Nutritionists assess the patient's nutritional and dietary status through:

- Detailed analysis of eating patterns, habits, and dietary records.
- Anthropometric measurements and weight parameters.
- Evaluation of body image satisfaction and the impact of nutritional deficiencies on physical and psychological health.

Psychological evaluation

Psychologists examine the patient's mental health and personality structure, addressing:

- Insight into their condition, defensive mechanisms, and conflict resolution capabilities.
- Anxiety patterns, reality testing, and acting-out behaviors.
- Capacity for symbolic thinking and overall structural personality diagnosis.
- Family dynamics, relational functioning, and their impact on the patient's recovery trajectory.

Occupational therapy evaluation

Occupational therapy plays a critical role in assessing and addressing both academic and vocational challenges. Key areas of focus include:

- Academic performance and the presence of learning difficulties or cognitive impairments.
- Work-related skills, productivity, and vocational interests.
- The patient's ability to engage in structured activities and manage daily responsibilities.
- Assessment of life skills and the development of strategies to improve functionality in academic and work settings. This evaluation ensures that patients receive tailored interventions to support their reintegration into educational or professional environments, aligning treatment goals with their life aspirations.
- Life history, current stressors, and global functioning, using tools such as the Global Assessment Scale (GAS) introduce by Lester Luborsky as health-sickness scale (HSRS) in 1962 (Armelius et al., 1991).

Nursing evaluation

Nurses provide a comprehensive assessment of the patient's overall condition, including:

- Monitoring of vital signs, symptoms, and general health status.
- Observation of the patient's environment, physical presentation, and treatment adherence.
- Evaluating the patient's expression and demeanor, identifying subtle behavioral patterns that may impact treatment outcomes.

As mentioned earlier, the nursing staff occupies a central and pivotal role in the structure of the day hospital, with their office strategically located at its core. This placement is not merely logistical but intentional, reflecting the vital role nurses play in the daily functioning of the therapeutic community. The nursing station serves as the primary point of contact for patients, making it the hub for immediate care, whether physical or emotional.

This is the place where first aid care is administered, ensuring that patients' urgent medical needs are promptly addressed. It is also where daily physical health monitoring occurs, such as checking vital signs, managing medication distribution, and providing support for any immediate concerns raised by patients. The nursing team often becomes the first to identify subtle changes in a patient's condition—whether physical, emotional, or behavioral—allowing for early interventions and informing the multidisciplinary team of potential issues that may require attention.

Moreover, the location of the nursing office facilitates accessibility, fostering a sense of safety and reassurance for patients. It acts as a bridge between the clinical and therapeutic aspects of the community, ensuring that patients feel cared for in a holistic and integrated manner. By being at the heart of the day hospital, the nursing staff not only delivers essential medical care but also plays an integral role in maintaining the therapeutic environment, supporting both patients and other staff members in the shared mission of recovery.

This central positioning underscores the critical importance of nursing professionals in the horizontal structure of the therapeutic community, reinforcing their role as key contributors to the healing process.

This interdisciplinary admission process ensures a detailed understanding of each patient's needs, addressing both their immediate clinical conditions and broader life challenges. By including occupational therapy in the evaluation, the program integrates strategies for improving academic and vocational performance, emphasizing the importance of functional recovery alongside medical and psychological stability.

This holistic approach not only sets the foundation for personalized treatment plans but also reinforces the therapeutic community's mission of fostering comprehensive, sustainable recovery.

Decision-making and staff supervision in treatment planning

After completing the diagnostic process, the case is thoroughly discussed in a multidisciplinary team meeting. This collaborative discussion ensures that the perspectives of all staff members—psychiatrists, clinical physicians, psychologists, nutritionists, occupational therapists, nurses, and others—are considered in developing a comprehensive treatment plan. Supervision by senior staff members plays a pivotal role in this process, offering guidance based on experience and ensuring that the chosen plan aligns with the patient's clinical and personal needs (Persano, 2014).

The therapeutic contract: Framing the process

In classical psychoanalysis, the treatment frame is essential for establishing the boundaries and structure within which therapeutic work occurs. Similarly, the "treatment contract" in EDs interventions provides a clear and mutually agreed-upon framework. This contract outlines the responsibilities and expectations of both the patient and the therapeutic team, serving as a guide throughout the process (Yeomans, Selzer, and Clarkin, 1992; Yeomans et al., 1994).

Key functions of the contract include:

- *Commitment to treatment goals*: The contract formalizes the patient's agreement to actively engage in the therapeutic process, adhere to the treatment plan, and work toward defined goals.
- *Establishing boundaries*: By explicitly defining acceptable behaviors and responsibilities, the contract minimizes the risk of acting-out behaviors, which are common in ED patients due to the ego-syntonic nature of their symptoms.
- *Providing a holding framework*: The contract offers a stable structure that supports the patient through the often-challenging process of change, fostering a sense of safety and predictability.

Informed consent: Empowering the patient

In addition to the therapeutic contract, obtaining informed consent is a critical component of ethical and effective treatment. Informed consent ensures that the patient:

- *Understands the nature of the treatment*: Patients receive detailed explanations about the therapeutic approach, the roles of various team members, and the expected course of treatment.
- *Acknowledges risks and responsibilities*: The patient is made aware of potential challenges, including emotional discomfort and the effort required to achieve progress.

- *Exercises autonomy*: Informed consent empowers patients by involving them in decision-making and establishing a collaborative relationship with the therapeutic team.

Contractual elements specific to EDs treatment

Given the complexity of EDs, the treatment contract incorporates elements tailored to the unique needs of this population:

- *Nutritional commitment*: Patients agree to participate in meal plans and nutritional education while adhering to guidelines for healthy eating habits.
- *Therapeutic participation*: Patients commit to attending group therapy sessions, workshops, and individual treatments consistently.
- *Safety agreements*: To address risks such as self-harm or purging, patients agree to communicate openly with the therapeutic team and follow safety protocols.
- *Family involvement*: Where appropriate, the contract includes family participation in workshops or family group therapy sessions to foster a supportive home environment.

Benefits of the treatment contract

The use of a treatment contract benefits both patients and the therapeutic team:

- For patients, it provides clarity, accountability, and a sense of partnership in the therapeutic process.
- For therapists, it creates a shared understanding of goals and boundaries, reducing ambiguities that may disrupt treatment.

By integrating the concepts of a treatment contract and informed consent, the therapeutic process is framed within a structured, collaborative, and ethical context. This approach aligns with psychoanalytic principles while addressing the specific challenges posed by EDs, ultimately fostering a more stable and effective therapeutic alliance.

When the team carefully evaluates the severity of the patient's condition to determine the most appropriate level of care:

- *Outpatient treatment*: For less severe cases, outpatient care may suffice, focusing on regular individual and group therapy sessions, nutritional guidance, and periodic medical evaluations.
- *Day hospital intensive care*: For more severe cases, admission to the day hospital program is recommended. This program is structured into two core modules:

1   *Health recovery*: The initial phase focuses on stabilizing the patient's physical and psychological health. This includes addressing immediate risks, normalizing eating behaviors, and fostering initial insight into their condition.

2   *Resocialization and integration*: The second phase aims to reintegrate the patient into daily life, emphasizing the development of life skills, social interactions, and preparation for academic or professional activities.

The treatment plan typically spans two years, with periodic evaluations and adjustments based on the patient's progress. Supervision meetings throughout the treatment process ensure that all staff members remain aligned in their approach, continuously refining the plan to address emerging challenges or needs.

This structured yet flexible approach combines interdisciplinary collaboration, clinical expertise, and ongoing supervision to deliver personalized care, supporting patients on their journey toward recovery and reintegration into their communities.

Inclusion criteria for day hospital admission

Before recommending a day hospital treatment, it is crucial to evaluate whether the patient meets the inclusion criteria, which are as follows:

- Patients unresponsive to outpatient treatment.
- Patients recovering from inpatient care.
- Patients require supervised mealtimes without needing full hospitalization.
- Patients are prone to acting-out behaviors.
- Patients from families lacking emotional containment.
- Patients with limited introspective capacity for outpatient psychotherapy.

Additionally, candidates must present a formal ED diagnosis, provide written informed consent adhering to ethical standards, and commit to attending and following the team's recommendations.

Exclusion criteria for day hospital admission

Exclusion criteria are equally important and include:

- Patients in clinical, nutritional, or psychiatric emergencies.
- Cases where the condition is secondary to another clinical disorder rather than a primary ED.
- Patients with a primary diagnosis of substance addiction, as they pose a significant risk of disrupting other patients and may inadvertently

lead to new disorders during recovery. Such cases require specialized addiction programs due to the fragility of eating disorder patients.

Risks of misunderstanding severity and delayed referrals to day hospital programs

Timely and accurate referral to a day hospital program is critical in the treatment of EDs. However, prolonged failures in outpatient treatments are frequently linked to several systemic and clinical shortcomings:

- *Inadequate personality evaluations*: Healthcare professionals may overlook or underestimate the complexity of personality structures and psychological vulnerabilities underlying EDs. This lack of comprehensive assessment can result in ineffective or inappropriate treatment strategies.
- *Minimized clinical risks*: The severity of clinical and nutritional parameters, including malnutrition, electrolyte imbalances, or cardiac risks, is often downplayed, delaying the necessary escalation of care.
- *Overly individualistic approaches*: A narrow focus on individual symptom management without considering the broader psychosocial and familial dynamics contributing to the disorder can limit the effectiveness of outpatient treatments.

The consequences of delayed referral

When healthcare professionals fail to recognize the holistic needs of patients, referrals to more intensive care settings like day hospitals are often delayed. This delay can have serious repercussions:

- *Escalation of severity*: Patients may deteriorate significantly, arriving at the day hospital in conditions better suited for inpatient care due to severe malnutrition, electrolyte imbalances, or psychological crises.
- *Life-threatening risks*: Prolonged outpatient treatments that fail to address imminent risks—such as self-harm behaviors, cardiac instability, or severe weight loss—can lead to life-threatening situations.
- *Compromised recovery*: Late intervention often means that the patient requires more intensive and prolonged treatment, reducing the chances of achieving a smooth recovery and increasing the burden on healthcare systems.

Systemic challenges and the need for holistic evaluation

The delays often stem from systemic challenges within healthcare systems, including:

- *Limited interdisciplinary collaboration*: A lack of coordination among medical, psychological, and nutritional professionals can lead to fragmented care, where critical risks are overlooked.
- *Inadequate training in EDs*: Many general practitioners and outpatient therapists lack specialized training in recognizing the early signs of medical and psychological risks in ED patients.
- *Naturalization of symptoms*: In some cases, the chronic nature of eating disorders (EDs) results in the normalization of symptoms, where dangerously low body weight or severe purging behaviors are incorrectly perceived as conditions that can be managed adequately within an outpatient care setting. This misjudgment can delay the initiation of more intensive and necessary interventions.

The importance of timely and holistic referrals

Effective referrals require a holistic and multidisciplinary assessment that goes beyond symptom management to consider the full scope of the patient's condition. This includes:

- *Personality and risk evaluation*: Assessing the psychological and personality structure to determine the patient's ability to engage with outpatient care versus the need for a more structured setting.
- *Comprehensive clinical assessment*: Monitoring vital signs, nutritional status, and medical risks to ensure timely identification of patients who require more intensive care.
- *Collaboration and communication*: Encouraging consistent communication among outpatient providers and day hospital teams to ensure patients are referred promptly when outpatient care is insufficient.

Prevention of delayed escalation

To mitigate the risks of delayed referral:

- *Training programs*: Equip outpatient providers with the tools and knowledge to identify high-risk ED patients early.
- *Standardized assessment protocols*: Implement uniform guidelines for evaluating medical, psychological, and nutritional risks.
- *Structured referral pathways*: Establish clear, efficient processes for transitioning patients from outpatient care to day hospital programs, minimizing delays.

By recognizing the risks of delayed referrals and addressing the systemic challenges that contribute to these delays, healthcare systems can ensure that ED patients receive timely, appropriate care. Early referral to day hospital programs provides patients with the structured, multidisciplinary approach they need, significantly improving treatment outcomes and reducing the likelihood of critical health crises.

Psychoanalytic framework for day hospital intensive care in eating disorders: Addressing eating disorders through group-based methodologies

EDs and body image conflicts, particularly prevalent among adolescents, are deeply entrenched in societal and cultural dynamics. The pervasive emphasis on perfection, hyper-individualism, and unattainable beauty standards exacerbates these struggles, rendering them highly egosyntonic. Patients often fail to perceive their behaviors as problematic, presenting significant challenges to individual therapeutic approaches. As Lipovetsky (1983) observes, the individualistic ethos of postmodernity magnifies these tensions, underscoring the need for collective therapeutic frameworks.

Challenges of hypermodern individualism in treatment

Failures in treatment often stem from the pervasive influence of hyper-modern individualism, which complicates patients' engagement with therapeutic processes. Marcel Gauchet describes "individuals in excess" as those increasingly disconnected from the fabric of society, navigating life in a state of profound uncertainty (Castel, 2009). These individuals frequently exhibit behaviors aligned with hypermodern values—excessive autonomy, consumerism, and self-focus—that further isolate them and hinder their ability to integrate into collective therapeutic settings.

Overcoming individualistic biases in therapeutic communities

To effectively address these challenges, professionals within therapeutic communities must actively recognize and transcend the individualistic biases often ingrained through traditional academic and clinical training. Hypermodern culture tends to valorize independence and self-reliance at the expense of relational and collective values, which can subtly influence therapeutic approaches.

Embracing a collective, interdisciplinary perspective becomes essential in counteracting these isolating forces. This shift not only enriches the therapeutic framework by incorporating diverse perspectives but also models the collaborative dynamics necessary to foster connection and belonging. Within the therapeutic community, such a perspective:

- *Encourages interdependence*: Patients are guided to explore the value of mutual support and shared experiences, counteracting hypermodern tendencies toward self-isolation.
- *Promotes collaboration among professionals*: By integrating knowledge from various disciplines, the community creates a holistic approach that mirrors the interconnectedness needed for patients to reengage with society.

- *Challenges cultural norms*: The therapeutic setting becomes a microcosm where hypermodern values of autonomy and consumerism are deconstructed, enabling patients to reconsider their relationship with themselves and others.

Role of therapeutic communities in a hypermodern world

In this context, therapeutic communities offer a critical counterbalance to the fragmented, individualistic ethos of hypermodernity. These communities emphasize shared responsibility, relational growth, and the importance of collective engagement, creating an environment where patients can reconnect with a sense of belonging and shared purpose.

By modeling these values, therapeutic professionals not only help patients recover but also challenge the broader societal patterns that contribute to their distress.

Through collective frameworks, therapeutic communities provide a path for patients to move beyond the isolating tendencies of hypermodern individualism, fostering meaningful connections and lasting recovery.

The question of therapeutic efficacy

Therapeutic efficacy must extend beyond short-term markers such as weight restoration or impulse control. The true measure of success lies in whether these changes translate into sustained and meaningful transformations in the patient's overall health, relationships, and quality of life. Genuine efficacy reflects holistic improvements, encompassing physical, emotional, and social well-being.

In our research on treatment efficacy and challenges, we have identified key areas of resistance that significantly impact outcomes. One of the most critical factors is body image distortion, which emerges as a primary point of resistance. This distortion not only determines the severity of the condition but also heavily influences treatment refractoriness.

Another important variable is excessive exercise, which remains resistant to change during recovery (Persano et al., 2022). Our hypothesis is that this behavior persists because it is often socially reinforced as a health-positive practice. Many healthcare professionals inadvertently support excessive exercise, viewing it as a beneficial recommendation without fully evaluating its maladaptive aspects in the context of EDs. This misjudgment leads to a lack of proper assessment and intervention for overexercise, undermining recovery efforts and prolonging the course of treatment.

An important consideration in the treatment of EDs is the widely documented poor recovery rates, chronic outcomes, and high mortality associated with these conditions in international literature. Numerous studies emphasize the significant challenges in achieving sustained recovery, highlighting the severe physical and psychological toll EDs take on individuals. However, our experience treating more than 3,000 patients over the course of 25 years offers a contrasting perspective, as we have observed notably low mortality rates within our population.

We hypothesize that this outcome is largely attributable to our treatment framework, which emphasizes community-based therapy, deep introspection, and the cultivation of embodied healthy experiences. By fostering a therapeutic environment where patients are not only encouraged to confront their inner conflicts but also provided with opportunities to reconnect with their bodies and their environments in meaningful ways, we believe our approach addresses the multifaceted nature of EDs more holistically. This model integrates relational support, introspective work, and experiential learning, creating a pathway for recovery that extends beyond symptomatic relief.

Community-based therapy plays a crucial role in this success, as it reinforces a sense of belonging and shared purpose, counteracting the isolation often experienced by individuals with EDs. Similarly, introspective recovery, guided by psychodynamic principles, enables patients to explore the deeper emotional and symbolic meanings tied to their eating behaviors, fostering long-term psychological resilience. Finally, embodied healthy experiences—such as reconnecting with food through cultivation, preparation, and shared meals—help patients rebuild a positive and grounded relationship with nourishment and their own physical selves.

While these observations are promising, we acknowledge the need for further research to confirm this hypothesis and better understand the mechanisms behind our outcomes. Rigorous studies comparing community-based, introspection-driven frameworks with more traditional approaches would be invaluable in exploring how these elements contribute to reduced mortality and improved recovery rates. Such investigations could not only validate our approach but also offer insights to enhance ED treatment on a broader scale.

Our public open to the community center frequently receives patients labeled as "treatment-resistant" in private healthcare settings. Often, these cases were deemed "success stories" due to initial progress, only to experience rapid deterioration upon treatment discontinuation. These failures highlight the limitations of commercialized healthcare models, where the focus is often on superficial outcomes rather than comprehensive recovery. The public health system is then left to address the long-term needs of these patients, revealing the societal cost of health systems driven by market dynamics. In such systems, health risks becoming a commodity rather than a fundamental right, perpetuating exclusion and inequality.

The sociocultural context of treatment

Healthcare professionals, as participants in the same sociocultural framework, may unconsciously adopt roles shaped by hypermodern values.

These roles can reinforce individualistic treatment approaches that fail to address the collective dimensions of EDs. Understanding these broader sociocultural forces is essential for designing effective therapeutic interventions.

The psychoanalytic group framework in our day hospital program explicitly confronts these dynamics by integrating sociocultural critique into treatment. Group settings encourage patients to explore the societal origins of their struggles, including the unrealistic standards imposed by media and cultural norms. Simultaneously, these settings foster shared experiences that counteract the isolation and disconnection characteristic of hypermodern life.

Toward lasting transformation

The integration of psychoanalytic principles within a group-based framework offers a pathway to holistic recovery. By addressing the interplay between societal influences and individual struggles, the day hospital program moves beyond symptom management to foster profound, lasting changes. This approach underscores the importance of seeing EDs not merely as individual pathologies but as manifestations of broader sociocultural dysfunctions.

Through collective therapeutic processes, interdisciplinary collaboration, and a commitment to addressing societal influences, the program creates a space where patients can achieve meaningful transformations. These transformations challenge the hypermodern ethos, promoting connection, resilience, and the rediscovery of health as a shared human right rather than an individualistic pursuit.

Key therapeutic approaches for the initial phase: Workshops and group therapy

The "initial phase" of treatment in the therapeutic community centers on workshops and group therapy, which provide a structured and supportive environment for addressing the complexities of EDs. These methodologies focus on fostering interpersonal connections, exploring sociocultural influences, and developing practical skills that contribute to recovery.

Key psychodynamic interventions in eating disorder treatment

This topic is also partially addressed in Chapter 3, where foundational concepts related to psychodynamic approaches are introduced and contextualized within broader treatment frameworks.

By revisiting and expanding upon these concepts, this section delves deeper into the specific applications of psychodynamic interventions in addressing the complex psychological and relational dimensions of eating disorders. It highlights the nuanced ways in which these techniques can be tailored to meet the unique needs of patients, reinforcing the connections established earlier in the book.

1 *Food and mealtime therapy*: Meals are utilized as therapeutic opportunities for patients to confront their fears and anxieties around food. Through psychodynamic principles, patients explore the symbolic meanings they attach to food—such as control, nurturing, and punishment—while working toward balanced eating within a supportive environment.

2 *Family therapy and conflict resolution*: Given the central role of family dynamics in the development and perpetuation of eating disorders, psychodynamic family therapy addresses unresolved relational issues and improves communication patterns. This approach helps mitigate familial factors that may reinforce disordered behaviors.

3 *Exploration of responsible sexuality and gender identity*: Sexuality and identity-related concerns often surface in the context of eating disorders, with patients projecting body-related anxieties onto issues of self-worth and gender. A psychodynamic framework provides a safe, non-judgmental space to explore these aspects, fostering a deeper understanding of identity and self-acceptance.

4 *Emotion-focused interventions*: By employing psychodynamic techniques, therapists assist patients in identifying and exploring distorted beliefs about body image and food. This process enables patients to recognize, process, and regulate emotions tied to their self-perception, reducing reliance on eating disorder behaviors and fostering healthier coping mechanisms.

5 *Cohabitation workshop: Building foundations of intersubjective tolerance*: At the heart of the therapeutic community is the "cohabitation workshop" where group dynamics are explored, and participants learn to navigate intersubjective relationships. This space serves as an entry point for new members, introducing them to community guidelines and emphasizing respect, empathy, and mutual accountability. The workshop fosters a sense of belonging and helps participants build the interpersonal skills necessary for engaging in the therapeutic process.

6 *Cultural workshop: Deconstructing harmful ideals*: The cultural workshop, as was extended presented in Chapter 10, addresses the societal roots of EDs, encouraging participants to examine the cultural ideals and pressures that contribute to their struggles. By critically analyzing these influences, participants begin to deconstruct harmful norms and develop a sense of solidarity with others. The workshop promotes a shift from the marginality of suffering to active social inclusion, challenging participants to rethink their relationships with societal expectations.

7   *Art workshop: Transitioning from image to articulation*: The "art workshop" combines visual stimuli, both from movies and designs, with group discussions, helping participants transition from passive image-based understanding to active verbal expression. By reflecting on cinematic themes and connecting them to personal experiences, participants gain insight into the narratives shaping their self-representations.

Therapeutic workshops: Nutrition, commensality, and family dynamics

Nutritional workshops: Rebuilding a relationship with food

Coordinated by nutritionists, nutritional workshops help participants reassess their attitudes toward food and develop healthier eating habits. These sessions provide education on balanced nutrition while addressing the emotional and psychological dimensions of eating.

Monthly "cooking workshops" add a hands-on, engaging component to the program, emphasizing the enjoyment and creativity of food preparation. This experiential approach counters the alienation often associated with rigid dietary rules and EDs, transforming food from a source of anxiety or control into a means of nourishment and connection. Participants gain practical culinary skills while learning to experience food as a positive and integral part of their lives.

Patients suffering from eating disorders (EDs) often have little awareness of how the food they consume is cultivated by farmers. In modern, urban societies, the connection to the continuous process of cultivating, cooking, and presenting food has been largely severed. Instead, these individuals frequently consume highly processed foods and are disconnected from the origins of what they eat. Ironically, many ED patients are overly involved in the commercial aspects of food—they often work in restaurants or stores—but they have lost the ability to perceive and appreciate the entire food cycle, from cultivation to preparation.

Our aim is to help patients reconnect with the natural processes of growing and preparing food. By encouraging them to cultivate food themselves and to present it in a communal, joyful environment, we strive to foster a deeper, more positive relationship with food. This approach not only addresses their disconnection but also promotes mindfulness, emotional grounding, and a renewed sense of appreciation for nourishment as a natural and fulfilling part of life.

Food and commensality: Shared mealtime as a therapeutic space

A unique feature of the therapeutic community approach is "commensality"—staff members and patients sharing lunch together. This communal mealtime serves dual purposes:

- *Supervising feeding processes*: Staff observe and support patients during meals, ensuring adherence to nutritional plans and addressing any anxieties or challenges.
- *Fostering shared experiences*: Many ED patients have a history of eating in isolation or within strained family dynamics. Sharing meals in a supportive, communal environment allows participants to embody new, positive experiences of eating. These mealtimes provide an opportunity to normalize feeding behaviors, promote relational growth, and rebuild trust around food and social interaction.

Family workshops: Strengthening support systems

Family workshops recognize the central role of familial dynamics in the development and maintenance of EDs. These sessions foster open communication, address misunderstandings, and explore family histories and relational roles. By identifying patterns that may contribute to the disorder, participants and their families gain valuable insights into how these dynamics influence behavior.

The workshops aim to:

- *Resolve conflict*: Encourage families to address unresolved tensions and promote empathy.
- *Build relational understanding*: Help family members understand the emotional and psychological needs of their loved ones.
- *Strengthen social support*: Provide families with the necessary tools to offer meaningful and sustainable support throughout the recovery process.

By fostering a stronger support network, family workshops create a foundation for sustained recovery and reinforce the importance of relational healing as part of the broader therapeutic process.

These workshops, whether focused on nutrition, shared meals, or family dynamics, collectively address the multifaceted nature of EDs. By integrating practical skills, relational growth, and emotional healing, they provide participants with a comprehensive framework for recovery and reintegration into healthier, more connected lives.

Supporting individual goals and social reintegration

To ensure sustained recovery, the therapeutic community places a strong emphasis on supporting participants' long-term goals and social reintegration:

- *Therapeutic companions*: These individuals work closely with severely affected patients, providing emotional support, fostering treatment adherence, and alleviating isolation.

- *Occupational therapy*: Occupational therapy helps participants identify realistic goals and transform ideas into actionable projects. This process encourages skill-building and self-confidence, preparing participants for reintegration into educational, professional, and social contexts.

Toward a health-oriented society

The therapeutic community model creates an environment that prioritizes health, offering a constructive alternative to societal contexts that exacerbate EDs. Through workshops and group therapy, participants are encouraged to engage in verbal expression, introspection, and mutual support, fostering lasting change.

Returning to Freud's concepts in *Civilization and Its Discontents*, the discontents of civilization arise from the tension between instinctual drives and societal constraints (Freud, 1930[1929]). While Freud does not explicitly advocate for solidarity, his exploration of human suffering invites consideration of its relational dimensions. His work suggests that psychic distress cannot be fully understood in isolation but must be examined within the context of human connections. This perspective opens the door for psychoanalysts and other thinkers to consider how shared experiences, collective efforts, and solidarity might play a role in alleviating the psychological tensions inherent in civilization.

By integrating these psychoanalytic principles with community-based interventions, the "therapeutic community model" offers a powerful approach to healing. This model emphasizes collective engagement, mutual support, and the creation of a shared space where individuals can explore and process their suffering. It moves beyond the isolated focus of individual therapy to embrace the broader social and relational dimensions of recovery.

In this framework, the therapeutic community fosters not only individual healing but also the reintegration of participants into a more health-oriented society. By addressing the roots of suffering—both personal and societal—it encourages participants to rebuild connections, challenge destructive cultural norms, and develop healthier relationships with themselves and others. This alignment of psychoanalytic insights with communal practices underscores the transformative potential of solidarity, offering a pathway to profound and lasting recovery.

Individual treatments in a community therapeutic framework

Having outlined the characteristics of our therapeutic device and the significance of group and community-based interventions in mental health, I now turn to the individual treatments offered within this broader framework. These individual approaches are designed to complement communal care by addressing the unique subjective experiences of each patient, as emphasized in the "Psychodynamic Diagnostic Manual, Second Edition" -PDM-2, (Lingiardi and McWilliams, 2017).

The PDM-2 framework underscores the importance of understanding the patient's internal world by focusing on personality patterns, emotional functioning, and mental processes. Central to this model is the subjective experience axis, which offers critical insights into the inner experiences of patients with EDs. By exploring affective states, cognitive patterns, somatic experiences, and relational dynamics (Mundo, Persano, and Moore, 2018; Persano, 2018), the framework helps to reveal how symptoms emerge as expressions of underlying psychological conflicts, maladaptive defenses, and relational patterns.

Integrating subjective experience into individual care

Incorporating the PDM-2 perspective into individual care enriches the therapeutic process by fostering a comprehensive understanding of the patient's subjective landscape. This approach ensures that each patient's psychological experience is not only acknowledged but also intricately explored. Key aspects of this integration include:

- *Affective states*: Recognizing and addressing the patient's emotional responses, including feelings of shame, guilt, fear, or anger, which often underpin ED behaviors.
- *Cognitive patterns*: Identifying distorted thought processes, such as perfectionism or dichotomous thinking, that sustain the disorder.
- *Somatic experiences*: Understanding how bodily sensations and symptoms are linked to unresolved psychological conflicts, reflecting the body-mind interplay characteristic of EDs.
- *Relational patterns*: Examining interpersonal dynamics and attachment styles that influence the patient's relationships and self-concept.

By systematically addressing these dimensions, the therapeutic team ensures that each patient's care is both individualized and deeply aligned with their unique needs and experiences.

The author's contribution to PDM-2 and further reading

I encourage readers to explore the subjective patterns of EDs in greater depth within the PDM-2, where I have contributed to this specific topic. By delving into the manual, readers can gain a more detailed understanding of the psychological underpinnings of EDs and how the subjective experience axis informs effective treatment. This resource provides a robust framework for clinicians seeking to integrate psychodynamic principles into the care of patients with complex mental health needs.

By emphasizing subjective experience through the lens of the PDM-2, individual treatments within the therapeutic community framework address the multifaceted psychological dimensions of EDs. This approach not only complements the communal interventions but also ensures a nuanced and compassionate understanding of each patient's inner world, fostering deeper and more sustained recovery.

Role of individual psychiatry approach in the specialized program context

Each patient in the therapeutic community receives individual care from a psychiatrist, who plays a pivotal role in monitoring clinical evolution and managing psychopharmacological interventions when needed. While the use of medication is discussed in greater depth in another chapter by contributing authors, it is important to briefly highlight its role in this context:

- *Stabilizing symptoms*: Medication is employed judiciously to manage severe symptoms such as mood instability, anxiety, or impulsivity, providing patients with the stability needed to engage fully in the therapeutic process.
- *Supporting psychotherapy*: Pharmacological treatments are viewed as adjuncts to psychoanalytic and psychotherapeutic work, creating a supportive baseline that allows patients to address deeper psychological conflicts.
- *Facilitating community engagement*: By mitigating overwhelming symptoms, medication can enhance the patient's ability to participate in group activities, workshops, and interpersonal relationships within the therapeutic community.

Integrating individual psychiatry and psychopharmacology in the community therapeutic framework

The integration of individual psychiatry within a community therapeutic framework exemplifies the program's holistic approach to EDs. While group therapy and communal workshops address the societal and relational dimensions of EDs, individual care focuses on the unique subjective experiences of each patient, delving into the personal histories, conflicts, and aspirations that shape their journey.

This dual approach ensures that patients are supported as both members of a therapeutic community and individuals with distinct needs. By incorporating the PDM-2 axis on subjective experience, the program provides a nuanced understanding of each patient's internal world, fostering a treatment environment that respects individuality while situating care within a collective healing process. This integration offers a model that is both expansive and deeply personalized, addressing the multifaceted nature of EDs with sensitivity and depth.

Assessing symptomatic dimensions to guide treatment

As previously highlighted in the discussion on the intersection of personality disorders and EDs, particularly the overlap between borderline personality disorder (BPD) and BN, identifying predominant symptomatic dimensions is essential for effective and tailored treatment. To support this process, the DIB-R (Diagnostic Interview for Borderlines-Revised) proves to be a valuable tool (Zanarini et al., 1989).

This instrument is particularly beneficial for:

- *Training junior therapists*: Providing a structured framework to develop diagnostic precision and clinical understanding.
- *Research purposes*: Offering standardized criteria to evaluate symptomatology and track treatment outcomes.
- *Symptom identification*: Enabling a nuanced assessment of patient presentations to inform individualized treatment plans.

The DIB-R assesses four core areas that are frequently impacted in patients with BPD and are also commonly observed in those with EDs:

1 *Affect regulation*: Examines emotional instability, mood shifts, and the intensity of affective responses.
2 *Cognitive functioning*: Identifies patterns of distorted thinking, dissociation, and identity disturbance.
3 *Impulse control*: Evaluates difficulties in managing impulsive behaviors, including binge-purge cycles and self-harm tendencies.
4 *Interpersonal relationships*: Explores the dynamics of relational instability, dependency, and conflicts.

By systematically addressing these dimensions, the DIB-R provides a comprehensive framework for understanding the patient's psychological profile. This tool enhances diagnostic accuracy and informs the development of targeted, multidimensional treatment approaches tailored to the individual's needs.

The first three dimensions—affect regulation, cognitive functioning, and impulse control—are particularly significant for determining appropriate psychopharmacological interventions. Medications can be adapted to address the predominant symptom profile, such as mood stabilization for emotional dysregulation, antipsychotics for cognitive distortions, or SSRIs and mood stabilizers for impulse-related behaviors like binge-purge cycles (Persano, 2014).

The fourth dimension—interpersonal relationships—is especially critical within the psychotherapeutic domain. Understanding relational instability and dynamics allows therapists to develop strategies that foster healthier attachments, improve communication patterns, and address dependency or conflict in relationships.

Together, these dimensions bridge the biological and psychological aspects of treatment, supporting a holistic and integrative approach to care. By combining psychopharmacological and psychotherapeutic interventions based on the insights provided by the DIB-R, clinicians can address the complexity of EDs and comorbid personality disorders more effectively.

Pharmacological interventions for specific symptom clusters

Impulse control and bulimia nervosa

For patients struggling with BN and impulse control issues, selective serotonin reuptake inhibitors (SSRIs) are often effective. SSRIs, such as fluoxetine and sertraline, are commonly prescribed to:

- *Reduce binge-purge cycles*: By modulating serotonin levels, these medications help diminish the frequency and intensity of binge-purge behaviors.
- *Improve impulse control*: SSRIs mitigate impulsivity, allowing patients to engage more effectively in therapeutic processes.
- *Alleviate comorbid anxiety or depression*: Given the high prevalence of mood disturbances in ED patients, SSRIs provide dual benefits for both impulse control and emotional regulation.

Severe body image disturbances in anorexia nervosa

For patients with AN experiencing severe body image disturbances or distorted perceptions, atypical antipsychotic drugs may be introduced. These medications, such as olanzapine, quetiapine or aripiprazole, are used to:

- *Address cognitive distortions*: Antipsychotics can reduce the rigidity of obsessive thoughts related to weight and body image.
- *Enhance emotional stability*: By modulating dopamine and serotonin pathways, these drugs help stabilize mood and reduce anxiety, making patients more receptive to psychotherapy.
- *Promote weight gain*: In some cases, atypical antipsychotics have been found to encourage appetite and support weight restoration efforts.

A comprehensive and adaptive framework

The integration of psychopharmacology into the therapeutic community framework significantly enhances the program's capacity to address a wide range of symptomatic presentations. Psychopharmacological interventions play a critical role in stabilizing symptoms, improving emotional regulation, and promoting cognitive clarity, creating a foundation for deeper therapeutic work. Simultaneously, the communal and group-based approaches within the therapeutic community foster relational healing, build emotional resilience, and support societal reintegration.

By employing specific tools, such as the DIB-R, to identify predominant symptomatic dimensions, the program ensures that interventions are tailored to meet each patient's unique needs. This collaborative and flexible treatment model integrates individual and collective care, addressing the complex interplay between personality disorders and EDs.

This dual approach not only tackles the psychological and biological dimensions of these disorders but also empowers patients to actively participate in their recovery. The emphasis on individualized care within a supportive and dynamic therapeutic environment encourages meaningful and sustained progress, helping patients rebuild their sense of self, strengthen interpersonal relationships, and reintegrate into their communities with greater confidence and stability.

Comprehensive medical and nutritional care in day hospital programs for eating disorders

Medical and nutritional care are cornerstones of the multidisciplinary treatment provided within the day hospital program for patients with eating disorders (EDs). These aspects of care address both the immediate physical complications of EDs and the longer-term challenges of restoring nutritional balance and overall health.

Given the wide range of medical complications associated with EDs, continuous medical monitoring is essential to ensure patient safety and guide effective interventions.

Key components of medical care include:

Cardiac evaluations in eating disorder treatment

These cardiac evaluations are vital components of the medical care provided within a multidisciplinary ED treatment framework. By integrating routine ECGs, QTc monitoring, and vital sign assessments, the care team can proactively identify and address potential cardiac risks. This ensures not only the patient's safety during treatment but also lays the groundwork for restoring overall physical health, enabling more effective participation in the therapeutic process.

Electrocardiograms (ECGs)

Patients in ED treatment undergo regular electrocardiograms (ECGs) to monitor their heart health, as cardiac complications are common in this population, particularly in individuals with severe malnutrition or purging behaviors. Specific concerns addressed through ECG monitoring include:

Bradycardia and arrhythmias: ED patients frequently experience bradycardia (low heart rate) and arrhythmias due to malnutrition and electrolyte imbalances, making regular ECGs crucial for early detection and management.

QTc interval monitoring: The QTc interval, which represents the heart's electrical recovery time, is often prolonged in patients with chronic hypokalemia (low potassium levels), a condition frequently observed in ED patients who purge. Prolongation of the QTc interval is a significant risk factor for arrhythmias such as torsade's pointes, which can lead to sudden cardiac death. Monitoring QTc is also essential when initiating or continuing psychopharmacological treatments, as many psychiatric medications can exacerbate QTc prolongation, increasing the risk of adverse cardiac events.

Blood pressure and heart rate monitoring

Continuous observation of blood pressure and heart rate plays a critical role in identifying early signs of cardiovascular instability, including heart failure. Severe malnutrition can weaken the heart muscle, leading to diminished cardiac output and signs of heart failure.

Electrolyte and metabolic assessments

Regular laboratory tests monitor levels of potassium, magnesium, calcium, and other vital electrolytes, which are often depleted due to purging or restrictive eating patterns. Metabolic evaluations help track organ function, such as kidney and liver performance, identifying early signs of dysfunction that may result from malnutrition.

Electrolyte imbalances such as irregularities in potassium, magnesium, and calcium levels, commonly seen in ED patients, can significantly impact cardiac function. Close monitoring ensures timely intervention to correct these imbalances and prevent complications.

Dental care

For patients with purging behaviors, dental check-ups are critical to assess and mitigate enamel erosion, gum disease, and other oral health issues caused by frequent exposure to stomach acid. Preventive dental care, combined with nutritional improvements, can reduce long-term damage and improve overall health.

Bone health assessments

Patients with prolonged malnutrition are at risk of osteoporosis or osteopenia. Periodic bone density scans and vitamin D/calcium supplementation plans are incorporated into care strategies.

Nutritional care and monitoring

Nutritional rehabilitation is a cornerstone of recovery in ED treatment, focusing on stabilizing patients' physical health, restoring metabolic function, and addressing their psychological relationship with food. Core aspects of nutritional care include:

1 *Individualized nutritional plans*:

- Tailored dietary plans are developed by registered nutritionists based on each patient's needs, addressing caloric intake, macronutrient balance, and specific deficiencies.
- Plans are flexible and adjust as patients' progress, ensuring that dietary goals remain achievable and non-threatening.
- Educational nutrition about healthy eating according to individual requirements.

2 *Guidance on eating behaviors*:

- Nutritional counseling emphasizes normalizing eating patterns, reducing anxiety around food, and introducing structure into mealtimes.
- Patients are encouraged to challenge food-related fears gradually, fostering a healthier and more sustainable relationship with eating.

3 *Practical skill development*:

- Monthly cooking workshops provide hands-on opportunities for patients to engage with food in a positive and communal setting.
- Participants learn to prepare balanced meals, explore diverse cuisines, and rediscover the joy of cooking and eating as part of daily life.

4 *Nutritional monitoring*

Comprehensive assessments: Patients undergo ongoing evaluations of their nutritional status and physical health indicators to monitor progress, ensure safety, and identify any signs of deterioration. These assessments include anthropometric measurements, dietary intake analysis, and tracking biochemical markers to maintain a holistic understanding of the patient's health.

Weekly check-ins with Nutritionists: Structured weekly sessions serve as a supportive and collaborative space for patients, particularly those with AN, to express concerns, celebrate progress, and address emerging challenges. These sessions aim to foster trust and create a safe environment for open dialogue about food and recovery. The focus is on promoting sustainable, healthy eating habits tailored to each patient's unique needs and goals, helping them reframe their relationship with food as a source of nourishment and well-being.

However, for patients with BN, weekly check-ins may sometimes introduce stress or exacerbate feelings of shame, guilt, or pressure related to food and weight discussions. In such cases, these sessions may be contraindicated or adapted to minimize stress. Flexible scheduling, alternative therapeutic approaches, or integrating these discussions within a broader treatment context can help create a more supportive environment. This ensures that the nutritional care plan remains patient-centered and sensitive to individual emotional and psychological needs.

By tailoring the frequency and structure of these check-ins to each patient's condition, the therapeutic process maintains its balance between fostering accountability and providing compassionate care (Personal communication, *Nutritionist* Paula Rodríguez, November, 2024).

Tailored interventions: Nutritionists work closely with patients to create individualized meal plans that address their specific needs, preferences, and goals. This process helps to reduce anxiety around food, reframe eating as a positive and nourishing experience, and build confidence in making balanced choices.

Education and empowerment: Nutritional monitoring is complemented by educational sessions aimed at increasing patients' understanding of their body's needs. By demystifying the physiological processes related to nutrition, patients are empowered to view food as an ally in their recovery rather than a source of fear or control.

This comprehensive approach ensures that nutritional monitoring goes beyond tracking numbers—it becomes an integral part of the therapeutic process, supporting physical recovery while addressing the psychological and emotional barriers tied to food and eating.

The role of nutritional and medical care in psychotherapeutic integration

Medical and nutritional monitoring is not merely about addressing physical health; it is also deeply intertwined with the therapeutic process. Restoring physical stability provides patients with the energy and cognitive clarity needed to engage more fully in psychotherapy, group activities, and other aspects of the day hospital program (Personal Communication, *Nutritionist* Sofía Soto, April, 2024).

Simultaneously, addressing the psychological barriers to healthy eating and body acceptance complements the physical care provided. Patients learn to view food not as a source of anxiety or control but as a vital aspect of life, health, and connection.

By integrating comprehensive medical care with personalized nutritional support, the day hospital program creates a robust framework for addressing both the physical and emotional dimensions of eating disorders. This approach ensures that patients receive the care they need to recover fully, fostering long-term resilience and well-being.

Emergencies requiring full hospitalization in eating disorder patients

Patients with EDs may encounter emergencies that necessitate suspension of day intensive care hospital treatment and require full hospitalization. These emergencies can be categorized into psychiatric emergencies and clinical-nutritional emergencies.

Psychiatric emergencies in eating disorder treatment

Psychiatric emergencies are critical situations that necessitate immediate intervention and, in many cases, hospitalization. Within the context of ED treatment, such emergencies often arise when the patient's psychological state or behavior poses a direct threat to their safety or the therapeutic process (Persano, 2014, 2022). Key psychiatric emergencies requiring hospitalization include:

1 *Suicide threats or attempts*

- Suicide is a leading cause of death among adolescents and young people, especially in individuals with EDs, particularly AN and BN, where the prevalence of comorbid mood disorders and hopelessness is high.
- Any expression of suicidal ideation, planning, or attempt warrants immediate assessment and intervention. In these cases, hospitalization provides a safe environment where the patient can be stabilized, monitored, and engaged in intensive therapeutic care.

2   *Severe substance abuse or alcohol addictions*

- Substance abuse disorders, including severe drug or alcohol addiction, frequently co-occur with EDs, complicating the treatment process.
- These addictions can disrupt participation in day hospital programs by impairing judgment, increasing impulsivity, and interfering with the therapeutic alliance.
- Hospitalization is necessary when substance use exacerbates medical risks, such as electrolyte imbalances or cardiac complications, or when detoxification in a controlled environment is required to ensure safety and facilitate engagement with ED treatment.

3   *Severe mood disorders*

- Patients presenting with extreme mood dysregulation, such as severe depression, mania, or mixed states, may require hospitalization for stabilization.
- Severe mood disorders can undermine the patient's ability to participate in day hospital programs and exacerbate ED behaviors, including restriction, binging, purging, or self-harm.
- Hospitalization allows for intensive psychiatric care, including medication adjustments, mood stabilization, and crisis intervention.

4   *Noncompliance in high-risk patients*

- Some patients, particularly those with severe ED symptoms or comorbid personality disorders, may exhibit behaviors that disrupt the therapeutic process or place themselves at heightened risk.
- Examples include persistent noncompliance with dietary plans, refusal to engage in treatment activities, or frequent absences from the program.
- For high-risk patients—such as those with life-threatening weight loss, severe purging, or impulsive self-harming behaviors—noncompliance can escalate into a medical or psychiatric emergency. Hospitalization in these cases provides a structured environment for re-engagement with treatment and the prevention of further deterioration.

Holistic management of psychiatric emergencies

Addressing psychiatric emergencies in ED treatment requires a multidisciplinary approach to ensure both safety and continuity of care:

- *Comprehensive assessment*: Immediate evaluation of the patient's mental and physical status is critical to determine the level of risk and appropriate intervention.
- *Crisis stabilization*: Hospitalization provides a controlled setting for addressing acute risks, including medical stabilization for co-occurring physical complications.
- *Integrated care*: Coordination between psychiatric, medical, and ED treatment teams ensures that hospitalization is seamlessly integrated into the broader therapeutic plan, supporting long-term recovery.
- *Reintegration into the day hospital program*: Once stabilized, patients can transition back into the day hospital program, where they receive ongoing care to address the underlying issues contributing to the emergency.

By recognizing and effectively managing psychiatric emergencies, treatment teams can safeguard the well-being of patients while maintaining the integrity of the therapeutic process. This proactive approach not only addresses immediate risks but also fosters a pathway for patients to re-engage with recovery in a structured and supportive environment.

Clinical-nutritional emergencies

Clinical or nutritional emergencies that may arise during day hospital treatment and necessitate full hospitalization include (Pasqualini, 2010; Pasqualini et al., 2007):

1 *Cardiac arrhythmias*:

- Significant bradycardia with a heart rate below 40 beats per minute or other arrhythmias, including prolonged QTc interval.

2 *Pulse and blood pressure abnormalities*:

- Pulse variations exceeding 20 beats per minute with postural changes.
- Hypotension with systolic blood pressure below 70 mmHg.
- Frequent syncopal episodes or repeated fainting spells.

3 *Dehydration and/or electrolyte imbalance*:

- Hypokalemia (serum potassium concentration below 3.2 mEq/L).
- Hyponatremia (serum sodium concentration below 88 mEq/L).
- Hypophosphatemia.

4 *Severe weight loss*:

- The body mass index (BMI) is below 14,5.
- Significant malnutrition (>30%) or weight loss exceeding 30% of initial weight within three months.

5 *Compulsive or uncontrollable vomiting*:

- Life-threatening episodes of recurrent vomiting.

6 *Gastrointestinal complications*:

- Hematemesis or esophageal tears.

7 *Infections in malnourished patients*:

- Infections compromise general health status.

8 *Seizures*
9 *Pancreatitis*

Behavioral issues requiring hospitalization

Behavioral disturbances necessitating full hospitalization include (Pasqualini, 2010; Pasqualini et al., 2007):

- Absolute refusal to ingest food.
- Uncontrollable binge eating and purging behaviors.

Situations beyond outpatient team capacity

Certain scenarios exceed the capabilities of any outpatient team, such as (Pasqualini, 2010; Pasqualini et al., 2007):

- Family dysfunction, including life-threatening risks to adolescent or domestic violence.
- Social factors hinder treatment adherence, such as excessive distance from home to the treatment center.
- Economic factors preventing continuation of outpatient care.

Hospitalization serves to stabilize the patient and provide a controlled environment while addressing these challenges.

Introducing individual psychotherapy in the context of eating disorders treatment

The decision to introduce individual psychotherapy in the treatment of ED patients is a carefully calibrated process within the broader therapeutic framework. While this topic is explored in depth in Chapter 9, it is worth emphasizing that individual psychotherapy in EDs is most effective when integrated into a larger communal and multidisciplinary approach.

Challenges and preconditions for individual psychotherapy

ED patients often do not seek treatment spontaneously, as their symptoms are frequently ego-syntonic, perceived not as pathological but as a way of life. Resistance to therapy is common, requiring a nuanced approach to engaging patients. As Professor Philippe Jeammet noted in a discussion during his visit to Argentina, imposing individual psychotherapy early in treatment risks undermining the psychoanalytic principles of patient autonomy and self-discovery and is generally ineffective in such cases (Personal communication, Philippe Jeammet, 1998).

In the context of partial hospitalization or day hospital programs, patients engage in group therapy and communal interventions, which serve as a foundational phase (Persano, 2022). These settings allow individuals to:

- Develop the capacity for representability, symbolization, and historization of their experiences.
- Shift from acting out behaviors to recognizing and verbalizing their internal conflicts.
- Transition from ego-syntonic functioning to experiencing anguish and a genuine desire for change.

When to introduce individual psychotherapy

Individual psychotherapy is best introduced during advanced stages of treatment when patients demonstrate:

- A shift from primitive defense mechanisms (e.g., acting out, splitting, withdrawal, idealization) to higher-level defenses, including "affiliation"—manifested in their willingness to ask for help.
- A demand for private therapeutic encounters, reflecting their readiness to explore their suffering and pursue deeper psychic change.

At this stage, the treatment focus transitions from intensive day hospital care to less frequent modalities, such as outpatient programs. The introduction of individual psychotherapy coincides with this shift, providing a structured and personalized space for patients to process their experiences and foster enduring change (Persano, 2022).

The psychotherapeutic process and its challenges

The psychotherapeutic process for ED patients is particularly challenging due to the persistence of archaic psychic functioning and primitive mental contents, which often emerge during therapy. These include feelings of loneliness, abandonment, and intense transference manifestations (Persano, 2022). Psychoanalytic psychotherapy must:

- Actively tolerate and address primitive transferences.
- Provide a framework that avoids excessive silences, which can exacerbate regressive defenses.
- Gradually promote psychic integration, allowing patients to process conflicts and develop a cohesive sense of self.

This process is not linear, as archaic defenses can persist and test the therapeutic alliance. However, over time, patients begin to exhibit subtle intrapsychic transformations, evidenced by:

- Improved emotional regulation.
- Healthier interpersonal relationships.
- Emerging desires, projects, and vocational attitudes.

Manualized psychoanalytic psychotherapies

In institutional settings, manualized psychoanalytic psychotherapies such as Mentalization-Based Treatment (MBT) (Allen and Fonagy, 2006) and Transference-Focused Psychotherapy (TFP) (Kernberg et al., 2008; Yeomans, Clarkin, and Kernberg, 2015) have proven particularly effective. These models provide structured strategies for addressing the complexities of EDs, offering both therapeutic rigor and training opportunities for mental health professionals.

MBT and TFP in clinical practice

- MBT is especially suited to patients with AN, focusing on enhancing their ability to mentalize and process emotions.
- TFP is more effective for patients with BN and borderline personality traits, addressing fragmentation and promoting integration of split self and object representations.

Both approaches aim to:

- Foster mentalization and symbolization processes.
- Rescue the individual from identity diffusion and psychic fragmentation.
- Reestablish ownership over the body, thoughts, and emotions, leading to stabilization and integration.

Outcomes of individual psychotherapy

Individual psychotherapy, when introduced at the right stage, facilitates a profound transformation in patients. By addressing the psychic roots of their suffering, therapy enables patients to:

- Move beyond dependence on external validation and societal ideals.
- Reconnect with their bodies and recognize the complexity of their emotions.
- Shift from living in the tyranny of perfection to embracing a more authentic and fulfilling life.

This process integrates both internal and external realities, allowing patients to rebuild their lives with a deeper sense of autonomy and well-being.

In summary, individual psychotherapy in the treatment of EDs is not a standalone intervention but a key component of a larger therapeutic strategy. Introduced at the appropriate phase of treatment, it offers patients the opportunity to achieve enduring psychic change and a more meaningful connection to themselves and the world around them (Persano, 2022).

Difficulties during the therapeutic process

Impulse control difficulties in eating disorder treatment

Impulse control difficulties present significant challenges in the treatment of EDs, often complicating the clinical picture and undermining the therapeutic process. These challenges are particularly prevalent in patients exhibiting multi-impulsive behaviors, which may include:

- Drug and alcohol dependency.
- Aggression and impulsive sexual behaviors.
- Irritability and dysregulated interpersonal relationships.
- Self-harming behaviors.
- Manipulative suicide threats and attempts.

Such behaviors are frequently observed in bulimic cases, where they exacerbate clinical complications and lead to poorer treatment outcomes.

Studies from German ED specialty hospitals demonstrate that bulimic symptoms, compounded by multi-impulsivity, additional anorexic symptoms, and a history of failed treatments, result in markedly poor prognoses (Kächele et al. unpublished).

Multi-impulsivity and addictive dimensions

The recurrent impulsivity observed in ED patients, particularly in BN, is often conceptualized within an addiction framework. This perspective highlights how binge behaviors, including binge-drinking during weekends, are reflective of an addictive predisposition. This predisposition is often linked to early relational dynamics that shape a psychic economy dominated by compulsive tendencies. These patterns underline the necessity of monitoring and addressing escalating addictive behaviors in ED patients as part of comprehensive care.

Identity disturbances and impulse dysregulation

Impulse control difficulties in EDs are closely tied to identity disturbances, often manifesting as identity diffusion, a characteristic commonly observed in individuals with borderline personality organization (Kernberg, 1984).

- These disturbances frequently involve depersonalization experiences, which further complicate the clinical presentation (Persano, 2005).
- The lack of internalized object constancy and a reliance on external validation create cycles of impulsivity and relational instability, perpetuating the psychopathological loop.

This dynamic reflects a fragile sense of self, where patients struggle to maintain stable internal representations and instead rely on external validation to regulate their emotions and sense of identity.

Implications for treatment

Impulse control difficulties, particularly when associated with multi-impulsivity, represent a critical challenge in ED treatment. To effectively address these complexities, clinicians must adopt a multidimensional approach that incorporates the following elements:

1 *Comprehensive assessment*:

- Identify underlying dynamics, including addiction-like behaviors, relational voracity, and identity diffusion.
- Monitor patterns of impulsive behaviors such as binge-drinking and self-harming tendencies to tailor interventions effectively.

2   *Tailored interventions*:

- Integrate psychodynamic, behavioral, and pharmacological strategies to stabilize impulse control.
- Foster internalized object representations to reduce reliance on external validation.

3   *Focus on transition dynamics*:

- Recognize and address the progression from AN to BN.
- Implement targeted interventions to rebuild identity, emotional regulation, and relational stability.

Building a path to recovery

By addressing the underlying mechanisms of impulse dysregulation and their connection to identity disturbances, clinicians can create a supportive therapeutic environment that promotes long-term recovery. Recognizing the continuum between AN and BN, as well as the interplay of identity and relational dynamics, allows for the development of more nuanced and effective therapeutic strategies.

This holistic approach not only stabilizes impulsive behaviors but also fosters deeper emotional and relational healing, enabling patients to achieve greater psychological resilience and sustainable recovery.

The transition from anorexia nervosa to bulimia nervosa

One of the most complex challenges in treating EDs is addressing the dynamic progression from AN to bulimic behaviors, a shift that can significantly complicate the therapeutic process.

1.   Anorexia nervosa: A defense against loss of control

AN often functions as a defensive response to profound fears of losing control over impulses. Patients with anorexia frequently report that their restrictive eating behaviors stem from a fear that, once they begin eating, they will be unable to stop (Persano, 2005). This hyper-control over food intake serves as a protective mechanism, allowing individuals to maintain a fragile sense of order in their lives.

2.   The breakdown of rigidity: Emergence of bulimic behaviors

Over time, the rigid control characteristic of AN can deteriorate, giving way to binge-eating episodes. This transition often reflects the collapse of the defensive structure, leading to cycles of binging and purging that define bulimia nervosa. The binge episodes are frequently accompanied by an overwhelming sense of loss of control, which contrasts sharply with the hyper-controlled patterns seen in anorexia.

3. The continuum of impulse control challenges

This shift from AN to BN underscores the continuum of impulse control challenges within EDs.

- AN, is typified by hyper-control and rigidity, where the individual exerts extreme restraint to avoid perceived chaos.
- BN, in contrast, represents an impulsive overcompensation, where the individual struggles with unregulated eating behaviors that they attempt to counteract through purging or other compensatory measures.

These contrasting behaviors highlight the complex interplay of control, identity, and relational dynamics that must be addressed during treatment. The transition reflects deeper disturbances in self-regulation, where the need for control gives way to cycles of overindulgence and self-punishment, perpetuating the psychopathological loop.

4. Implications for treatment

Recognizing and addressing this progression is critical for developing effective therapeutic strategies:

- *Comprehensive assessment*: Early identification of emerging bulimic patterns in AN can allow for timely intervention.
- *Addressing fear of loss of control:* Therapeutic approaches must help patients explore and process the fears underlying their restrictive eating behaviors, paving the way for healthier coping mechanisms.
- *Building impulse regulation*: Interventions should focus on fostering emotional regulation and impulse control, helping patients transition from destructive cycles of rigidity and binge-purge patterns to more stable relational and emotional functioning.

The transition from AN to BN represents a critical complication in the treatment of EDs, requiring nuanced and dynamic therapeutic approaches. Understanding the underlying fears and relational dynamics driving this shift allows clinicians to better address the continuum of impulse control challenges, facilitating recovery and promoting long-term psychological stability.

A patient-led reframing: From "Day Hospital" to "Hospital of Life"

The renaming of the "day hospital" to the "Hospital of Life" by the patients themselves, as discussed in Chapter 10, signifies a profound shift in their understanding of their recovery journey and their role within the therapeutic process. This change in terminology is far more than a symbolic gesture; it represents a transformative reframing of their experiences, identities, and relationships—with themselves, their bodies, and the broader society. It encapsulates a move from seeing the treatment space as solely a site of illness management to a place of growth, renewal, and reconnection with life and community.

Challenging and changing overall functioning

The concept of the "Hospital of Life" underscores the therapeutic community's ability to foster functional changes beyond symptom reduction. Through group interactions, shared activities, and communal goals, patients begin to reconstruct their internal and external worlds. These shifts are evident in several domains:

- *Emotional functioning*: Patients move from emotional rigidity or suppression toward greater flexibility and emotional expression, supported by the safety of the therapeutic space.
- *Relational dynamics*: By engaging with peers and staff in a shared environment, patients challenge patterns of isolation, mistrust, and alienation, replacing them with mutual support and collaboration.
- *Life engagement*: The focus shifts from survival and symptom management to living with intention, building meaningful relationships, and contributing to the broader social fabric.

The role of mentalization and embodiment

Central to this transformation is the interplay between mentalization and embodiment experiences:

- *Mentalization*: Patients learn to interpret their internal states and those of others with greater nuance. This process allows them to recognize their emotions, motivations, and relational patterns, fostering a more coherent sense of self.
- *Embodiment*: For patients with EDs, reconnecting with their bodies as integral parts of their identities is a vital step. The therapeutic process facilitates a shift from viewing the body as an object to be controlled or punished to experiencing it as a living, feeling subject. This change is reinforced through activities that encourage bodily awareness, such as art therapy, physical relaxation practices, and communal meals.

Reframing cultural views

The "Hospital of Life" concept also challenges and redefines cultural narratives surrounding EDs and recovery:

- *Beyond labels*: By shedding the identity of "anorexic" or "bulimic", patients resist the societal tendency to define individuals solely by their diagnoses. They embrace a more holistic view of themselves as individuals striving to live fully, beyond the confines of illness.
- *Cultural critique*: The therapeutic community offers a space to deconstruct harmful cultural ideals, such as perfectionism, hyper-individualism, and unrealistic beauty standards. Workshops and group discussions enable patients to critically analyze and challenge these narratives, empowering them to adopt healthier perspectives.

A catalyst for societal reintegration

The term "Hospital of Life" encapsulates the program's goal of reintegrating patients into society with a renewed sense of agency and purpose. Patients begin to envision themselves not as passive recipients of care but as active participants in their own lives and communities. This perspective aligns with the broader psychoanalytic and therapeutic aims of fostering autonomy, resilience, and social engagement.

Conclusion: A transformative journey

The patient-led redefinition of the day hospital as the "Hospital of Life" symbolizes a profound transformation in their recovery journey. This reframing not only highlights the program's success in fostering mentalization, embodiment, and cultural reframing, but it also challenges the isolating and reductive labels often associated with eating disorders. By envisioning the therapeutic space as a "Hospital of Life", patients reclaim their agency, shifting their focus from survival to actively participating in and contributing to society.

This terminology captures the transformative potential of therapeutic communities, where healing extends beyond the resolution of symptoms. It reflects the program's holistic approach, integrating individual growth with communal support, and emphasizing that recovery is not just about overcoming illness but also about rediscovering purpose, connection, and identity.

The "Hospital of Life" encapsulates the essence of recovery as an opportunity to reconstruct one's narrative, heal relational dynamics, and build a more fulfilling life. It serves as a testament to the power of community, the importance of reclaiming identity, and the possibility of embracing life anew. This patient-led initiative highlights the collaborative and empowering ethos of the program, demonstrating that, at its core, recovery is about living, not just existing.

Implications of psychoanalytic understanding for prevention and early intervention outreach in the community context

Primary level of care: A foundational framework for mental health services

The primary level of care represents the social sphere where individuals live, work, and interact daily, forming the foundation of the healthcare network. According to international evidence and scientific consensus, mental health interventions embedded in this framework have proven more effective, enhancing both the responsiveness and resolution capacity of healthcare systems (PAHO/WHO, 2010).

From a psychoanalytic perspective, the primary level of care can be seen as a space where early relational dynamics are echoed within community interactions. Drawing on attachment theory and the psychoanalytic understanding of early development, primary care offers an opportunity to address vulnerabilities rooted in early relational deficits before they evolve into entrenched psychopathologies. In the case of EDs, this includes addressing object relations, early disruptions in self-representation, and cultural influences on identity formation.

Key features of primary care in mental health

Primary care in mental health plays a foundational role in promoting well-being and preventing the escalation of psychological vulnerabilities. As developed in "The Program for Eating Disorders in Mental Health Services", led in collaboration with Psychologist Violeta Salusky and Nutritionist Paula Rodríguez, a population-centered approach is essential. This approach is informed by both epidemiological insights and psychoanalytic understandings of subjective experience (Persano, Rodríguez, and Salusky, 2021).

Core objectives of primary care in mental health

1 *Detecting vulnerabilities early*: Early identification is crucial for individuals at risk due to familial, relational, or societal stressors. Psychoanalytic frameworks, emphasizing unconscious processes and transgenerational dynamics, enable a deeper understanding of latent vulnerabilities before they manifest as severe psychopathology.

2 *Promoting resilience*: Community-based initiatives aim to foster healthier emotional and relational dynamics. Drawing on psychoanalytic concepts like object relations theory and attachment dynamics, these

interventions address the underlying relational patterns that contribute to mental health challenges. For instance, promoting secure attachment in educational and familial contexts can mitigate the relational fragility often associated with EDs.

3 *Preventing escalation*: By intervening proactively, primary care can prevent the progression of mild symptoms into severe mental health conditions. Psychoanalytic insights into defensive mechanisms—such as denial, splitting, and idealization—equip primary care providers to detect and address early maladaptive coping strategies.

The integration of psychoanalytic perspective in primary care

Incorporating psychoanalytic principles within primary care not only addresses surface-level symptoms but also engages with the emotional and relational underpinnings of mental health vulnerabilities. This includes:

- *Addressing unconscious processes*: Uncovering the hidden emotional conflicts and anxieties driving maladaptive behaviors, particularly in populations prone to EDs.
- *Recognizing transgenerational dynamics*: Identifying patterns of emotional transmission across generations that may predispose individuals to mental health challenges.
- *Strengthening subjective experience*: Fostering the development of a cohesive sense of self through reflective practices that enhance mentalization and emotional regulation.

Primary care as a first line of defense for eating disorders

Populations at risk for EDs, including adolescents, high-performance athletes, dancers, and young women, benefit significantly from a primary care approach that integrates epidemiological data with psychoanalytic insights. Through a combination of training, collaboration, and proactive interventions, primary care providers can address:

- *Body image distortions*: Helping individuals develop healthier relationships with their bodies by addressing unconscious associations and societal pressures.
- *Relational vulnerabilities*: Mitigating the impact of familial and cultural dynamics that may contribute to disordered eating patterns.
- *Early symptomatology*: Using screening tools and psychoeducational strategies to identify and intervene in the early stages of ED development.

By adopting a population-centered approach informed by psychoanalytic perspectives, primary care can serve as a transformative platform for mental health interventions. It provides the tools to detect vulnerabilities, promote resilience, and prevent escalation, particularly in high-risk populations. Integrating these principles ensures a nuanced and comprehensive approach that addresses both the visible symptoms and the deeper emotional conflicts underlying mental health challenges. This framework not only enhances the efficacy of primary care but also contributes to a more compassionate and responsive mental health system.

Primary care actions in eating disorders (EDs)

1   *Building dialogue with educational communities*: Psychoanalytic concepts of symbolization and mentalization highlight the importance of fostering reflective capacities within educational settings. By training primary and secondary school educators to identify early signs of EDs, schools become pivotal in preventing the alienation and stigmatization that often accompany these conditions.
2   *Training primary care providers*: Providers must be equipped to recognize EDs not only as physical conditions but also as expressions of underlying psychic conflicts. Training programs should incorporate tools to discern body image distortions, identity diffusion, and relational fragility, all of which are hallmarks of EDs.
3   *Coordination with nutritional programs*: By integrating nutritional education with psychoanalytic insights, providers can address the symbolic meanings attached to food and eating behaviors. These collaborations promote early identification and non-stigmatizing interventions.
4   *Awareness of stigmatization risks*: Stigmatization can exacerbate shame and self-criticism, perpetuating the cycles of ED pathology. Psychoanalytic training can sensitize providers to the unconscious dynamics of projection and introjection, fostering empathetic and supportive care.
5   *Improving communication across care levels*: Digital health tools such as electronic health records (EHRs) can facilitate the seamless exchange of clinical observations and psychoanalytic formulations across different levels of care. This ensures continuity and depth in case management.
6   *Promoting intersectoral collaboration*: Psychoanalytic insights into family dynamics and systemic influences underscore the need for collaboration with social services, violence prevention programs, and the justice system. Such intersectoral efforts can address the broader socio-emotional contexts contributing to EDs.

Specific actions for primary care providers in EDs

1   *Training healthcare professionals*: Training should include psychoanalytic concepts such as defensive mechanisms (e.g., denial, splitting, and

omnipotence) and the symbolic function of ED behaviors, helping professionals recognize deeper dynamics behind presenting symptoms.

2   *Screening tools for early detection*: Screening tools should not only identify physical symptoms but also assess emotional and relational vulnerabilities, drawing on psychodynamic frameworks for a comprehensive understanding of risk factors.

3   *Emergency intervention training*: Providers must be trained to manage acute crises—including self-harming behaviors, suicidal ideation, and multi-impulsive behaviors—using approaches informed by both medical and psychoanalytic principles.

4   *Specialized ED teams*: Establishing dedicated teams within "Outreach Centers for Mental Health Services" can provide a consistent framework for addressing the multifaceted nature of EDs, incorporating insights from psychoanalysis, family therapy, and nutritional science.

Community reintegration initiatives

Reintegration programs, informed by psychoanalytic theories of transference and relational dynamics, are critical for fostering long-term recovery. Specific actions include:

- *Emotional support spaces*
  Accessible spaces are designed for individuals to explore their emotional experiences and relational patterns with trained primary care professionals, such as psychologists, social workers, or general practitioners with specialized training in mental health. These spaces focus on providing empathetic listening, and guidance to address emotional and relational challenges effectively.
- *Community leader roles*
  Assigning roles to leaders trained in psychoanalytic principles of group dynamics and symbol formation, enabling them to coordinate workshops and promote preventive measures.
- *Strengthening community bonds*
  Programs are designed to rebuild trust and connection within communities, countering the isolation and fragmentation often seen in ED patients.

Conclusion: A psychoanalytic lens on primary care

The primary level of care serves as both a preventive and transformative platform, where psychoanalytic principles can enrich existing public health strategies. By addressing early relational deficits, fostering mentalization and emotional resilience, and challenging cultural narratives surrounding body image and identity, primary care can significantly mitigate the development and progression of EDs.

As Freud's exploration of civilization and discontent reminds us (Freud, 1930), the roots of psychic suffering often lie in social and relational contexts. A primary care framework informed by psychoanalytic insights bridges the gap between individual vulnerabilities and collective responsibility, paving the way for more holistic, inclusive, and effective mental health interventions.

Bibliography

Allen, J. G. and Fonagy, P. (eds.) (2006). *The Handbook of Mentalization-based Treatment*. New York: John Wiley & Sons.

Ammon, G. (1995). Theoretical aspects of milieu therapy. *Dynamische Psychiatrie. Int. Zeitschrift für Psychiatrie und Psychoanalyse*, 3(6): 282–311.

Armelius, B. Å., Gerin, P., Luborsky, L., and Alexander, L. (1991). Clinicians' judgment of mental mealth: An international validation of HSRS. *Psychotherapy Research*, 1(1): 31–38.

Birot, E., Chabert, S., and Jeammet, P. (2006). *Soigner l'Anorexie et la Boulimie: Des Psychanalystes à l'Hôpital*. Paris: Le fil rouge PUF, Press Universitaries de France.

Bauman, Z. (2013). *Liquid Modernity*. New York: John Wiley & Sons.

Bialakowsky, A., Franco, D., Lusnich, C., Persano, H., Bardi, N., Santilan, P., Miguez, R., Aquila, S., Haimovici, N. and staff (2009). El encuentrode saberes en la coproducción de conocimientos en salud mental y trabajo. In P. E. Martins and R. De Souza Medeiros (eds.) *América Latina e Brasilem Perspectiva*. Recife, Brazil: Editora Universitaria Universidade Federal de Pernambuco UFPE, 171–188.

Castel, R. (2009). *El Ascenso de las Incertidumbres: Trabajo, Protecciones, Estatuto del Individuo*. Buenos Aires: Ed. Fondo de Cultura Económica, Sociología (2012 edition).

Fonagy, P. and Bateman, A. W. (2007). Mentalizing and borderline personality disorder. *Journal of Mental Health*, 16(1), 83–101.

Fonagy, P., Gergely, G., Jurist, E. L., and Target, M. (2002). *Affect Regulation, Mentalization and the Development of the Self*. New York: Other Press.

Freud, S. (1912). The dynamics of transference. *The Standard Edition of the Complete Psychological Works of Sigmund Freud, (12)*. London: The Hogarth Press, 97–108 (1991 edition).

Freud, S. (1930) [1929]. Civilization and Its Discontents. *The Standard Edition of the Complete Psychological Works of Sigmund Freud, (21)*. London: The Hogarth Press, 59–145 (1991 edition).

García Badaracco, J. (1990): *Comunidad Terapéutica Psicoanalítica de Estructura Multifamiliar*. Madrid: Tecnipublicaciones, S.A.

Gómez-Candela, C., Palma-Milla, S., Miján-de-la-Torre, A., Rodríguez-Ortega, P., Matía-Martín, P., Loria-Kohen, V., *et al.* (2016). Consenso sobre la evaluación y el tratamiento nutricional de los trastornos de la conducta alimentaria: Bulimia nerviosa, trastorno por atracón y otros. *Nutrición Hospitalaria*, 35(2): 49–97.

Hoek, H. W. and Van Hoeken, D. (2003). Review of the prevalence and incidence of eating disorders. *International Journal of Eating Disorders*, 34(4): 383–396.

Jeammet, P. (1984). L'Anorexie mentale. *Encycl. Med. Chir. Psychiatrie, 37350 A10-A15*: A10–A15. Paris: Elsevier.

Jones, M. (1953). *The Therapeutic Community: A New Treatment Method in Psychiatry.* New York: Basic Book, Inc.

Kächele, H., Kordy, H., Richard, M. and ResearchGroup TR-EAT. *Outcome of Psychodynamic Therapy of Eating Disorders.* Stuttgart: Center for Psychotherapy Research, 1–39 (Unpublished).

Kernberg, O. F. (1984). *Severe Personality Disorders: Psychotherapeutic Strategies.* New Haven, CT: Yale University Press.

Kernberg, O. F., Yeomans, F. E., Clarkin, J. F., and Levy, K. N. (2008). Transference focused psychotherapy: Overview and update. *The International Journal of Psychoanalysis*, 89(3): 601–620.

Leuzinger-Bohleber, M. (2015). *Finding the Body in the Mind: Embodied Memories, Trauma, and Depression.* London and New York: Routledge (2018 edition).

Lingiardi, V. and McWilliams, N. (2017). *Psychodynamic Diagnostic Manual* (2nd ed.). New York: The Guilford Press.

Lipovetsky, G. (1983). *La Era del Vacío. Ensayos Sobre el Individualismo Contemporáneo.* Barcelona: Anagrama.

Morando, S., Robinson, P., Skårderud, F., and Sommerfeldt, B. (2023). Mentalization based therapy for eating disorders. In P. Robinson, T. Wade, B. Herpertz-Dahlmann, F. Fernandez-Aranda, J. Treasure, and S. Wonderlich (eds.) *Eating Disorders: An International Comprehensive View.* Cham: Springer International Publishing, 1215–1238.

Mundo, E., Persano, H., and Moore, K. (2018). The S Axis in PDM-2. Symptom patterns: The subjective experience. *Psychoanalytic Psychology*, 35(3), 315–319.

PAHO/WHO (2010). Organización Panamericana de la Salud (OPS). *Redes Integradas de Servicios de Salud: Conceptos, Opciones de Política y Hoja de Ruta para su Implementación en las Américas.* Pan American Health Organization.

Pasqualini, D. (2010). Abordaje clínico nutricional de los trastornos de la conducta alimentaria. In D. Pasqualini and A. Llorens(eds.) *Salud y Bienestar de adolescentes y jóvenes.* Buenos Aires:OPS/OMS. Facultad de Medicina, Universidad de Buenos Aires, 297–305.

Pasqualini, D., Toporosi, S., Caballero, M., Miklarski, G., Salgado, P., and Hiebra, M. C. (2007). Atención de adolescentes: Los múltiples diagnósticos y las estrategias terapéuticas. *Revista del Hospital de Niños BAires*, 49(222): 99–108.

Pérez, J. A. H., Botina, A. D. M., Hormiga, M. P., and Bastidas, B. E. (2017). Trastornos de la alimentación: Anorexia y bulimia nerviosa. *Revista Facultad de Salud*, 9(1): 9–19.

Persano, H. (2005). Abordagem psicodinâmica do paciente com trastornos alimentares. In C. L. Eizirik, R. W. Aguiar, and S. S. Schestatsky (eds.) *Psicoterapia de Orientação Analítica: Fundamentos Teóricos e Clínicos, (49).* Porto Alegre: Artmed Editora, 674–688.

Persano, H. L. (2014). El hospital de día para sujetos con trastornos de la conducta alimentaria: Abordaje interdisciplinario en la comunidad terapéutica con enfoque psicodinámico. *PROAPSI*, 3(1): 129–168.

Persano, H. L. (2018). The importance of psychodynamic diagnosis in patients with severe mental illness. In C. L. Eizirik and G. Foresti *(eds.) Psychoanalysis and Psychiatry: Partners and Competitors in the Mental Health Field.* London: Routledge, 187–201.

Persano, H. L. (2022). Day hospital intensive care for patients with eating disorders. In H. Schwartz (ed.) *Applying Psychoanalysis in Medical Care.* London: Routledge, 71–90 (chapter 5).

Persano, H. L., Bialakowsky, A., Franco, D., Cuesta, M., and Patrouilleau, M. (2003). Exclusión social y nuevos padecimientos en la cultura contemporánea, Abordaje Interdisciplinario en Dispositivos Colectivos. In *X Jornada Psicoanálisis y Comunidad, "Angustia Social E Incertidumbre: Fragilización Existencial, Exclusión y Marginalidad"*, Sept. 2003. Buenos Aires: Asociación Psicoanalítica Argentina.

Persano, H. L., Rodríguez, P. Y., and Salusky, V. (2021). Proyecto de actualización del programa en red integrada de cuidados progresivos en desórdenes del comportamiento alimentario. *DGSAM, Ministerio de Salud*. Ciudad Autónoma de Buenos Aires.

Persano, H. L., Soto, S. L., García Méndez, C. S., and Kremer, C. D. (2022). *Evaluación de la eficacia de un dispositivo de hospital de día para pacientes con desórdenes del comportamiento alimentario persistentes en el sistema público de salud*. Poster, May 2022, XXXV Congreso Argentino de Psiquiatría, Mar del Plata.

Racamier, P. C. (1970). *Le Psychanalyste Sans Divan*. Paris: Ed. Payot.

Skårderud, F. and Fonagy, P. (2012). Eating disorders. In A. Bateman and P. Fonagy (eds.) *Handbook of Mentalizing in Mental Health Practice*. Arlington, VA: American Psychiatric Publishing, 347–384.

Schwartz, H. (2022). *Applying Psychoanalysis in Medical Care*. London: Routledge.

Stice, E., Marti, C. N., and Rohde, P. (2013). Prevalence, incidence, impairment, and course of the proposed DSM-5 eating disorder diagnoses in an 8-year prospective community study of young women. *Journal of Abnormal Psychology*, 122(2): 445–457.

WHO (World Health Organization) (2022). *World Mental Health Report: Transforming Mental Health for All*. Geneva: World Health Organization. https://www.who.int/publications/i/item/9789240049338.

Yeomans, F. E., Selzer, M. A., and Clarkin, J. F. (1992). *Treating the Borderline Patient: A Contract-based Approach*. New York: Basic Books.

Yeomans, F. E., Clarkin, J. F., and Kernberg, O. F. (2015). *Transference-focused Psychotherapy for Borderline Personality Disorder: A Clinical Guide*. Arlington, VA: American Psychiatric Publishing.

Yeomans, F., Gutfreund, J., Selzer, M., Clarkin, J., Hull, J., and Smith, T. (1994). Factors related to dropouts by borderline patients: Treatment contract and therapeutic alliance. *The Journal of Psychotherapy Practice and Research*, 3(1): 16–24.

Zanarini, M. C., Gunderson, J. G., Frankenburg, F. R., and Chauncey, D. L. (1989). The revised diagnostic interview for borderlines: Discriminating BPD from other axis II disorders. *Journal of Personality Disorders*, 3(1): 10–18.

Zipfel, S., Reas, D. L., Thornton, C., Olmsted, M. P., Williamson, D. A., Gerlinghoff, M., … and Beumont, P. J. (2002). Day hospitalization programs for eating disorders: A systematic review of the literature. *International Journal of Eating Disorders*, 31(2): 105–117.

Epilogue
Conclusion—The journey toward healing

Opening: A metaphor for the journey

Jean-Paul Sartre's existentialist philosophy profoundly shaped my adolescence and has likely guided my entire life. His ideas about the necessity of coherence between feelings, thoughts, and actions resonated deeply with me, offering a framework that aligns closely with my understanding of human experience and the path to healing. Sartre's assertion that "man is nothing else but what he makes of himself"[1] and it could be added "commitment is an act, not a word" underscores the responsibility and freedom each of us holds to shape our lives through authentic choices and deliberate actions. The notion of commitment in Sartre's work transcends the literal meaning of words and focuses on the congruence between intention and action. Sartre, as an existentialist, argues that we are responsible for giving meaning to our existence through our actions, which entails a rejection of self-deception and "bad faith".

In *Being and Nothingness* [2], although the exact phrase "Commitment is an act, not a word" does not appear, the idea is developed that human beings are free and responsible for their choices, and that these choices gain reality and authenticity only through actions. This is closely related to his critique of those who live in "bad faith", that is, those who deny their freedom by making excuses based on external circumstances or mere words to avoid taking responsibility for their actions. In summary, Sartre's philosophy consistently emphasizes that authentic commitment is defined not by words but by actions. It serves as a powerful reminder that our deeds are the ultimate measure of both our freedom and our responsibility.

This philosophy mirrors the complex, courageous journey of recovery from eating disorders, where thoughts, emotions, and behaviors must harmonize to forge a path toward health and wholeness.

1 Jean-Paul Sartre (1946). *L'existentialisme est un humanisme*, Paris: Les Éditions Nagel.
2 Jean-Paul Sartre (1943). *L'Être et le Néant*, Paris: Ed. Gallimard.

DOI: 10.4324/9781032724997-12

The process of healing from eating disorders is akin to traversing an intricate, winding path through a dense forest. It is not a straightforward road but one marked by struggles and triumphs, moments of shadow and light. Obstacles abound, demanding courage to navigate and persistence to continue moving forward. Yet, with each step—no matter how small—progress is made. Each forward movement becomes a victory, no matter how incremental, affirming the resilience and strength inherent in the human spirit.

Sartre's belief in human freedom and responsibility finds a powerful echo here. The journey of healing demands the courage to embrace hope, to believe in the possibility of change, and to act with intention. Like the forest path, recovery can feel overwhelming at times, with periods of darkness where the destination seems unclear. However, as one perseveres, small openings of light begin to emerge, illuminating the way forward. These glimmers of progress, though subtle, serve as reminders that even the most challenging journeys can lead to profound transformation and renewal.

In the same way that Sartre's existentialism calls for an authentic commitment to being, the journey toward healing requires an unwavering dedication to reconciling one's inner world with outward action. This alignment fosters not just recovery but also the rediscovery of a life imbued with purpose, connection, and the freedom to become one's truest self.

The process of healing: A holistic vision

Complexity and small victories

Healing from eating disorders is not merely about symptom reduction; it is a deeply personal and transformative journey. Eating disorders are multifaceted conditions that intertwine biological vulnerabilities, psychological conflicts, and societal pressures. Acknowledging this complexity is crucial, as it helps patients and caregivers approach recovery with realistic expectations and compassion.

Within this intricate process, small victories hold immense significance. These milestones—whether a shift in behavior, a moment of self-awareness, or progress in nutritional health—are powerful reminders of growth. They affirm that healing is not a race but a gradual process of rebuilding, brick by brick, toward psychic stability and emotional resilience. Celebrating these achievements fosters motivation and reinforces the belief that recovery is possible, even in the face of setbacks.

Every small step forward is like placing a stone on a path that leads to stability and strength. Each stone matters, building a foundation for a brighter future.

Embodied memories and integration

Healing is not solely an intellectual exercise; it involves a profound reconnection with the body. Eating disorders often emerge as coping mechanisms for unresolved emotions, relational disruptions, or sensory experiences that are stored as embodied memories. These memories, rooted in early interactions and lived experiences, are not always accessible through words. They live in the body—in patterns of tension, avoidance, or distress.

True recovery requires transforming these embodied memories through new, healing interactions. Relationships that are safe and nurturing, meaningful activities that foster self-expression, and therapeutic environments that provide containment all contribute to this process.

By addressing the mind-body connection, patients can begin to experience their bodies not as sources of pain or control but as integral parts of their identity and well-being. This integration is a cornerstone of recovery, fostering a sense of wholeness and connection.

The body remembers what the mind cannot express. Healing involves teaching the body to trust, to release, and to reconnect with the self.

Reintegration into society

True healing extends beyond the boundaries of individual recovery. It involves reintegrating the person into society not as a chronic patient defined by their disorder but dynamic individual with agency and purpose. Eating disorders often isolate individuals, leaving them feeling disconnected from the world. Recovery, therefore, must restore not only health but also a sense of belonging.

This reintegration means empowering individuals to reclaim their roles as engaged citizens—whether as family members, friends, professionals, or creators. It involves rebuilding confidence, nurturing relationships, and fostering a sense of purpose that extends beyond the self. Healing, in this sense, is not just about reclaiming life but about rejoining the larger fabric of humanity with a renewed sense of connection and meaning.

Reintegration is about stepping back into the world with a renewed sense of self, belonging, and purpose—moving from isolation to connection, and from survival to living fully.

Transformative spaces

The spaces in which healing takes place have a profound impact on recovery. Day hospital programs and therapeutic environments exemplify the application of psychoanalytic principles to create spaces that transform trauma into growth. These programs offer patients more than just clinical treatment; they provide havens where vulnerability is met with safety, and where suffering is acknowledged and held with compassion.

In these transformative spaces, individuals are supported in reconnecting with their bodies, processing their emotions, and rebuilding their identities. These environments nurture self-discovery, foster connection, and offer tools for resilience. They are not merely treatment centers but havens of hope and renewal, where individuals can take meaningful steps toward reclaiming their lives.

In spaces designed for healing, patients can feel safe exploring their vulnerabilities, rediscover their strengths, and envision a future beyond their disorder. These sanctuaries are where hope takes root and transformation begins.

A unified vision of healing

The journey of healing is both deeply personal and profoundly universal. It is a delicate interplay of small victories, embodied transformation, societal reintegration, and the creation of nurturing spaces that foster growth. Together, these elements form a holistic vision of recovery—one that honors the individuality of each person's struggle while recognizing the collective effort and shared humanity required to support them.

Healing is not a linear process, but a tapestry woven from moments of struggle and triumph. It is the emergence of light from darkness, the gradual clearing of paths through a dense forest of pain and uncertainty. It is a process of rediscovery and renewal, where resilience is cultivated, hope rekindled, and transformation unfolds step by step. In this journey, each milestone, no matter how small, becomes a testament to the enduring strength of the human spirit.

At its core, healing is a relational endeavor. It requires the interplay of introspection, connection, and community. The individual must confront their inner conflicts and fears, but the presence of others—be it through family, therapeutic alliances, or supportive communities—creates the scaffolding necessary for true change. This process highlights the importance of shared spaces, where vulnerability is met with compassion and progress is celebrated collectively.

Societal reintegration is another vital aspect of this journey. Recovery is not just about resolving internal struggles; it is also about reestablishing a sense of belonging and purpose in the broader world. Healing requires opportunities for individuals to engage meaningfully with their environment, to feel seen and valued, and to rebuild their identity in a way that aligns with their evolving sense of self.

Ultimately, healing affirms the boundless potential for transformation inherent in every human being. It is an act of courage and perseverance, of choosing growth over stagnation and hope over despair. By embracing this journey, we honor not only the individual's unique path but also the shared human capacity for resilience and renewal. In doing so, we illuminate the profound interconnectedness that underpins the process of healing and the enduring power of collective support.

Integration with interdisciplinary approaches

While psychoanalysis offers a profound understanding of the inner world, its power is amplified when integrated with other disciplines. Eating disorders are multifaceted conditions that affect not only the mind but also the body and social environment. Collaborating with fields such as medicine, nutrition, sociology, and even architecture enriches the psychoanalytic framework, ensuring a comprehensive approach to recovery.

Medicine and Nutrition: Addressing the physical health consequences of EDs is essential for stabilizing patients and creating a foundation for psychological work. Nutritionists and medical professionals provide crucial interventions that complement psychoanalytic exploration, ensuring patients' immediate safety and long-term well-being.

Sociology: Understanding the societal and cultural pressures that contribute to EDs—such as beauty ideals, gender norms, and social media influences—enables psychoanalysis to address the broader context of these disorders. This interdisciplinary lens ensures that patients' struggles are understood not in isolation but as part of a larger social framework.

Architecture and therapeutic spaces: The design of therapeutic environments plays a significant role in the healing process. Psychoanalysis, when combined with insights from architecture, can create spaces that support recovery by fostering a sense of safety, warmth, and connection. These environments help patients feel contained and understood, facilitating the deep emotional work required for healing.

Psychoanalysis as a transformative tool in the journey toward healing in eating disorders

Psychoanalysis offers a unique and profound perspective on the treatment of eating disorders (EDs). It goes beyond surface-level symptoms to explore the intricate narratives of pain, longing, and disruption that underlie these conditions. In doing so, psychoanalysis transforms the therapeutic process into a journey of self-discovery, emotional integration, and personal growth.

The stories beneath symptoms

Eating disorders are not random behaviors but deeply meaningful expressions of unconscious conflicts. Psychoanalysis teaches us that behind every symptom lies a story—a story of unprocessed emotions, unmet needs, and fractured connections. These symptoms serve as both shields and signals, protecting individuals from overwhelming feelings while also expressing their inner turmoil.

Through the psychoanalytic process, these hidden stories come to light. Whether it is the perfectionism rooted in a yearning for validation, the compulsive control of food masking a fear of abandonment, or the destructive behaviors driven by unresolved trauma, psychoanalysis enables patients to uncover the origins of their suffering. This understanding provides not only relief but also the foundation for building healthier, more cohesive selves.

Behind every symptom lies a story—a yearning for connection, a struggle for meaning. Uncovering these stories provides a pathway to lasting transformation.

By reframing symptoms as messages from the unconscious, psychoanalysis empowers individuals to see their eating disorders not as flaws or failures but as meaningful expressions of their internal world. This shift in perspective fosters self-compassion and opens the door to genuine healing.

The transformative power of self-awareness

One of psychoanalysis's greatest contributions to the treatment of EDs is its emphasis on fostering self-awareness. As patients gain insight into their unconscious motivations and the emotional roots of their behaviors, they become active participants in their healing journey. This process of discovery enables them to break free from destructive cycles and reclaim a sense of agency in their lives.

Through therapeutic relationships, patients are provided with a safe and non-judgmental space to explore their vulnerabilities, fears, and desires. This environment fosters a sense of trust and connection that is often missing in the lives of individuals with eating disorders. It is within this relational context that true transformation occurs.

A bridge between past and present

Psychoanalysis is uniquely equipped to help patients bridge their past and present experiences. By revisiting early relational patterns, developmental disruptions, and unresolved traumas, individuals can gain clarity about how these factors shape their current struggles with food, body image, and self-worth. This understanding allows them to rewrite their narratives and envision a future that is not defined by their eating disorder.

The therapeutic process also emphasizes the role of the present—particularly the dynamics within the therapeutic relationship. The interactions between patient and therapist provide a microcosm of the patient's broader relational patterns, offering valuable opportunities for insight and growth.

From treatment to transformation

Psychoanalysis does not simply aim to reduce symptoms; it seeks to transform lives. It helps individuals reconnect with their authentic selves, repair damaged relationships, and build a more stable and resilient sense of identity. This holistic approach ensures that healing extends beyond the clinical setting, empowering patients to engage with the world in healthier and more fulfilling ways.

Psychoanalysis remains a cornerstone of the healing journey in eating disorders, offering a pathway that is both profound and transformative. By uncovering the stories beneath symptoms and integrating insights from multiple disciplines, it creates a comprehensive framework for recovery. Through this process, patients are not just treated—they are understood, supported, and empowered to reclaim their lives.

The transformative power of psychoanalysis lies in its ability to illuminate the hidden narratives that shape our struggles and to provide a roadmap for healing. It reminds us that beyond every symptom is a story waiting to be heard—and through understanding, connection, and compassion, we can help individuals write a new chapter filled with hope and resilience.

The power of collective healing

The interdisciplinary approach reminds us that healing is not a solitary endeavor. It is a collective process, forged through the collaboration of diverse disciplines—psychiatry, psychology, nutrition, nursing, sociology, and more. These efforts create bridges where there were once barriers, crafting spaces for recovery that are grounded in connection, mutual respect, and shared responsibility.

This holistic approach opens the door to more effective and sustainable outcomes, fostering recovery that is as individualized as the patients themselves.

Ultimately, this evolving understanding underscores the importance of viewing eating disorders not simply as behavioral issues, but as multi-faceted conditions influenced by a confluence of genetic, biological, psychological, and environmental factors. Through this lens, treatment can evolve into a more compassionate and effective process, grounded in science and attuned to the unique needs of everyone.

If societal pressures contribute to the emergence of eating disorders, then societal structures must be part of the solution. Community-based interventions, public health initiatives, and systemic changes in care accessibility are essential. Prevention and early intervention must remain at the forefront, ensuring that help is available before suffering becomes entrenched.

Healing is a collective endeavor. When disciplines unite, they transform obstacles into opportunities, fostering environments of growth and renewal.

New directions in research and treatment

Recent research on genetic and temperamental factors has significantly deepened our understanding of EDs, highlighting their complex nature as biologically influenced conditions. Traits such as perfectionism and heightened sensitivity to criticism, often associated with individuals struggling with eating disorders, are now understood not solely as character developments shaped by life experiences but also as part of a genetic and temperamental legacy. Recognizing these inherited traits is crucial for fostering a therapeutic alliance that respects and works with, rather than against, these intrinsic aspects of the individual's personality.

Advances in neurobiology and brain imaging have further illuminated the underlying mechanisms of these disorders. For instance, research has revealed alterations in brain regions involved in reward processing, impulse control, and emotional regulation, offering insight into why certain individuals may be more vulnerable to disordered eating behaviors. These findings emphasize the need for therapies that address both the psychological and neurobiological dimensions of eating disorders.

Temperament-based therapies have emerged as a promising approach, tailoring interventions to align with an individual's unique genetic predispositions and personality traits. Such therapies may focus on helping individuals manage traits like rigidity, emotional dysregulation, or a heightened fear of failure, which are often amplified in those with perfectionistic tendencies. By addressing these temperamental vulnerabilities, treatment can support patients in building emotional resilience and developing healthier coping mechanisms.

This integration of scientific research and therapeutic practice marks a significant shift toward personalized care in eating disorder treatment. By considering both inherited biological factors and environmental influences, clinicians can create interventions that not only target symptoms but also address the deeper temperamental and neurobiological underpinnings of these disorders.

Hope and gratitude: A reflection on healing

Over the years, I have had the privilege of witnessing profound transformations—individuals reclaiming their voices, their bodies, and their lives. These moments are powerful reminders of the extraordinary strength inherent in the human capacity for change. Recovery is not merely the absence of symptoms; it is the reclamation of identity, purpose, and connection. It is the rekindling of hope, a process that reaffirms life's potential even in the face of profound suffering.

The journey of healing

Healing is not a straight path, nor is it free of challenges. It is a journey—a deeply personal voyage that requires patience, perseverance, and courage. Each step, no matter how small, is a testament to the resilience of the human spirit. Recovery is about more than achieving a specific outcome; it is about rediscovering one's voice, reuniting with the body, and rebuilding relationships with oneself and the world.

Healing is possible. It is the journey of rediscovering one's voice, reuniting with one's body, and reclaiming one's life—a journey of resilience, growth, and hope.

This book reflects not only my professional journey but also the countless individuals who have shaped it. The patients I have worked with have taught me about courage, vulnerability, and the power of persistence. Their strength in confronting their struggles and their willingness to embark on the uncertain path of recovery are profound sources of inspiration. From them, I have learned that healing is as much about growth and self-discovery as it is about overcoming challenges.

My colleagues, too, were integral to this journey. They have pushed me to think deeper, to question assumptions, and to continuously grow as a clinician and as a person. Their expertise, collaboration, and unwavering commitment to the shared vision of healing have enriched my understanding and enhanced the care we provide together.

The institutions that supported our work—public health systems, hospitals, and academic settings—have been foundational in turning hope into action. They provided the platforms to innovate, collaborate, and bring new approaches to life. It is within these spaces that collective efforts have transformed visions into realities, impacting the lives of thousands.

Hope is a universal force that connects us all. It is the belief that no matter how dark the moment, there is light ahead—a belief that fuels resilience and inspires action. As we walk alongside those on the path of recovery, we carry the hope that they will find peace within themselves, strength to confront challenges, and joy in reclaiming their lives.

Every step forward, however small, deserves to be celebrated. Progress may come slowly, but each moment of growth signifies movement toward a fuller, more connected life. It is in these steps—small victories, renewed perspectives, and deeper self-awareness—that the essence of healing is found.

This book is more than a compilation of my experiences; it is a tribute to the collective effort of everyone who has made healing possible. To the patients who bravely faced their fears, the colleagues who stood by my side, and the institutions that trusted in our vision—I offer my deepest gratitude. It is through these shared efforts that healing becomes more than an abstract idea; it becomes a tangible reality, achieved one step at a time.

Hope is not just a feeling; it is a practice. It is the quiet assurance that transformation is possible, the gentle reminder that even in the face of struggle, life holds the promise of renewal.

A universal call for empathy

Let us approach eating disorders—and mental health as a whole—with empathy and understanding, recognizing that behind every disorder is a person with hopes, fears, and a longing to heal. These conditions are not merely medical diagnoses or psychological puzzles; they are deeply human experiences, marked by struggles that touch the core of identity, relationships, and existence itself. To truly support those on their journey, we must look beyond the symptoms and see the individual—their pain, their resilience, and their potential for growth.

Empathy is not only a tool for connection but also a transformative force. It allows us to bridge divides, whether between patient and clinician, family members, or within society itself. In understanding the pain of others, we cultivate a deeper awareness of our shared humanity, transcending the labels and stigmas that too often isolate those with mental health challenges. As we extend compassion, we create a space for trust, safety, and healing—a space where individuals feel seen and valued not for their struggles but for their intrinsic worth.

Empathy transforms not only others but ourselves. In recognizing the struggles of others, we learn more about our own vulnerabilities and strengths. It is through this shared understanding that we find a connection to the greater fabric of humanity.

The process of healing is never solitary. It is woven through the relationships we build, the support we offer, and the understanding we extend. Empathy is the cornerstone of these connections, reminding us that recovery is not simply an individual achievement but a collective endeavor. Families, friends, clinicians, and communities all play a vital role in creating environments where individuals feel empowered to heal and thrive. By embracing empathy, we foster a culture of inclusion, acceptance, and hope that extends far beyond the individual.

To approach EDs and mental health with empathy is also to challenge societal perceptions. It is to reject the stigmas that cast these struggles as weaknesses and instead honor the courage it takes to confront them. It is to recognize the interconnectedness of all human suffering and the collective responsibility we bear to support one another. In this sense, empathy becomes not only an individual virtue but a societal imperative—a way of transforming how we view and respond to mental health challenges on every level.

The journey toward healing is like the gradual emergence of dawn after a long, dark night. At first, the changes are subtle—soft glimmers of light that seem almost imperceptible. But with time, the light grows stronger, illuminating the path ahead and bringing clarity to what was once obscured by shadow. Healing, too, is a process of steady unfolding—a series of small but significant steps that together create the warmth, clarity, and promise of a new day.

Each sunrise reminds us that no matter how long or dark the night, light will always return. Healing may not come all at once, but with patience and care, it will come—bringing with it the possibility of renewal and transformation.

As we close this journey through the complexities of EDs and mental health, let us carry forward a universal call to empathy. Let us approach those who are struggling not with judgment but with understanding, not with pity but with compassion. In doing so, we contribute not only to their healing but also to the healing of a world that desperately needs more kindness, more connection, and more hope.

Let us be the light that helps others find their way out of the darkness. In extending empathy, we ignite the spark of healing—not just for individuals, but for the collective humanity that binds us all.

Index

For Product Safety Concerns and Information please contact our EU
representative GPSR@taylorandfrancis.com
Taylor & Francis Verlag GmbH, Kaufingerstraße 24, 80331 München, Germany